Health Economics: Concepts, Tools and Applications

Health Economics: Concepts, Tools and Applications

Edited by Robert Martin

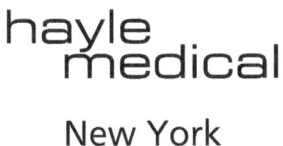

hayle
medical

New York

Hayle Medical,
750 Third Avenue, 9th Floor,
New York, NY 10017, USA

Visit us on the World Wide Web at:
www.haylemedical.com

ISBN: 978-1-63241-849-4

Cataloging-in-Publication Data

Health economics : concepts, tools and applications / edited by Robert Martin.
    p. cm.
Includes bibliographical references and index.
ISBN 978-1-63241-849-4
1. Medical economics. 2. Medical care, Cost of. 3. Health care rationing. I. Martin, Robert.
R728 .H43 2020
338.473 621--dc21

Table of Contents

Preface

Health economics is a branch of economics, which is concerned with the rigorous and systematic examination of the problems of healthcare. It strives to develop a comprehension of the behavior of individuals, health care providers and governments by applying economic theories of producer and consumer. Multiple types of financial information are evaluated, such as charges, costs and expenditures. Health economics seeks to optimize the allocation of available health resources for fair distribution, health promotion and disease prevention. It applies economic theory, economic models and empirical techniques for decision-making by health care providers, individuals and governments relative to health and health care. Health economics is crucial for promoting healthy lifestyles and positive health outcomes. This book aims to shed light on some of the unexplored aspects of health economics and the recent researches in this field. Most of the topics introduced herein cover new concepts, tools and applications of health economics. It will help new researchers by foregrounding their knowledge in this field.

The information contained in this book is the result of intensive hard work done by researchers in this field. All due efforts have been made to make this book serve as a complete guiding source for students and researchers. The topics in this book have been comprehensively explained to help readers understand the growing trends in the field.

I would like to thank the entire group of writers who made sincere efforts in this book and my family who supported me in my efforts of working on this book. I take this opportunity to thank all those who have been a guiding force throughout my life.

Editor

Cost-utility analysis of dynamic intraligamentary stabilization versus early reconstruction after rupture of the anterior cruciate ligament

Martin Bierbaum[1][*] [ID], Oliver Schöffski[1], Benedikt Schliemann[2] and Clemens Kösters[2]

Abstract

Objectives: The aim of this study was to evaluate the cost-effectiveness of the dynamic intraligamentary stabilization (DIS) technique in comparison with reconstructive surgery (ACLR) in the treatment of isolated anterior cruciate ligament (ACL) ruptures from the perspective of the community of insured citizens in Germany.

Methods: Because of the specific decision problem at hand, namely that with DIS the procedure has to take place within 21 days after the initial trauma, a decision tree was developed.
The time horizon of the model was set to 3 years. Input data was taken from official tariffs, payer data, the literature and assumptions based on expert opinion when necessary.

Results: The decision tree analysis identified the DIS strategy as the superior one with 2.34 QALY versus 2.26 QALY for the ACLR branch. The higher QALY also came with higher costs of 5,398.05 € for the DIS branch versus 4,632.68 € for the ACLR branch respectively, leading to an ICER of 9,092.66 € per QALY. Results were robust after sensitivity analysis. Uncertainty was examined via probabilistic sensitivity analysis resulting in a slightly higher ICER of 9,567.13 € per QALY gained.

Conclusion: The DIS technology delivers an effective treatment for the ACL rupture at a favorable incremental cost-effectiveness ratio.

Background

The main cause for a rupture of the anterior cruciate ligament (ACL) are non-contact injuries during football, basketball, soccer and downhill skiing [1]. The US alone spend over $1 billion on anterior cruciate ligament reconstructions (ACLR) annually [2, 3]. In Germany more than 30,000 ACLs are reconstructed every year leading to about 113.3 Million € in hospital costs. In addition, ACL tears lead to an array of indirect costs such as personal loss of income, government-funded injury leaves, absence from school or university and the loss of conditioning due to reduced activity [3]. Furthermore, rupture of the ACL is strongly linked to osteoarthrosis with many patients showing osteoarthritic changes and

related functional disability as early as 10 to 15 years after initial injury [3]. Since mostly young people are affected, the prevention of long-term results becomes vitally important [4].

The current standard of care for an isolated rupture of the ACL consists of two different strategies. The first one is a wait and see strategy, also known as early rehabilitation with delayed reconstruction if needed. Here the patient tries to compensate the instability caused by the torn ACL with muscular training. This treatment is considered suitable for older and/or less active people. If the patient is not satisfied with the outcome, he can still choose reconstructive surgery later on [5, 6]. The second strategy is early reconstructive surgery (ACLR in the model). Hereby the torn ligament is reconstructed as early as six weeks after the trauma [3]. For surgical reconstruction a variety of procedures and techniques (i.e. single bundle, double bundle, allo- or autograft)

* Correspondence: martin.bierbaum@fau.de
[1]Friedrich-Alexander-Universität Erlangen-Nürnberg (FAU), Nuremberg, Germany
Full list of author information is available at the end of the article

exist, but recent studies show no significant differences regarding outcomes [2, 3, 6–8]. In practice younger patients are often treated surgically whereas older patients are more often treated conservatively due to their lesser demand to perform on a high activity level. Regarding different age groups and sex, current study data suggests that there is little difference in outcome between current treatment strategies [9, 10].

With the dynamic intraligamentary stabilization (DIS) a new treatment option became available. This technique makes use of the healing potential of the ligament. The surgical procedure is similar to the reconstruction, but instead of removing and replacing the original ligament, a supportive mechanism is set into the knee. With this technology an intraarticular stabilization of the knee is achieved which is accompanied by the healing of the augmented ligament. A spring system (with 8 mm deflection) compensates the anisometry of the anterior cruciate ligament. This mechanism fulfills the task of the original ligament for the time of healing. Besides the repair of the original ligament the technique has additional advantages. It potentially preserves the proprioceptive ability of the ligament, which may decrease the incidence of re-tears and the development of posttraumatic osteoarthrosis. Another advantage comes with the timing of the technique. Surgery needs to take place within 21 days after trauma. During the procedure, meniscal tears can be acutely repaired at the same time, increasing the probability of healing. This is especially important since available evidence suggests that the meniscal status is the main driver for the development of osteoarthrosis [3, 11–22].

Whereas before, wait and see was a viable strategy and reconstructions could be performed as needed, decision makers now face another strategy where time is critical. Thus the aim of our study is to analyze the cost-effectiveness of the dynamic intraligamentary stabilization technology in comparison to early reconstructive surgery as a benchmark of the current standard of care after the rupture of the anterior cruciate ligament. Our purpose is to provide decision makers with information for reimbursement decision concerning this new technology.

Methods

Setting and perspective

The target population of our study are patients with an isolated rupture of the anterior cruciate ligament with or without meniscal injury who are eligible for the treatment with the dynamic intraligamentary stabilization system according to the instructions of use [23]. Study setting is the German public healthcare sector with patients covered by the statutory health insurance. As far as surgical procedures are concerned the analysis is

limited to the inpatient setting, because only a small number of patients are treated ambulatory. We chose the perspective of the community of insured citizens. It is the preferred perspective of the German HTA-body IQWiG when evaluating interventions. The perspective includes all direct costs, including reimbursable and out-of-pocket medical costs [24]. In contrast to the societal perspective it does not account for other social security costs and indirect costs.

Input data

To gather the relevant information about the indication as well as the data to populate the model we performed a systematic literature search in the following databases: Medline/PubMed, Cochrane Library, NHS-EED, Science-Direct Navigator and Scopus. The findings about the indication were then summarized into an influence diagram (see Additional file 1) which served as the basis for model development. Due to the strong heterogeneity of the study populations of the literature search it was not possible to consolidate the relevant data in the form of a meta-analysis. Instead we used the best evidence available (i.e. Cochrane review) as baseline values wherever possible. Findings from other sources were then used for the parameter ranges in the sensitivity analysis. Reimbursement rates were taken from the official tariffs. The model calculates patient copayments accordingly. Additional sources were statutory health fund data and hospital data. Health fund data was analyzed and contributed by one of the largest health funds in Germany. Hospital data was obtained from the participating hospitals in the DIS study. Parameter uncertainty in the model is addressed via one-way and probabilistic sensitivity analysis. Table 1 gives an overview of the input parameters and its sources.

Costs

Since the costs for surgical treatment in the inpatient sector are covered by a case based lump sum (flat fee) we did not distinguish between different surgical approaches like single-bundle or double-bundle technique or the use of allografts vs. autografts. In the outpatient sector the situation is quite similar as well because the operational procedures are covered by a case based lump sum. Differences only occur in the coverage of the implant, which might be reimbursed in some cases [25].

All prices are reported in 2014 Euros. Cost data is based on sources assessed between 2012 and 2014, hence there is no need for adjusting unit costs. The initial treatment costs such as hospital charges, co-payments and rehabilitation charges are all incurred within a few months after the trauma. All other costs are discounted accordingly. Discount rate is set as 3% and varied between 0%

Table 1 Input parameters

input parameter	baseline-value	SA/PSA	Source
cost inpatient surgery (DIS & ACLR)	3,605.09€	-	G-DRG catalogue
cost DIS (Ligamys)	1,284.00€	-	Mathys AG, Bettlach
cost monobloc removal (DIS)	398.85 €	2,190.83€	Eggli et al. (2016) [33], expert opinion, G-DRG catalogue
cost medical devices (ACLR)	532.00€	-	payer data
average costs of rehab per cycle	82.00€	-	payer data
cost medication (ACLR)	117.92€	-	official tariff (Lauer Taxe)
cost medication (DIS)	58.86€	-	official tariff (Lauer Taxe)
disutility for revision surgery	0.05	0–0.1	Mather et al. (2014) [6]
monobloc removal rate (DIS)	0.241	0.05	Henle et al. (2015) [11]
probability of revision surgery (DIS)	0.029	-	Henle et al. (2015) [11]
probability of revision surgery (ACLR)	0.025	0.0025–0.14	Janssen et al. (2012); Magnussen et al. (2010); Lind et al. (2012); Frobell et al. (2013) [1, 4, 15, 31]
days in hospital (DIS)	2	-	Henle et al. (2015) [11]
days in hospital (ACLR)	5	-	Geiger et al. (2013) [25]
discount rate	0.03	0–0.05%	german HTA guidelines [26]
number of prescriptions for rehab	2	-	payer data
hrQoL baseline (DIS)	0.85	beta dist. 0.85 +/- 0.09	study data on file
hrQoL baseline (ACLR)	0.80	beta dist. 0.80 +/- 0.11	Mather et al. (2014) [6]
hrQoL first 12 m (DIS)	0.79375	beta dist. 0.79375 +/- 0.1	study data on file
hrQoL first 12 m (ACLR)	0.79813	beta dist. 0.79813 +/- 0.11	Mather et al. (2014) [6]
hrQoL after revision (DIS)	lq_ACLR_norm		Assumption; equals the baseline hrQoL of ACLR because ACLR treatment is the revision therapy for DIS
hrQoL after revision (ACLR)	0.755	0.71–0.8	Lind/Menhert et al. (2012); Spindler et al. (2011); Lind/Lund et al. (2012); Wright et al.(2011) [15, 17, 27, 30]
time to revision surgery in months (ACLR)	21.6	9.6–33.6	Lind/Menhert et al. (2012) [15]
time to revision surgery in months (DIS)	11.1	3.5–24.3	Henle et al. (2015) [11]

and 5% for sensitivity analysis. Outcomes are discounted accordingly [26].

Quality of life

Treatment effects after ACL-rupture are often measured with objective tests which do not necessarily reflect the patient's subjective health related quality of life (hrQoL) [9, 15, 17, 27]. While many objective tests report significant differences between treatment strategies, studies assessing patient reported outcomes fail to support these findings. Therefore, we decided to use quality adjusted life years as the measure of benefit in our analysis.

To measure patient relevant outcomes, the SF-12 questionnaire was used to assess patient reported outcomes in a prospective open label study comparing DIS and ACLR. The study took place at the university hospital of Münster, Germany and was approved by the universities ethics committee. Informed consent to participate in the study was obtained from all participants. Questionnaires had to be filled out before surgery, at 6 weeks and at 6 and 12 months after surgery. Utilities

were derived from the SF-12 data with use of the Short Form−6 dimensions (SF-6D) [28]. Due to the low enrollment rates in the ACLR group the number of returned questionnaires was insufficient for analysis ($n = 9$ at six months and $n = 2$ at twelve months). So utilities for the ACLR group had to be derived from the literature [6].

To make DIS study data and literature data comparable, hrQoL values were standardized for the first 12 months after injury. The input values and results are shown in Table 2. The values for DIS are taken from the study data. The values for ACLR where derived from Mather et al [6] where we assumed the utility value for an unstable knee to be equivalent to the quality of life before surgery which incidentally equals the pre-op utility value from our study data. The utility value for week 10 is directly taken from the literature. For the remaining months we linearly approximated the 0,81 value from the literature. Since no high quality data is available for hrQoL after revision surgery we assume the hrQoL not to be worse than an unstable knee in the ACLR group, which is a very conservative assumption in favor of the ACLR strategy.

Table 2 QALY calculation for the first year after surgery

DIS		ACLR	
Time	hrQoL	Time	hrQoL
Injury to surgery (3 weeks)	0.71	Injury to surgery (6 weeks)	0.71
Surgery to week 6	0.71 -> 0.75	Surgery to week 10	0.71 -> 0.82
Week 6 to 6 months	0.75 -> 0.81	Week 10 to 12 month	0.82 -> 0.81
6 months to 12 months	0.81 -> 0.85		
QALY for first year	0.79317		0.79813

Model development

In practice the decision in question has to be made within 21 days after the trauma occurs and cannot be redeemed afterwards. Given the decision problem at hand we decided to use a decision tree [29]. Figure 1 shows the structure of the decision tree.

When early reconstruction and DIS are compared, the initial physician contact and diagnostics after trauma are basically the same in both strategies, hence they are not incorporated into the model. Regarding the postoperative care, we limited the analysis to the differences between treatment strategies. Adverse events are not taken into account too. They are very rare and available study data suggests that they do not differ significantly between treatment strategies. The same states for chondral lesions, which occur seldom and do affect the outcome only in severe cases, which are not treatable with the strategies under scrutiny anyway [14, 16, 17].

Regarding revision surgery after treatment failure, the model does distinguish between treatment strategies. Revision in the DIS branch of the tree leads to costs of an ACLR and subsequently to the hrQoL of ACLR for the remaining time horizon. Revision in the ACLR branch also leads to costs of an ACLR but is assigned a lower health related quality of life for the remaining time horizon because outcomes deteriorate significantly after a second reconstruction [15, 17, 27, 30]. Re-revisions are not incorporated into the model due to high uncertainty and wide range of possible outcomes. Anyway, outcomes deteriorate even further after re-revisions irrespective of treatment strategy [15, 27].

Results

The decision tree analysis identified the DIS strategy as the superior one with 2.34 QALY versus 2.26 QALY for the ACLR branch. The higher QALY also came with higher costs of 5,398.05€ for the DIS branch and 4,632.68€ for the ACLR branch respectively. The resulting ICER is 9,092.66€ per QALY.

Figure 2 shows the results of the univariate sensitivity analysis. The main influencing variables are the probability of revision surgery in the ACLR group and the costs associated with the removal of the DIS monobloc. In case of the incidence of revision surgery and the timeframe within a revision surgery becomes necessary a lot of inconsistent data exists, e.g. the reported rates for revision surgery after an reconstruction of the anterior cruciate ligament lie between 2.5% and 14%. So in the base-case we used the lowest reported value of revision incidence for ACLR. So it comes with no surprise that the higher the rate of revision surgery in the ACLR group, the more favorable the DIS strategy becomes. Regarding the removal costs of the DIS monobloc it is the other way around. Basically the procedure can be performed with local anesthesia within 5 min in an ambulatory setting. Nevertheless some physicians prefer to perform the procedure in a hospital where the costs are much higher and the ICER becomes less favorable. All the remaining variables only have a marginal effect on the ICER.

Table 3 shows the results of the probabilistic sensitivity analysis for the utilities, which are in line with the decision tree results besides a slightly higher ICER of 9,567.13 €/QALY. The cost-effectiveness acceptability curve shows

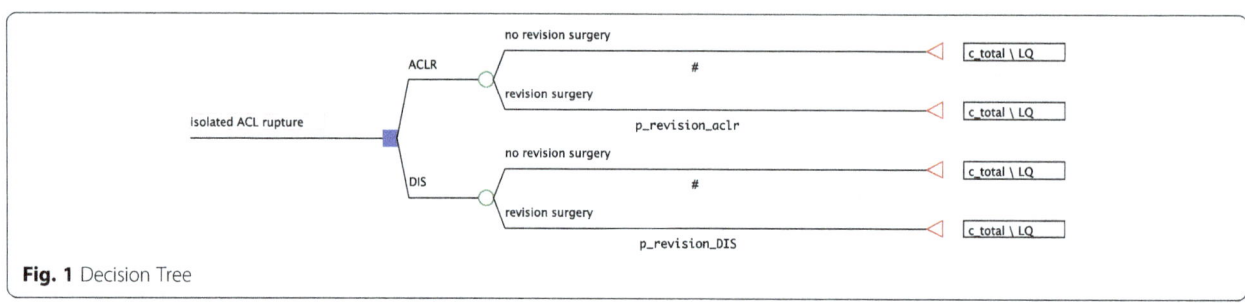

Fig. 1 Decision Tree

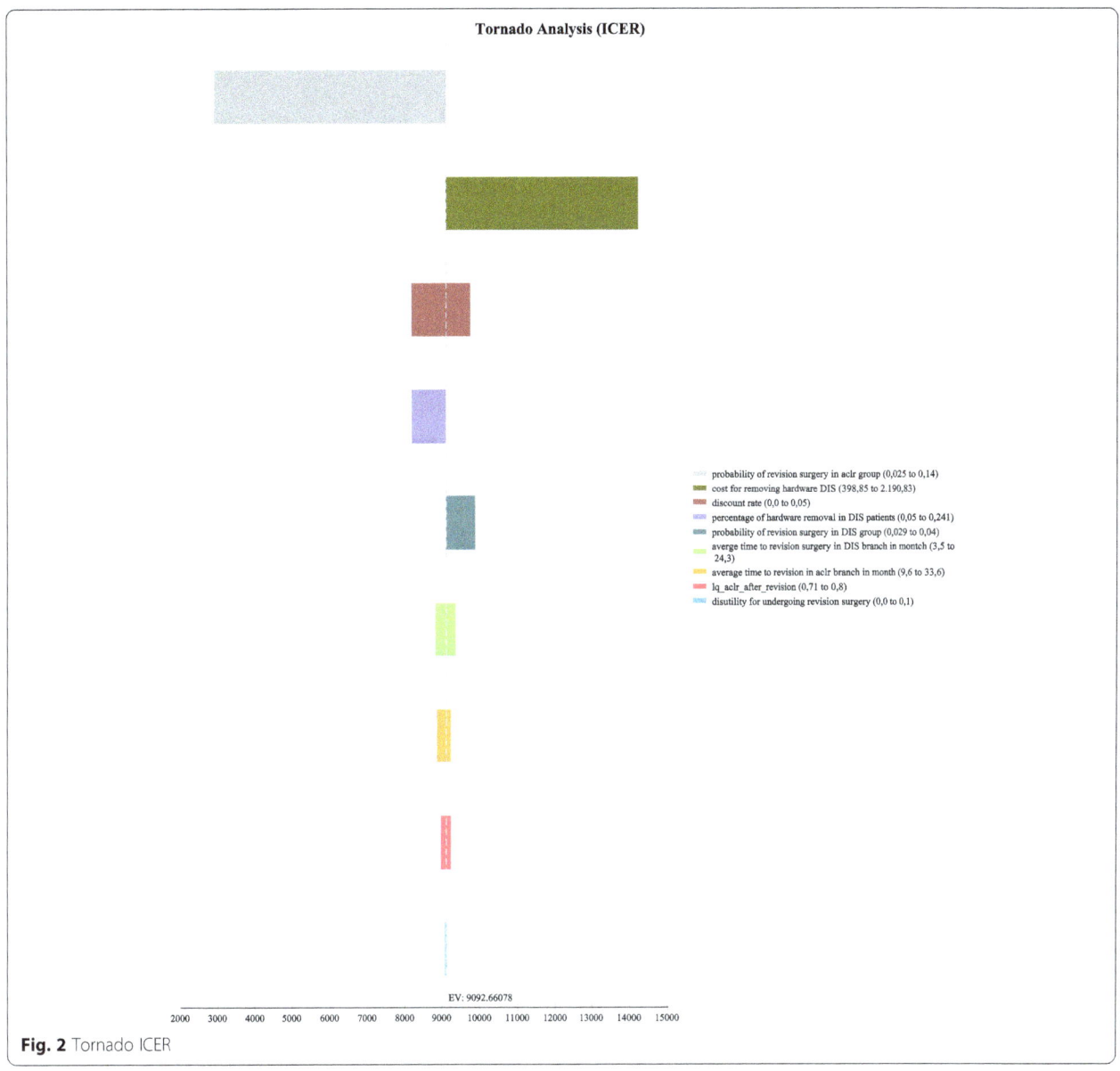

Fig. 2 Tornado ICER

that beginning from a willingness to pay of 9,000 € per QALY the DIS strategy is more likely to be cost-effective (see Fig. 3).

Discussion

At present there is no concluding evidence available whether wait and see or early intervention is the dominant strategy [5, 31, 32]. Thus we started our modeling approach by incorporating both strategies into our model. While gathering the input data we had to realize that there is no hrQoL data available for the wait and see strategy. As a result, we limited our study to a comparison between early reconstructive surgery and dynamic intraligamentary stabilization. At first sight this seems to be a severe limitation but regarding routine practice our study still is of particular relevance. Although it cannot be known a priori if a patient will benefit from an early reconstruction, with today's treatment strategies patients are undergoing such procedures notwithstanding. So if a patient decides against the wait and see approach the question remains which early intervention should be applied.

Table 3 PSA analysis for effectiveness (1 Mio. runs)

	Cost (SD)	Effectiveness (SD)
ACLR	4,632.68€	2.26 QALY (+/- 0.23)
		95% CI: 1.75–2.63 QALY
DIS	5,398.05€	2.34 QALY (+/- 0.19)
		95% CI: 1.92–2.65 QALY

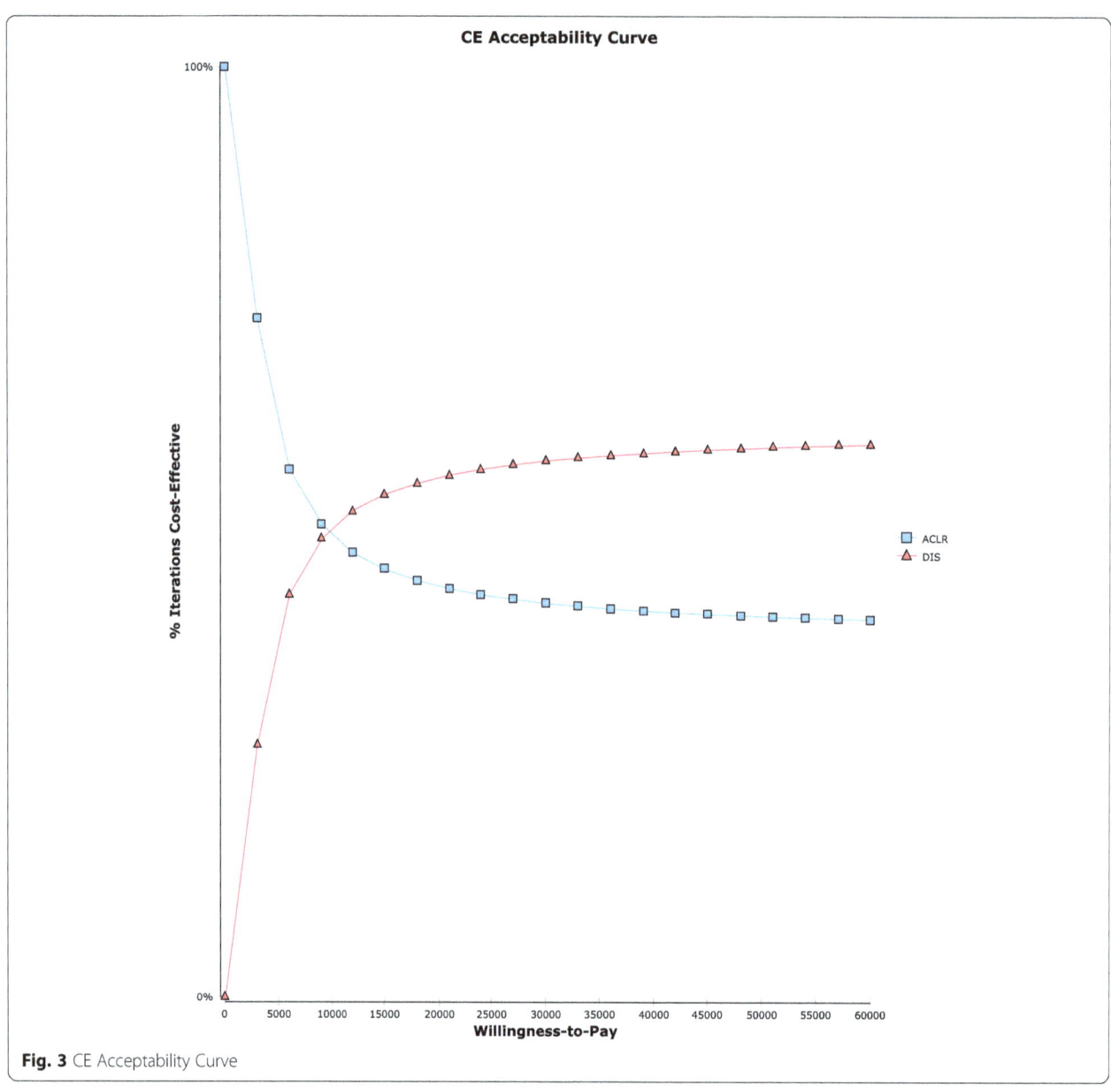

Fig. 3 CE Acceptability Curve

The scope of our analysis is limited to the inpatient setting due to data availability. Nevertheless, results should not be affected whether surgical treatment is performed out- or inpatient because overall reimbursement does not differ significantly and literature does not indicate differences in outcome. Furthermore, in Germany the majority of procedures are performed at a hospital. Moreover age and sex are not incorporated into the model. Incidence of ACL rupture has its peak between 18 and 34 years of age, so long term consequences are most likely to actually occur during the patients remaining lifetime [10, 14, 16, 17]. Studies investigating outcomes did not find clinical meaningful differences between sexes [9, 10, 17].

The time horizon of the model is limited to 3 years and cannot provide information about the long term consequences. Ultimately the patient relevant consequences are determined with the strategy chosen at the time of the ACL rupture. A knee set to develop osteoarthrosis will deteriorate further the longer the time horizon. Some of the patients will receive total knee endoprothesis, which would definitely increase costs and lower quality of life. So given today's knowledge the results would shift in favor of the DIS strategy the longer the time horizon of the model.

Until today it is still unclear what biomechanical effects lead to osteoarthrosis after an ACL-injury, whether it is the ruptured ligament or the meniscal and cartilage injuries. If it is the latter, every form of reconstruction is meaningless regarding the long term effects of osteoarthrosis. Nevertheless, some therapies can provide better quality of life in the meantime. The uncertainty surrounding the connection between biomechanical effects and outcomes is reflected in the large span between extreme values for the probabilistic sensitivity analysis for the hrQoL. As a consequence, the probability of DIS being cost-effective for a given willingness to pay is only slightly above 50%. Therefore, payers are advised to implement health services research alongside reimbursement of the DIS technology. Irrespective of the model results, the DIS technology additionally offers some advantages in the short term. First of all, with DIS there is no need of harvesting tendons from the patient thus resulting in a lower morbidity and preserving the hamstring tendon for knee stability. Furthermore, it potentially preserves the proprioceptive ability of the ligament. Another advantage is the full weight bearing capacity after surgery allowing a more aggressive rehabilitation strategy leading to significant shorter time to work (31 vs. 65 days) respectively sports (141 vs. 185 days). Depending on the patient's demand this might lead to a considerably higher quality of life shortly after the trauma.

Conclusion

Overall our findings fit with the current knowledge. There is very strong evidence, that the long term outcomes are mainly dependent on the meniscal status and some studies point out that early intervention seems to have the ability to delay or prevent further degradation of the menisci [10]. Since the DIS technology by its nature offers the earliest possible moment of intervention, the probability of saving the menisci is much higher than with the other treatment strategies and consequently a lesser number of patients are likely to develop osteoarthrosis in the long term. Since until today reconstructive surgery has not been able to reduce the rate of development of osteoarthrosis, it is rather probable that a successful preventative treatment must be delivered rapidly after injury to address the early pattern of joint damage changes [3]. But not only does the DIS technology offer such an early intervention with the potential to benefit patients with an ACL rupture in long term, it also delivers a higher hrQoL in the short term at a favorable ICER of 9092.66€ when it is compared to early reconstruction.

Acknowledgement
The authors wish to thank Stefanie Dickmänken for coordinating and supervising the collection of the SF-12 questionnaires. The project was funded by Mathys Medical AG.

Authors' contributions
MB developed and analysed the decision model, carried out the literature search and drafted the manuscript. OS participated in the development of the decision model and helped revising the manuscript. BS and CK supplied the input data for the DIS technology and assisted in the medical sections of the manuscript. All authors read and approved the final manuscript.

Competing interests
Financial support for this study was provided entirely by a grant from Mathys Medical AG. The funding agreement ensured the authors' independence in designing the study, interpreting the data, writing, and publishing the report.

Author details
[1]Friedrich-Alexander-Universität Erlangen-Nürnberg (FAU), Nuremberg, Germany. [2]Department of Trauma, Hand and Reconstructive Surgery, University Hospital Münster, Münster, Germany.

References
1. Magnussen RA, Granan L-P, Dunn WR, et al. Cross-cultural comparison of patients undergoing ACL reconstruction in the United States and Norway. Knee Surg Sports Traumatol Arthrosc. 2010;18(1):98–105. doi:10.1007/s00167-009-0919-5.
2. Greis PE, Koch BS, Adams B. Tibialis anterior or posterior allograft anterior cruciate ligament reconstruction versus hamstring autograft reconstruction: an economic analysis in a hospital-based outpatient setting. Arthroscopy. 2012;28(11):1695–701. doi:10.1016/j.arthro.2012.04.144.
3. Riordan EA, Frobell RB, Roemer FW, Hunter DJ. The health and structural consequences of acute knee injuries involving rupture of the anterior cruciate ligament. Rheum Dis Clin North Am. 2013;39(1):107–22. doi:10.1016/j.rdc.2012.10.002.
4. Janssen KW, Orchard JW, Driscoll TR, van Mechelen W. High incidence and costs for anterior cruciate ligament reconstructions performed in Australia from 2003-2004 to 2007-2008: time for an anterior cruciate ligament register by Scandinavian model? Scand J Med Sci Sports. 2012;22(4):495–501. doi:10.1111/j.1600-0838.2010.01253.x.
5. Linko E, Harilainen A, Malmivaara A, Seitsalo S. Surgical versus conservative interventions for anterior cruciate ligament ruptures in adults. Cochrane Database Syst Rev. 2005:CD001356. doi:10.1002/14651858.CD001356.pub3.
6. Mather RC, Hettrich CM, Dunn WR, et al. Cost-effectiveness Analysis of Early Reconstruction Versus Rehabilitation and Delayed Reconstruction for Anterior Cruciate Ligament Tears. Am J Sports Med. 2014. doi:10.1177/0363546514530866.
7. Baer GS, Harner CD. Clinical outcomes of allograft versus autograft in anterior cruciate ligament reconstruction. Clin Sports Med. 2007;26(4):661–81. doi:10.1016/j.csm.2007.06.010.
8. Núñez M, Sastre S, Núñez E, Lozano L, Nicodemo C, Segur JM. Health-related quality of life and direct costs in patients with anterior cruciate ligament injury: single-bundle versus double-bundle reconstruction in a low-demand cohort–a randomized trial with 2 years of follow-up. Arthroscopy. 2012;28(7):929–35. doi:10.1016/j.arthro.2011.11.034.
9. Månsson O, Kartus J, Sernert N. Health-related quality of life after anterior cruciate ligament reconstruction. Knee Surg Sports Traumatol Arthrosc. 2011;19(3):479–87. doi:10.1007/s00167-010-1303-1.
10. Barenius B, Forssblad M, Engström B, Eriksson K. Functional recovery after anterior cruciate ligament reconstruction, a study of health-related quality of life based on the Swedish National Knee Ligament Register. Knee Surg Sports Traumatol Arthrosc. 2013;21(4):914–27. doi:10.1007/s00167-012-2162-8.
11. Henle P, Röder C, Perler G, Heitkemper S, Eggli S. Dynamic Intraligamentary Stabilization (DIS) for treatment of acute anterior cruciate ligament ruptures: case series experience of the first three years. BMC Musculoskelet Disord. 2015;16(1):27. doi:10.1186/s12891-015-0484-7.
12. Kösters C, Herbort M, Schliemann B, Raschke MJ, Lenschow S. Dynamische intraligamentäre Stabilisierung des vorderen Kreuzbandes. Unfallchirurg. 2015;118(4):364–71. doi:10.1007/s00113-015-2745-1.
13. Kohl S, Ahmad S. Die Vordere Kreuzbandruptur – «… und sie heilt doch !». Swiss Med Forum. 2014;14(3):41–2.
14. Røtterud JH, Sivertsen EA, Forssblad M, Engebretsen L, Arøen A. Effect of meniscal and focal cartilage lesions on patient-reported outcome after anterior cruciate ligament reconstruction: a nationwide cohort study from Norway and Sweden of 8476 patients with 2-year follow-up. Am J Sports Med. 2013;41(3):535–43. doi:10.1177/0363546512473571.

15. Lind M, Menhert F, Pedersen AB. Incidence and outcome after revision anterior cruciate ligament reconstruction: results from the Danish registry for knee ligament reconstructions. Am J Sports Med. 2012;40(7):1551–7. doi:10.1177/0363546512446000.

16. Oiestad BE, Holm I, Engebretsen L, Risberg MA. The association between radiographic knee osteoarthritis and knee symptoms, function and quality of life 10-15 years after anterior cruciate ligament reconstruction. Br J Sports Med. 2011;45(7):583–8. doi:10.1136/bjsm.2010.073130.

17. Spindler KP, Huston LJ, Wright RW, et al. The prognosis and predictors of sports function and activity at minimum 6 years after anterior cruciate ligament reconstruction: a population cohort study. Am J Sports Med. 2011;39(2):348–59. doi:10.1177/0363546510383481.

18. Frobell RB, Roos EM, Roos HP, Ranstam J, Lohmander LS. A randomized trial of treatment for acute anterior cruciate ligament tears. N Engl J Med. 2010;363(4):331–42. doi:10.1056/NEJMoa0907797.

19. Neuman P, Englund M, Kostogiannis I, Fridén T, Roos H, Dahlberg LE. Prevalence of tibiofemoral osteoarthritis 15 years after nonoperative treatment of anterior cruciate ligament injury: a prospective cohort study. Am J Sports Med. 2008;36(9):1717–25. doi:10.1177/0363546508316770.

20. Oiestad BE, Engebretsen L, Storheim K, Risberg MA. Knee osteoarthritis after anterior cruciate ligament injury: a systematic review. Am J Sports Med. 2009;37:1434–43. doi:10.1177/0363546509338827.

21. Claes S, Hermie L, Verdonk R, Bellemans J, Verdonk P. Is osteoarthritis an inevitable consequence of anterior cruciate ligament reconstruction? A meta-analysis. Knee Surg Sport Traumatol Arthrosc. 2013;21:1967–76. doi:10.1007/s00167-012-2251-8.

22. Schliemann B, Lenschow S, Domnick C, et al. Knee joint kinematics after dynamic intraligamentary stabilization: cadaveric study on a novel anterior cruciate ligament repair technique. Knee Surg Sports Traumatol Arthrosc. August 2015. doi:10.1007/s00167-015-3735-0.

23. (Mathys European Orthopaedics). Instructions for use. 2012. http://ligamys. com/pdf/BZ-Booklet_Ligamys_95x85_75951_V01.pdf.

24. IQWiG. Arbeitspapier Kostenbestimmung. IQWiG; 2009. https://www.iqwig. de/download/Arbeitspapier_Kostenbestimmung_v_1_0.pdf.

25. Geiger EV, Laurer HL, Jakob H, Frank JM, Marzi I. Treatment costs for anterior cruciate ligament reconstruction: procedure related cost analysis in an university hospital. Unfallchirurg. 2013;116(6):517–23. doi:10.1007/s00113-011-2114-7.

26. IQWiG. Allgemeine Methoden. 2014. https://www.iqwig.de/download/ IQWiG_Methoden_Version_4-2.pdf.

27. Lind M, Lund B, Faunø P, Said S, Miller LL, Christiansen SE. Medium to long-term follow-up after ACL revision. Knee Surg Sports Traumatol Arthrosc. 2012;20(1):166–72. doi:10.1007/s00167-011-1629-3.

28. Brazier J, Roberts J. The estimation of a preference-based measure of health from the SF-12. Med Care. 2004;42(9):851–9.

29. Roberts M, Russell LB, Paltiel AD, Chambers M, McEwan P, Krahn M. Conceptualizing a model: a report of the ISPOR-SMDM Modeling Good Research Practices Task Force–2. Value Health. 2012;15(6):804–11. doi:10. 1016/j.jval.2012.06.016.

30. Wright R, Spindler K, Huston L, et al. Revision ACL reconstruction outcomes: MOON cohort. J Knee Surg. 2011;24(4):289–94. http://www.ncbi.nlm.nih.gov/ pubmed/24140144.

31. Frobell RB, Roos HP, Roos EM, Roemer FW, Ranstam J, Lohmander LS. Treatment for acute anterior cruciate ligament tear: five year outcome of randomised trial. BMJ. 2013;346(January):f232. doi:10.1136/bmj.f232.

32. Taylor DC, Posner M, Curl WW, Feagin JA. Isolated tears of the anterior cruciate ligament: over 30-year follow-up of patients treated with arthrotomy and primary repair. Am J Sports Med. 2009;37(1):65–71. doi:10.1177/ 0363546508325660.

33. Eggli S, Röder C, Perler G, Henle P. Five year results of the first ten ACL patients treated with dynamic intraligamentary stabilisation. BMC Musculoskelet Disord. 2016;17(1):105. doi:10.1186/s12891-016-0961-7.

2

Regional disparities in medical equipment distribution in the Slovak Republic – a platform for a health policy regulatory mechanism

Beáta Gavurová[1*] ⓘ, Viliam Kováč[2] and Ján Fedačko[3,4]

Abstract

Background: This study aims to examine the localisation of selected parameters in the deployment and use of medical equipment in the Slovak Republic and to verify potential regional disparities. The study evaluates the benefits of an analytical platform for regulatory mechanisms in the healthcare system.

Methods: The correspondence analysis is applied to the entire data set containing information regarding medical equipment distribution and mortality.

Results: The results highlight regional differences in the use of medical equipment throughout the analysed period from 2008 to 2014. The total amount of medical equipment increased slightly to 9192 devices during the time span. In 2014, there was a significant decrease of 16.44%. Disparities are found in the frequencies and structure of medical equipment. In some regions, medical equipment is not present or is present in low numbers.

Conclusions: The results regarding regional disparities demonstrate the regional development of the amount of medical equipment. The deployment of medical equipment is not proportional, and not all of the analysed devices are available in each region. The tests also indicate the appropriateness of the amount of medical equipment and create a platform for further investigation. The results of the analysis suggest the unsuitable distribution of medical equipment throughout the Slovak regions, where there are significant regional disparities. These findings can serve as a monitoring platform to evaluate the accessibility and efficiency of medical equipment usage.

Keywords: Medical equipment, Healthcare, Health facility, Region, Regional disparity

Background

In recent decades, the field of medical equipment and the promotion of medical and economic potential have received attention in terms of detecting the increase in the efficiency of health systems as well as rapid progress in the development and implementation of new knowledge from science and research. New medical equipment must be evaluated before it is introduced. This process is called health technology assessment. This multidisciplinary process summarises information regarding the medical, economic, social and ethical issues associated with the use of particular medical equipment. Health technology assessment has a specific position in scientific research [1–3]. It creates a link between science and decisions in health policy [4–6]. As evidenced by the International Monetary Fund studies comparing the effectiveness of health technology, this process has been ongoing in Europe for approximately a decade [7]. The Slovak Republic possesses great potential for eliminating inefficiencies [8] and determining the efficient allocation of financial resources for the health system. In some countries, health technology assessment involves a measurement process for safety and efficiency [9]. The Slovak Republic significantly lags behind in the implementation process. The

---
* Correspondence: beata.gavurova@tuke.sk
[1]Department of Banking and Investment, Faculty of Economics, Technical University of Košice, Němcovej 32, 04001 Košice, Slovak Republic

process of evaluating medical equipment directly relates to the many regulatory processes in the health system sector that are built on the pillars of the existence, acceptability, accessibility and quality of healthcare [10]. These aspects are determined by the sustainability of healthcare costs, which is a priority in the creation of a state budget. Transparent regulatory processes in healthcare along with product innovations and services and increased efficiency can greatly eliminate the disparity between resources and the cost of healthcare in a country. Studies have examined possibilities for increasing productivity in the interest of sustainable healthcare costs at optimal limits [11, 12]. Within the European Union as well as the Organisation for Economic Co-operation and Development, significant differences in the availability of resources for mental healthcare are evident. Over the past three decades, the most common causes of death changed from infectious diseases to chronic diseases, putting further pressure on the efficiency and effectiveness of healthcare [13, 14].

Management of spending on the healthcare system became a major health policy goal after the global financial crisis in 2008. Although these expenditures turned out to be stabilised after 2010, they remained considerably below the European average. There are several health indicators that can serve as evaluating points. The health care system in the Slovak Republic is based on universal coverage. It means health insurance is compulsory for each individual. General coverage is provided by basic benefit package. On the other hand, a competitive insurance model with selective contracting of health care providers by health insurers and flexible pricing of health services is offered too. After fulfilling certain explicit criteria, there are no barriers to entry the healthcare provision market or the health insurance market. Generally, healthcare is provided free of charge. It is paid by the health insurers and also some additional payments are delivered by them.

There are three health insurance companies which compete for clients based on the quality and variety of their contracted services. They are obliged to ensure accessible healthcare regulated by legislation – this means to contract a sufficient network of providers as determined by the Ministry of Health. The Health Care Surveillance Authority (Úrad pre dohľad nad zdravotnou starostlivosťou) is responsible for surveillance over the health insurance and healthcare provision. Since 2005, all the health insurance companies are joint stock companies. There is one state-owned health insurer and two privately owned health insurance companies. The first one possess roughly a 65-per-cent share of the market.

The Slovak healthcare system is now in a process of adopting new strategic planning framework. Firstly, it was introduced by the government in July 2014. This framework aims to ensure integrated outpatient care, to contain overutilization, and to restructure inpatient health care. In 2014, total expenditure in the health system was 8.1% of the gross domestic product. This figure is still significantly lower than the European Union average of 9.5%. Public resources brought 72.5% of total expenditure in the health system in that year – slightly lower than the European Union average of 76.2%. The main source of revenue of the health system is represented contributions from employees and employers, self-employed, voluntarily unemployed, publicly financed contributions on behalf of economically inactive persons and dividends. Compulsory health insurance contributions are collected by the health insurance companies. The main issue in field of financing is continually rising substantial debt of the healthcare facilities. On the other hand, the sole investments come only from the European Union structural funds [15].

From a demographic point of view, the situation in Europe is not appropriate in its current state. According to forecasts, in 2030, up to 30% of the European population will be over 65 years old, and fewer people will be in the age range for economic activity – over 15 and under 65 [16, 17]. This situation is caused by the projected decrease from 67% to 56% in the share of the population in the economically active age range. These reported demographic changes will have a significant impact on public finances in the European Union and will put pressure on health policies. It is important to give consideration to public spending linked to the issue of age, such as pensions, health and long-term care. These expenditures are expected to grow by 4.1% of the gross domestic product in 2060 compared to 2010. This represents an increase of approximately 25% to 29% of the gross domestic product. For expenditures on pensions, an increase from 11.3% to approximately 13% of the gross domestic product is expected. There will be significant differences determined by the structure and methods of implementation of potential pension reforms among the European countries. Because there are large discrepancies in the resources available for healthcare, the extent of differences and the rate of diffusion of new medical practices and equipment will play an important role. These aspects are optimally evaluated by a particular measurement system, avoidable mortality, which is the subject of development and review by many research teams around the world [8, 18–23]. This measurement system considers the extent of the implementation of modern healthcare technologies in the context of interventions that are the basis for recovery and the inclusion or exclusion of individual diagnoses of avoidable mortality. It is sometimes called treatable or preventable mortality. Negative values for avoidable mortality in a country may also reflect the significant non-availability of appropriate medical equipment, poor quality of provided healthcare services, or a combination of both. From a macroeconomic perspective, the smallest volume 872.9 USD of financial resources in healthcare per capita is spent in Romania, where the standardised mortality rate of 304 per 100,000 inhabitants is the highest among the European Union members. In contrast, Luxembourg is characterised by the highest amount 6340.6 USD, and its standardised mortality rate of 89 per 100,000 inhabitants is one of the lowest among the surveyed countries. The lowest treatable mortality rates are found in Denmark, Sweden, the Netherlands, Spain, and France. There are minimal differences in the values of treatable mortality among these countries; the significant differences are in the volume of expenditures on their national health systems per capita – for instance, Spain's expenditure is 3144.9 USD [10].

These facts prompted us to explore the situation in a field related to mortality in the Slovak Republic. Usage of the medical equipment influences mortality rate in general. Therefore, the primary aim of this study is to examine the localisation of the selected parameters in the deployment and use of selected medical equipment in the Slovak Republic and to verify the potential regional disparities. This study also evaluates the benefits of a quantitative analytical platform for regulatory and stabilising mechanisms in the health system. The unordinary methodical approaches are able to reveal the desired objective – a comprehensive evaluation of the observed equipment. It is not only to pick up advantages or disadvantages, but also to prepare a platform for further research. That is why, not multifaceted outputs are shown in the analysis, but rather significant points are addressed to be investigated in the subsequent steps. The study also assesses a position of an analytical platform in field of the healthcare system not only for the running regulatory mechanisms, but also to prepare new types of regulatory mechanisms.

Methods

The data is provided by the National Health Information Center (Národné centrum zdravotníckych informácií). The dataset involves numbers of the individual type of medical equipment in the particular healthcare facilities. There are twenty-nine medical equipment types included in this analysis. Their labels in the subsequent tables and figures are as follows: angiograph – 1; brachytherapy apparatus – 2; bronchoscope – 3; cystoscope – 4; dialysis monitor – 5; electrocardiograph – 6; electroencephalograph – 7; electromyograph – 8; endoscope – 9; laparoscope, arthroscope – 10; gamma camera – 11; gastroscope, duodenoscope – 12; isotope irradiator – 13; colonoscope, sigmoidoscope, proctoscope – 14; colposcope – 15; cryogenic device – 16; laryngoscope – 17; laser – 18; linear accelerator – 19; lithotripter – 20; magnetic resonance imaging device – 21; mammograph – 22; monitoring device – 23; positron tomograph – 24; x-ray – 25; tomograph – 26; ultraviolet

and infrared emitter – 27; ultrasound device – 28; uretroscope – 29; high-frequency device – 30.

Regional disparities are observed according to the third level of the nomenclature of territorial units for statistics. This administrative level of the territorial division of the Slovak Republic represents the highest tier of the administrative division of the country. This division is applied from the perspective of self-government because these self-governing regions also manage the health facilities in their territory.

There are eight self-governing regions in the Slovak Republic, which have the following labels in the subsequent tables and figures: the Banská Bystrica Self-governing Region – BC; the Bratislava Self-governing Region – BL; the Košice Self-governing Region – KI; the Nitra Self-governing Region – NI; the Prešov Self-governing Region – PV; the Trenčín Self-governing Region – TC; the Trnava Self-governing Region – TA; the Žilina Self-governing Region – ZI.

Several mathematical relations are applied in the analytical part of the study. They are mentioned in their applied forms for the purposes of this analysis. The majority of the analysis is conducted in the form of a correspondence analysis. The rest of the analysis involves identifying similarities between the types of medical equipment. All the analytical outputs are executed in the statistical software environment R using among others the package vcd handling visualising categorical data.

The equipment profile is calculated as follows [24]:

$$EP_{e;r} = \frac{n_{e;r}}{\sum\limits_{r=1}^{c} n_{e;r}}, \tag{1}$$

where the variables are as follows:

- $EP_{e;\,r}$ – equipment profile of the e equipment type in the r self-governing region;
- e – the equipment type;
- r – the self-governing region;
- $n_{e;\,r}$ – number of the e equipment type in the r self-governing region;
- c – number of the self-governing regions.

The quantification of the regional equipment profile is performed in the following way [24]:

$$REP_r = \frac{\sum\limits_{e=1}^{t} n_{e;r}}{\sum\limits_{e=1}^{t} \sum\limits_{r=1}^{c} n_{e;r}}, \tag{2}$$

where the variables are as follows:

- REP_r – regional equipment profile of the r self-governing region;

- t – number of the equipment types;
- e – the equipment type;
- r – the self-governing region;
- $n_{e;\,r}$ – number of the e equipment type in the r self-governing region;
- c – number of the self-governing regions.

There are 8 regions in the Slovak Republic, which is why c is equal to 8. In our case, there are 29 types of equipment, so t is equal to 29. To compute the ratio of the amount of equipment to the number of inhabitants, the population as of 31 December 2014 is used.

The chi-square distance is calculated as follows [25]:

$$D_{e_1:e_2} = \frac{EP_{e_1;r} - EP_{e_2;r}}{REP_r}, \tag{3}$$

where the variables are as follows:

- e_1 – the equipment type;
- e_2 – the equipment type;
- $D_{e_1:e_2}$ – regional equipment profile of the r self-governing region;
- r – the self-governing region;
- $EP_{e_1;r}$ – equipment profile of the e_1 equipment type in the r self-governing region;
- $EP_{e_2;r}$ – equipment profile of the e_2 equipment type in the r self-governing region;
- REP_r – regional equipment profile of the r self-governing region.

The output of the analysis is demonstrated on the plots which visualise localisation of the observed types of the medical equipment too. The applied types of the diagrams are mosaic plot and association plot. The first one introduces a multidimensional graphical method to envision the data from several qualitative variables. This method represents visualisation of contingency table involving discrete values in general. A standard way is to demonstrate two-dimensional contingency table. Dependence between parts of mosaic plot is found horizontally and vertically too. One reliance represents a proportion among categories of the particular variable, whilst the other one relation among the variables of the same category. Each cell pictured by rectangle created by rectangle exhibits a proportion of the particular category for the particular variable. Appropriate dimension of rectangle is determined by its share of the total for the variable [26, 27]. This type of diagram is also called mekko chart.

On the other hand, the association plot represents another way of visualisation of two-dimensional contingency table. Every cell visualised like rectangle represents one category of the individual variable. All the cells for each category and each variable are localised relative to a baseline representing an independent state. On the one hand, a case with observed frequency higher than expected frequency is demonstrated by cell rising above the line. On the other hand, a case, which shows smaller observed frequency than is expected, falls below the line. Comparison of observed and expected frequency is measured under the null hypothesis of independence [28, 29]. Sometimes, this type of diagram is referred to as Cohen-Friendly association plot.

Results

An initial look at the dataset demonstrates the localisation of the individual types of equipment in the particular self-governing regions in Fig.1.

Equipment	1	2	3	4	5	6	7	8	9	10	11	12	13	14	15	16	17	18	19	20	21	22	23	24	25	26	27	28	29	
Region																														
BC	5	1	9	7	53	11	196	5	46	1	28	1	21	6	6	6	27		2	2	8	312	1	61	10	7	145	1	30	1008
BL	5	1	18	17	100	15	283	14	113	7	54	3	36	16	19	24	43	6	5	9	22	404	3	108	15	18	278	16	68	1720
KI	7		16	4	151	10	233	11	77	8	29	3	25	2	6	17	25	3	1	2	11	292	1	65	8	10	131	4	36	1188
NI	3		19	8	109	9	157	8	46	2	16	3	14	6	2	8	19	1	3	4	10	185	2	76	9	3	116	6	42	886
PV	8	2	27	8	83	11	144	8	76	3	27	3	19	4	3	9	29	2	7	6	10	407		74	11	14	151	8	40	1194
TC	3		11	9	125	13	155	4	72		15		21	3	1	4	21	2	2	4	9	147		60	11	13	107	5	25	842
TA	1		7	13	87	12	113	9	65		21		17		6	7	17		5	4	8	214		61	7	7	90	21	21	813
ZI	5	3	20	11	108	14	243	5	110	4	36	6	20	9	6	9	33	3	5	5	11	519		96	13	14	170	11	52	1541
	37	7	127	77	816	95	1524	64	605	25	226	19	173	46	49	84	214	17	30	36	89	2480	7	601	84	86	1188	72	314	9192

Fig. 1 Equipment distribution according to the self-governing region and its type

The localisation of the equipment types in the separate self-governing regions is demonstrated in Fig. 1. The x-axis shows the order of all the equipment types recognised by the dataset from the National Centre of Health Information of the Slovak Republic, and the y-axis represents the administrative division of the Slovak Republic at the level of the territory units – the self-governing regions. The shading of the x-axis tags represents the share of the amount of equipment of that type to the total number of equipment of all 29 types on the x-axis and the share of the equipment located in the particular self-governing regions to the total amount of the equipment in the entire Slovak Republic on the y-axis. The size of the rings in the individual cells and their shading are determined by the chi-square distance. The larger the ring is, the larger the distance is between the given rows. This indicates that these types of equipment are more dissimilar. We have chosen this visualisation because more equipment types are similar rather than different. To analyse the distribution of the devices throughout the Slovak Republic, we quantify an equipment profile for each type of equipment in 2008 and in 2014. This profile presents the share of that type of equipment localised in the particular self-governing region to the total amount of equipment in the entire country. The equipment profiles in 2008 are shown in Table 1.

The unsuitable localisation of the devices among the self-governing regions in 2008 is seen mainly in the case of the least numerous types that are mentioned above in Table 1. Two exceptions appeared. The first one is the colposcope, which has 44 pieces and is the 18th most numerous device; however, 16 of them – 36.36% – are localised in one self-governing region. The second one is the laryngoscope, the 14th most numerous type of equipment. Its total number of 77 includes a 25.97% share and a 24.68% share in the two most abundant regions and zero in one region. The state at the end of the observed period is shown in Table 2.

The equipment profiles perform very similarly in 2014 in comparison to 2008, as seen in Table 2. The colposcope is still an instance of unsuitably located equipment, although with the increase of its total number to 46, its share in the same self-governing region fell to 34.78%. The share of laryngoscopes in the most abundant region increased to 28.57%, and the zero number in another region disappeared.

To examine the profile of the self-governing regions from with regard to equipment type, a regional equipment profile is applied. It characterises the particular type of medical device in light of all the self-governing regions. The regional equipment profile expresses the mean share of all the equipment profiles in each region, as shown in Table 3.

Table 1 Equipment profiles in 2008

Profile	BC	BL	KI	NI	PV	TC	TA	ZI
1	0.125	0.2	0.225	0.025	0.175	0.075	0	0.175
2	0.1818	0.0909	0.3636	0	0	0.0909	0	0.2727
3	0.0922	0.0922	0.1844	0.156	0.1773	0.078	0.0567	0.1631
4	0.0532	0.2234	0.1596	0.117	0.0957	0.1064	0.1064	0.1383
5	0.0669	0.6642	0.0291	0.0436	0.0392	0.0218	0.0567	0.0785
6	0.1342	0.2067	0.1902	0.0797	0.084	0.0926	0.0632	0.1493
7	0.1827	0.1731	0.1154	0.0865	0.1058	0.1154	0.1154	0.1058
8	0.1304	0.2174	0.2174	0.1449	0.1159	0.029	0.0435	0.1014
9	0.1084	0.1756	0.1979	0.0912	0.1188	0.0706	0.0826	0.1549
10	0.0909	0.2955	0.2273	0.0455	0.2273	0	0.0455	0.0682
11	0.1348	0.2348	0.187	0.0609	0.0652	0.0522	0.0739	0.1913
12	0.1481	0.1111	0.2222	0.1481	0.0741	0.037	0	0.2593
13	0.1045	0.204	0.194	0.0995	0.1045	0.0995	0.0796	0.1144
14	0.1136	0.3636	0.1364	0.0682	0.0455	0.0682	0	0.2045
15	0.0625	0.25	0.25	0.0625	0.0625	0.0312	0.1562	0.125
16	0.0909	0.2597	0.2468	0.0779	0.0779	0.026	0.1039	0.1169
17	0.1923	0.2564	0.1496	0.0684	0.1026	0.0556	0.0513	0.1239
18	0.1429	0.3571	0.1429	0	0.0714	0.1429	0	0.1429
19	0.1212	0.1818	0.1212	0.1515	0.1212	0.0606	0.1212	0.1212
20	0.1212	0.2121	0.303	0.1515	0.1515	0	0.0303	0.0303
21	0.0972	0.2639	0.1806	0.0833	0.125	0.0694	0.0694	0.1111
22	0.1275	0.2064	0.1779	0.0834	0.1209	0.0491	0.0615	0.1733
23	0	0.6667	0	0.3333	0	0	0	0
24	0.1212	0.1812	0.15	0.1288	0.1038	0.0762	0.0938	0.145
25	0.1714	0.2	0.1286	0.0857	0.1143	0.0571	0.0857	0.1571
26	0.0333	0.2	0.0667	0.1333	0.2333	0.1667	0	0.1667
27	0.1164	0.2578	0.1362	0.1185	0.105	0.0759	0.0613	0.1289
28	0.0448	0.2687	0.1642	0.0746	0.1045	0.0448	0.1791	0.1194
29	0.0989	0.1943	0.2792	0.0777	0.0954	0.0742	0.0424	0.1378

The regional equipment profiles demonstrate the average localisation of the equipment types according to the self-governing regions, as shown in Table 4.

The equipment average row profile shown in Table 4 reveals quite large regional disparities in this field in the Slovak Republic. For instance, the highest average row profile belongs to the BL Region, where its value reaches 0.1871, whereas the lowest one is associated with the TA Region at 0.884, which is less than half of the previous number. These values represent the share of the entire amount of equipment in the Slovak Republic according to localisation in the self-governing regions. They express the average share of all the equipment types in the individual self-governing regions.

The equipment to population ratio represents the amount of medical equipment per 1000 inhabitants. The

Table 2 Equipment profiles in 2014

Profile	BC	BL	KI	NI	PV	TC	TA	ZI
1	0.1351	0.1351	0.1892	0.0811	0.2162	0.0811	0.027	0.1351
2	0.1429	0.1429	0	0	0.2857	0	0	0.4286
3	0.0709	0.1417	0.126	0.1496	0.2126	0.0866	0.0551	0.1575
4	0.0909	0.2208	0.0519	0.1039	0.1039	0.1169	0.1688	0.1429
5	0.065	0.1225	0.185	0.1336	0.1017	0.1532	0.1066	0.1324
6	0.1286	0.1857	0.1529	0.103	0.0945	0.1017	0.0741	0.1594
7	0.1158	0.1579	0.1053	0.0947	0.1158	0.1368	0.1263	0.1474
8	0.0781	0.2188	0.1719	0.125	0.125	0.0625	0.1406	0.0781
9	0.076	0.1868	0.1273	0.076	0.1256	0.119	0.1074	0.1818
10	0.04	0.28	0.32	0.08	0.12	0	0	0.16
11	0.1239	0.2389	0.1283	0.0708	0.1195	0.0664	0.0929	0.1593
12	0.0526	0.1579	0.1579	0.1579	0.1579	0	0	0.3158
13	0.1214	0.2081	0.1445	0.0809	0.1098	0.1214	0.0983	0.1156
14	0.1304	0.3478	0.0435	0.1304	0.087	0.0652	0	0.1957
15	0.1224	0.3878	0.1224	0.0408	0.0612	0.0204	0.1224	0.1224
16	0.0714	0.2857	0.2024	0.0952	0.1071	0.0476	0.0833	0.1071
17	0.1262	0.2009	0.1168	0.0888	0.1355	0.0981	0.0794	0.1542
18	0	0.3529	0.1765	0.0588	0.1176	0.1176	0	0.1765
19	0.0667	0.1667	0.0333	0.1	0.2333	0.0667	0.1667	0.1667
20	0.0556	0.25	0.0556	0.1111	0.1667	0.1111	0.1111	0.1389
21	0.0899	0.2472	0.1236	0.1124	0.1124	0.1011	0.0899	0.1236
22	0.1258	0.1629	0.1177	0.0746	0.1641	0.0593	0.0863	0.2093
23	0.1429	0.4286	0.1429	0.2857	0	0	0	0
24	0.1015	0.1797	0.1082	0.1265	0.1231	0.0998	0.1015	0.1597
25	0.119	0.1786	0.0952	0.1071	0.131	0.131	0.0833	0.1548
26	0.0814	0.2093	0.1163	0.0349	0.1628	0.1512	0.0814	0.1628
27	0.1221	0.234	0.1103	0.0976	0.1271	0.0901	0.0758	0.1431
28	0.0139	0.2222	0.0556	0.0833	0.1111	0.0694	0.2917	0.1528
29	0.0955	0.2166	0.1146	0.1338	0.1274	0.0796	0.0669	0.1656

highest figure belongs to the BL Region, with a value of 0.2118, whereas the lowest ratio, at 0.0647, is assigned to the TA Region. This indicates that every thousand inhabitants are served by less than one-third of the medical equipment available in the best-equipped region.

Table 3 Regional equipment profiles

Year	BC	BL	KI	NI	PV	TC	TA	ZI
2008	0.119	0.2458	0.1658	0.0894	0.1023	0.0649	0.0672	0.1457
2009	0.1246	0.2118	0.1756	0.0875	0.1107	0.0719	0.0647	0.1533
2010	0.1178	0.2043	0.1939	0.0828	0.1092	0.0751	0.0696	0.1473
2011	0.117	0.2024	0.1978	0.0798	0.1091	0.0744	0.0684	0.151
2012	0.1187	0.2011	0.1956	0.0818	0.1093	0.073	0.0753	0.1452
2013	0.1173	0.1992	0.1963	0.0804	0.113	0.075	0.0747	0.1441
2014	0.1097	0.1871	0.1292	0.0964	0.1299	0.0916	0.0884	0.1676

Equipment density is calculated as the ratio of the average row profile and the equipment to population ratio. It expresses the proportion of whether a share of the equipment localised in a particular region is higher than the ratio of all the medical equipment to the population of the given region. The highest value, 1.1605, is reached by the BL Region, whereas the lowest value, 0.9026, belongs to the TC Region. This finding reveals that the most-equipped region also has the best density of medical equipment.

One of the most frequently applied methods to determine how much information is available in the examined data is to use the eigenvalue with its attributes as the indicator [30]. For this purpose, we have quantified the eigenvalues of the dimensions according to the correspondence analysis, as shown in Table 5.

According to the output of the executed correspondence analysis as seen in Table 5, there are eight dimensions, but the last one has a share of only $4.14 \cdot 10^{-30}\%$, which can be considered equal to 0. These eight dimensions represent the individual self-governing regions of the Slovak Republic. The main dimension explains 39.75% of the data inertia. This could be presented as the most representative self-governing region. The second and third dimensions add approximately the same share of inertia –20.85% and 16.98%, respectively. The fourth dimension and the successive dimensions individually produce less than a half of the inertia produced by the previous dimension. The fourth one explains 7.62%, which is only 44.84% of the inertia clarified by the previous dimension. Because the first three dimensions provide a 77.59% share of the data inertia together, we can set the number of statistically significant dimensions to three [31]. It means the three strongest self-governing regions – in terms of the strength from an angle of view of this analysis – are able to perform as the whole dataset. The rest of the analysis is concerned with this setting.

The situation of the localisation of health facilities is varied in the Slovak Republic. To measure regional disparities, the similarity of the equipment row profiles is used. We compute similarity as the chi-square distance. The output, which reflects the chi-square distances from the end of the explored period subtracted from the beginning of the explored period, is shown in Table 6.

If we compare individual distances between the equipment types at the beginning and at the end of the observed period, we can observe changes in the similarities of the same equipment type pairs. There are two cases in which no change occurred after the analysed period: between the angiograph and the group of colonoscopes, sigmoidoscopes and proctoscopes and between the laryngoscope and mammograph.

Table 4 Regional equipment profiles

Indicator	BC	BL	KI	NI	PV	TC	TA	ZI
average row profile	0.119	0.2458	0.1658	0.0894	0.1023	0.0649	0.0672	0.1457
equipment to population ratio	0.1246	0.2118	0.1756	0.0875	0.1107	0.0719	0.0647	0.1533
equipment density	0.9551	1.1605	0.9442	1.0217	0.9241	0.9026	1.0386	0.9504

Figure 2 presents an analysis of the equipment row profiles.

Figure 2 displays the chi-square distances of the equipment row profiles. If we consider this table matrix, we can observe that the matrix is symmetrical because the similarity of the equipment types based on the chi-square distance quantification is not directional or causal. Zeros in the main diagonal represent the identity of the same equipment row profiles. The smaller the distance between two row profiles is, the more similar they are. In our case, this indicates that the lower similarity values are between the two equipment row profiles. The most analogous localisation of these two equipment types is in the Slovak Republic. The largest distance can be seen between the brachytherapy apparatus and the positron tomograph, which indicates that the localisation of equipment for brachytherapy and the positron tomograph is the most different with a chi-square distance of 3.17. This is followed by the pair of the uretroscope and brachytherapy apparatus, which are distant from each other by 1.98. Generally, brachytherapy apparatus is the most distant one from all the equipment because as the only one device it is not nearer to any remaining equipment than distance of 1 is. Dependence between a number of the equipment and its localisation is demonstrated in Fig. 3.

The mosaic diagram in Fig. 3 presents the localisation of the equipment shown in the y-axis types according to the separate self-governing regions presented on the x-axis in such a way that the quadrilateral area represents the share of the number of the particular type of equipment to the total number of all equipment in the entire Slovak Republic or in the particular self-governing region. Blue shading

represents a situation in which the number of equipment of a particular type is higher than in the case of their uniform distribution among all the healthcare facilities in the Slovak Republic. The red shading indicates a state in which there is a smaller number of equipment of that type localised in the specific self-governing regions than in the case of uniform localisation.

These statements can be formulated into the two following hypotheses:

– H_0: there is no dependence between the number of equipment of the same type and its localisation;
– H_1: there is a dependence between the number of the equipment of the same type and its localisation.

To determine which statement is statistically true, we use standardised Pearson's residuals. Pearson's chi-square test statistics reach a value of 532.08 at 196 degrees of freedom. The p-value stands at $7.82 \cdot 10^{-33}$, which can be regarded as 0, so we do not reject the zero hypothesis H_0. This indicates that there is no evidence that dependence between the equipment type and its localisation is present according to this analysis. The most numerous equipment localisation is demonstrated in Fig. 4.

To visualise the most numerous equipment, we have chosen four types of equipment with the highest absolute quantities: monitoring devices, electrocardiographs, ultrasound devices and dialysis monitors. The association diagram in Fig. 4 shows the relationship between the type of equipment demonstrated on the y-axis and its location region visualised on the x-axis.

The hypotheses are as follows:

– H_0: there is no association between the number of equipment of a particular type and its localisation;
– H_1: there is an association between the number of equipment of a particular type and its localisation.

To verify the relationship between the types of equipment and the self-governing regions, we applied Pearson's chi-square test. The statistics reached a value of 265.30 at 21 degrees of freedom with a p-value of $2.2 \cdot 10^{-16}$, which can be considered to be 0. According to this result, we do not reject the zero hypothesis H_0, which says that there is no association between equipment type and its localisation.

Table 5 Eigenvalues of the dimensions of the medical equipment distribution

Dimension	Eigenvalue	Percentage of variance	Cumulative percentage of variance
1	0.0230	39.75%	39.75%
2	0.0121	20.85%	60.61%
3	0.0098	16.98%	77.59%
4	0.0044	7.62%	85.20%
5	0.0040	6.85%	92.06%
6	0.0029	4.98%	97.04%
7	0.0017	2.96%	100%
8	$2.40 \cdot 10^{-33}$	$4.14 \cdot 10^{-30}$%	100%

Table 6 Subtraction of chi-square distances of equipment profiles between 2014 and 2008

	1	2	3	4	5	6	7	8	9	10	11	12	13	14	15	16	17	18	19	20	21	22	23	24	25	26	27	28	29
1	0	0.474	0.18	0.188	1.1	0.022	0.105	0.085	0.083	0.198	0.006	0.124	0	0.194	0.138	0.055	0.059	0.157	0.018	0.098	0.079	0.012	1.455	0.085	0.038	0.261	0.082	0.733	0.059
2	0.474	0	0.133	0.701	0.617	0.806	0.534	0.99	0.592	0.293	0.636	0.269	0.805	0.433	0.772	0.846	0.412	0.701	0.061	0.218	0.638	0.13	0.878	0.455	0.498	0.434	0.305	1.055	0.747
3	0.18	0.133	0	0.187	1.65	0.014	0.062	0.093	0.081	0.114	0.098	0.095	0.085	0.171	0.216	0.078	0.21	0.333	0.105	0.207	0.037	0.01	1.242	0.005	0.074	0.1	0.038	0.544	0.133
4	0.188	0.701	0.187	0	0.918	0.108	0.11	0.06	0.034	0.565	0.001	0.488	0.096	0.188	0.17	0.163	0.106	0.201	0.114	0.445	0.041	0.121	0.566	0.044	0.041	0.228	0.087	0.145	0.018
5	1.1	0.617	1.65	0.918	0	1.064	1.299	1.03	1.217	0.364	0.78	1.125	1.107	0.029	0.44	0.717	0.796	0.325	0.81	1.353	0.788	0.849	0.36	1.165	1.057	1.555	0.721	0.233	1.203
6	0.022	0.806	0.014	0.108	1.064	0	0.041	0.031	0.032	0.072	0.008	0.246	0.009	0.072	0.101	0.003	0.053	0.094	0.28	0.231	0.011	0.065	1.244	0.019	0.022	0.409	0.024	0.568	0.021
7	0.105	0.534	0.062	0.11	1.299	0.041	0	0.139	0.067	0.259	0.095	0.521	0.073	0.003	0.035	0.051	0.088	0.091	0.16	0.548	0.101	0.026	1.096	0.053	0.054	0.534	0.054	0.247	0.195
8	0.085	0.99	0.093	0.06	1.03	0.031	0.139	0	0.067	0.292	0.046	0.329	0.024	0.226	0.035	0.051	0.084	0.026	0.144	0.076	0.008	0.156	0.832	0.002	0.059	0.357	0.051	0.09	0.032
9	0.083	0.592	0.081	0.034	1.217	0.032	0.067	0.067	0	0.31	0.005	0.024	0.241	0.094	0.207	0.096	0.084	0.109	0.162	0.254	0.015	0.079	0.913	0.01	0.051	0.483	0.001	0.381	0.019
10	0.198	0.293	0.114	0.565	0.364	0.072	0.259	0.292	0.31	0	0.027	0.347	0.241	0.03	0.123	0.061	0.227	0.345	0.641	0.571	0.326	0.263	1.278	0.186	0.354	0.057	0.162	1.267	0.136
11	0.006	0.636	0.098	0.001	0.78	0.008	0.095	0.046	0.005	0.027	0	0.264	0.051	0.102	0.019	0.008	0.06	0.03	0.091	0.348	0.048	0.017	1.192	0.043	0.025	0.636	0.085	0.431	0.055
12	0.124	0.269	0.095	0.488	1.125	0.246	0.521	0.329	0.024	0.347	0.264	0	0.396	0.07	0.151	0.003	0.16	0.144	0.355	0.172	0.188	0.146	1.179	0.22	0.308	0.048	0.187	0.806	0.098
13	0	0.805	0.085	0.096	1.107	0.009	0.073	0.024	0.207	0.241	0.019	0.16	0	0.076	0.106	0.138	0.105	0.017	0.275	0.222	0.003	0.085	0.994	0.017	0.061	0.395	0.008	0.5	0.019
14	0.194	0.433	0.171	0.188	0.029	0.072	0.003	0.226	0.094	0.03	0.102	0.07	0.076	0	0.151	0.003	0.067	0.183	0.27	0.352	0.028	0.139	1.001	0.026	0.026	0.236	0.017	0.838	0.122
15	0.138	0.772	0.216	0.17	0.44	0.101	0.076	0.035	0.207	0.123	0.019	0.278	0.106	0.151	0	0.138	0.042	0.2	0.375	0.094	0.069	0.15	1.407	0.148	0.175	0.674	0.034	0.674	0.114
16	0.055	0.846	0.078	0.163	0.717	0.003	0.038	0.051	0.096	0.061	0.008	0.11	0.138	0.003	0.138	0	0.043	0.277	0.29	0.222	0.003	0.113	1.282	0.015	0.067	0.664	0.046	0.687	0.013
17	0.059	0.412	0.21	0.106	0.796	0.053	0.088	0.021	0.084	0.227	0.06	0.16	0.105	0.067	0.042	0.043	0	0.083	0.077	0.299	0.058	0.014	0.975	0.111	0.023	0.622	0.078	0.39	0.159
18	0.157	0.701	0.333	0.201	0.325	0.094	0.091	0.088	0.109	0.345	0.03	0.144	0.017	0.183	0.2	0.277	0.083	0	0.167	0.574	0.023	0.093	1.092	0.077	0.013	0.399	0.009	0.654	0.08
19	0.018	0.061	0.105	0.114	0.81	0.28	0.16	0.144	0.162	0.641	0.091	0.355	0.275	0.27	0.375	0.29	0.077	0.167	0	0.289	0.197	0.088	0.067	0.219	0.218	0.252	0.229	0.208	0.01
20	0.098	0.218	0.207	0.445	1.353	0.231	0.548	0.076	0.254	0.571	0.348	0.172	0.222	0.352	0.094	0.037	0.299	0.574	0.289	0	0.23	0.153	0.773	0.331	0.378	0.899	0.281	0.111	0.158
21	0.079	0.638	0.037	0.041	0.788	0.011	0.101	0.008	0.015	0.326	0.048	0.188	0.003	0.028	0.069	0	0.058	0.023	0.197	0.23	0	0.105	1.017	0.048	0.045	0.361	0.015	0.497	0.064
22	0.012	0.13	0.01	0.121	0.849	0.065	0.026	0.156	0.079	0.263	0.017	0.146	0.085	0.139	0.15	0.113	0.014	0.093	0.088	0.153	0.105	0	0.81	0.033	0.084	0.382	0.024	0.518	0.003
23	1.455	0.878	1.242	0.566	0.36	1.244	1.096	0.832	0.913	1.278	1.192	1.179	0.994	1.001	1.407	1.282	0.975	1.092	0.067	0.773	1.017	0.81	0	0.968	1.046	0.693	0.72	0.153	1.546
24	0.085	0.455	0.005	0.044	1.165	0.019	0.053	0.002	0.01	0.186	0.043	0.22	0.017	0.026	0.148	0.015	0.111	0.077	0.219	0.331	0.048	0.033	0.968	0	0.027	0.37	0.006	0.421	0.144
25	0.038	0.498	0.074	0.041	1.057	0.022	0.054	0.059	0.019	0.354	0.025	0.308	0.061	0.026	0.175	0.067	0.023	0.013	0.218	0.378	0.045	0.084	1.046	0.027	0	0.548	0.029	0.519	0.154
26	0.261	0.434	0.1	0.228	1.555	0.409	0.534	0.357	0.483	0.057	0.636	0.048	0.395	0.236	0.674	0.664	0.622	0.399	0.252	0.899	0.361	0.382	0.693	0.37	0.548	0	0.323	0.125	0.487
27	0.082	0.305	0.038	0.087	0.721	0.024	0.054	0.051	0.001	0.162	0.085	0.187	0.008	0.017	0.034	0.046	0.078	0.009	0.229	0.281	0.015	0.024	0.72	0.006	0.029	0.323	0	0.531	0.14
28	0.733	1.055	0.544	0.145	0.233	0.568	0.247	0.09	0.381	1.267	0.431	0.806	0.5	0.838	0.674	0.687	0.39	0.654	0.208	0.111	0.497	0.518	0.153	0.421	0.519	0.125	0.531	0	0.441
29	0.059	0.747	0.133	0.018	1.203	0.021	0.195	0.032	0.019	0.136	0.055	0.098	0.019	0.122	0.114	0.013	0.159	0.08	0.01	0.158	0.064	0.003	1.546	0.144	0.154	0.487	0.14	0.441	0

Legend: figures written in the upper right half of the matrix belong to year 2008, and numbers displayed in the lower left half of the matrix belong to year 2014; main diagonal is the same for both years because of its characteristic; figures written in black are positive numbers, and numbers written in red are negative numbers

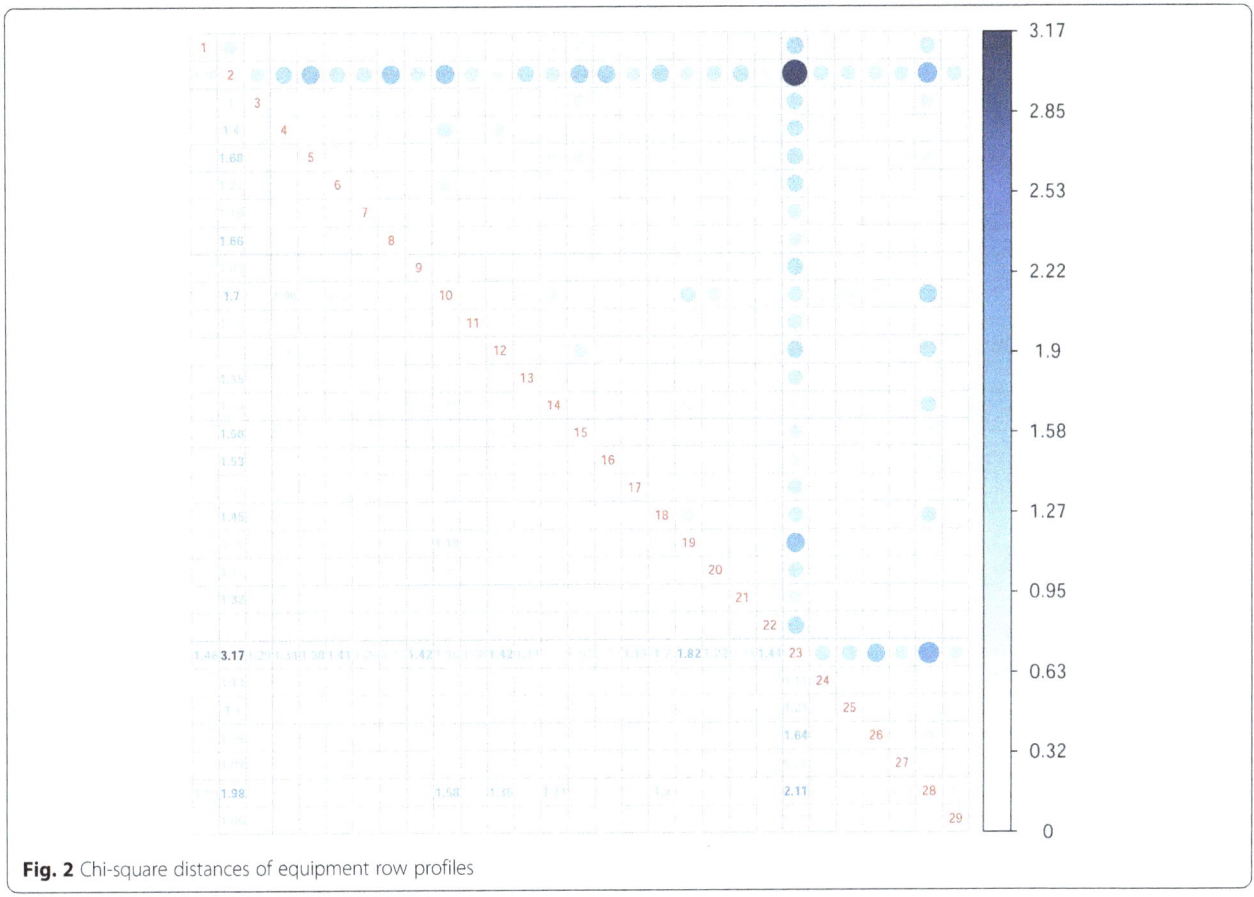

Fig. 2 Chi-square distances of equipment row profiles

Another analytical dimension is represented by causality between mortality and the localisation of the medical equipment. Our goal is to examine the relation between the health policy platform with a preference for the diagnoses of the circulatory system in the ninth chapter of the International Statistical Classification of Diseases and Related Health Problems maintained by the World Health Organization and the distribution of medical equipment throughout the Slovak regions.

The most common diagnoses causing death are the ones assigned to the circulatory system group. For the time span from 2008 to 2013, the correlation of the standardised mortality rate and the localisation of healthcare equipment according to the self-governing regions is calculated. The BL Region is the only one that shows a very weak correlation at the level of –0.1280. The TC Region and the TA Region are characterised by a low positive correlation reaching 0.3891 and 0.4017, respectively, whereas the NR Region is represented by a low negative correlation at –0.3787. The remaining four regions demonstrate cases with high correlations. The PV Region and the BC Region have a high positive correlation at 0.6209 and 0.8310, respectively, whereas the ZI Region and the KI Region have a high negative correlation at –0.7976 and –0.8615, respectively. A low correlation

indicates that there is no association between the amount of healthcare equipment and the decreasing standardised mortality rate. The most desirable occurrence happens when the increasing number of healthcare equipment helps to lower the standardised mortality rate.

Discussion

The medical equipment in the health facilities all over the Slovak Republic is localised very unproportionally. Its distribution does not follow the optimal localisation according to the map of the health facilities.

Several health facilities have limited access to tomography or magnetic resonance imaging devices. Situations may occur in which a patient in need must wait several months to be examined by x-ray computed tomograph. The origin of this situation is debatable. The most probable cause is the absence of financial resources that should be provided by health insurance companies. Currently, the Slovak economy and the related health system are established in a way that does not allow the natural reproduction of health technologies. Healthcare providers are not able to gather the financial resources to purchase new equipment. Therefore, it is necessary to address this issue and to communicate it at the

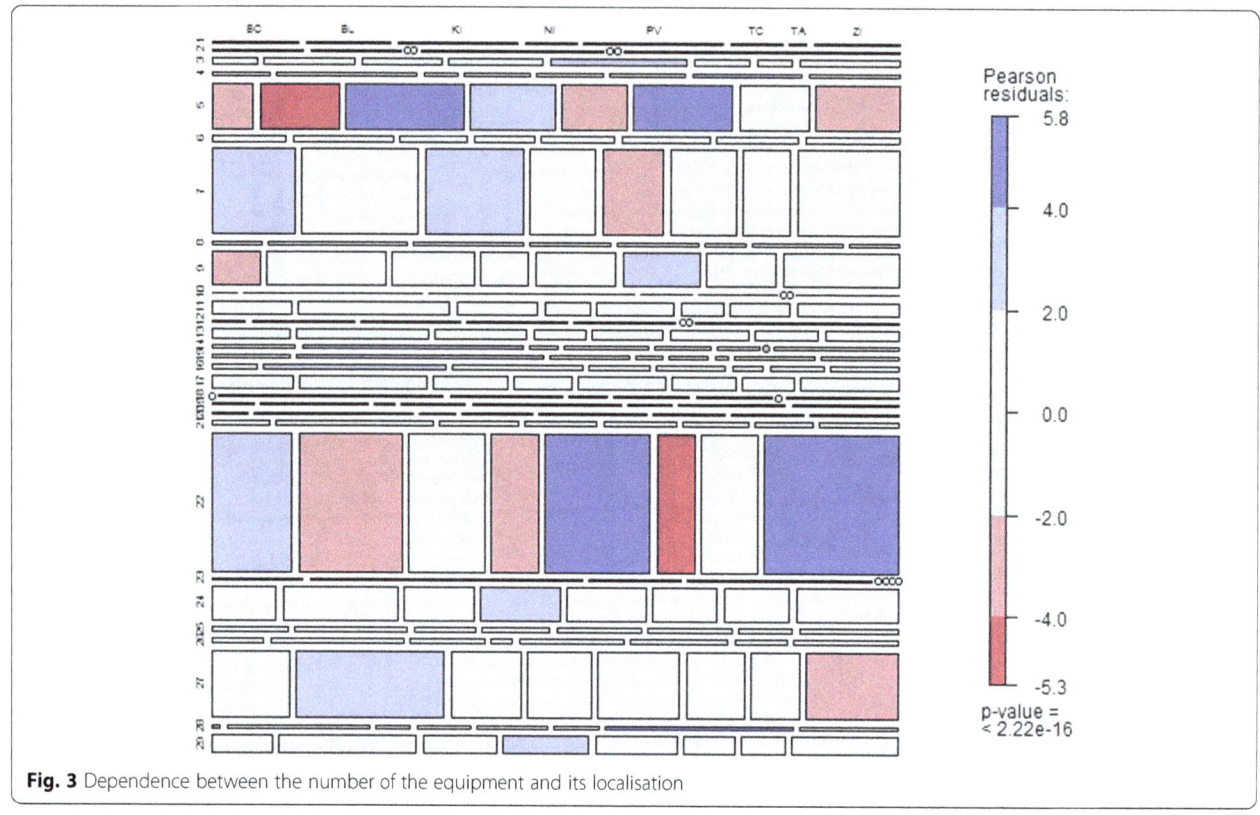

Fig. 3 Dependence between the number of the equipment and its localisation

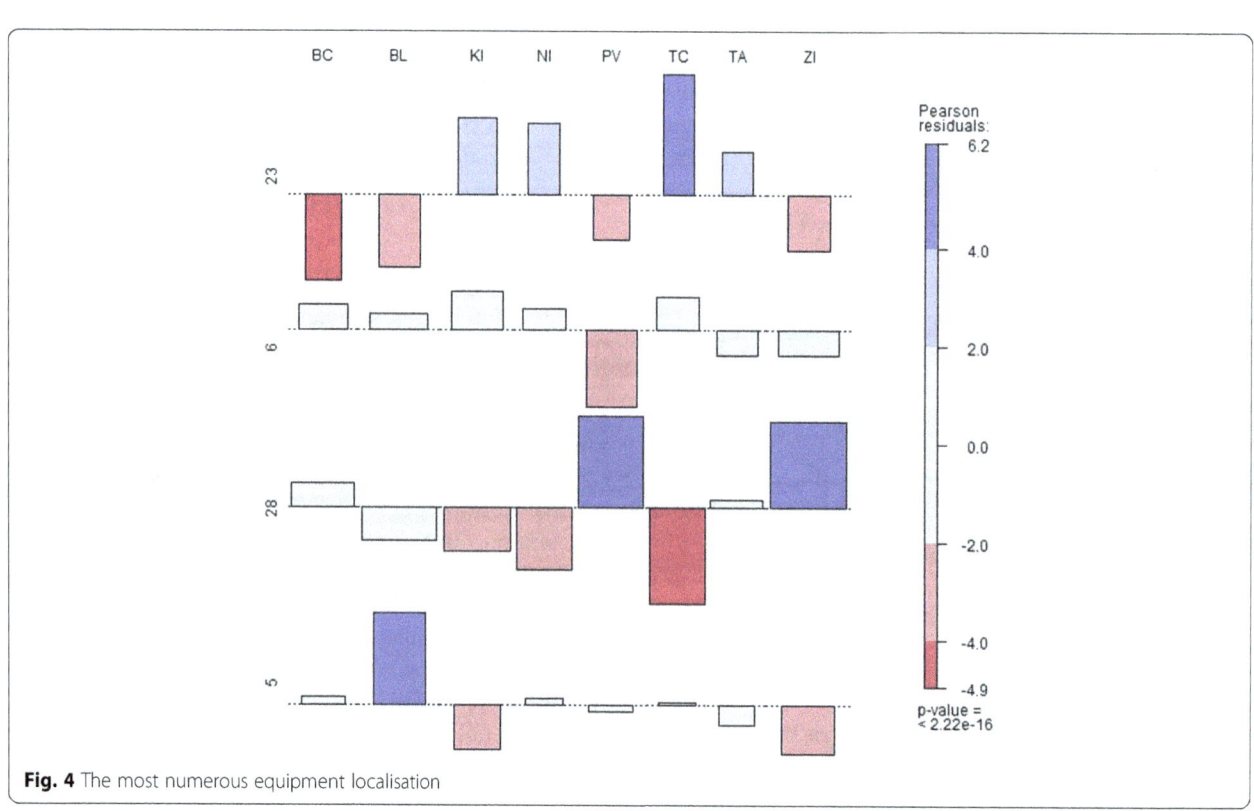

Fig. 4 The most numerous equipment localisation

government level. The need to acquire diagnostic equipment to coordinate public health departments is also an important issue. One solution could be the initiation of an adequate norm that would force healthcare providers to renovate medical equipment in the corresponding time period. An alternative to resolve this problem would be to introduce the process of financing the acquired health equipment from the state budget or by reimbursement from the health insurance companies. For instance, investments in radiological technology should be one of the most important indicators monitored within the strategic framework of the Slovak health service. Another issue is the inappropriate distribution of medical equipment throughout the Slovak regions, which have significant regional disparities between healthcare providers. This issue is closely tied to the autonomy of the self-governing regions of the Slovak Republic because they are also responsible for the management of healthcare providers supported by the state budget.

Many research teams have analysed medical equipment and the quantification of its causalities. Similarly, many scientific studies have focused on the status of medical equipment as part of a country's informatisation process in the context of various reforms or in research on regional disparities in terms of health [32–35]. Other authors focus on selected aspects of the health system and examine the influence of medical equipment on economic categories, the availability of healthcare and its real impact on regions [36–42]. Several studies that have conducted research on the geographical distribution of medical equipment and its causalities are heterogeneous in terms of the research targets as well as their methodological mechanisms that significantly limit international comparison. There are visible the considerable different results than obtained from this analysis. The main evidence may be provided by a study that analyses medical equipment in Japan. The paradox is that even in Japan, which has the highest number of computed tomographs and magnetic resonance imaging devices per inhabitant in the world, the geographic distribution of these technologies is currently unknown. Moreover, nothing is known regarding the cause and effect relationship between the number of diagnostic devices and their geographic distribution [43]. These facts create a wide platform for subsequent studies, whose findings are necessary for various types of policies in individual countries. The main strength of the study lies in a combination of an investigation that has not been yet done and usage of the new modern type of analysis. There is a lack of such studies in the Slovak Republic. The potential weakness is hide in a short period that is observed in the analysis. This is due the fact that there had been no such data before the beginning of the explored period.

Conclusion

Global ageing is a process that is related to the development of the standardised mortality rate. These two factors have a significant impact on the health system of a country and are influenced by a number of socio-economic determinants. Moreover, several aspects influence the processes discussed here. For instance, the health insurance system, with its excessive expenses that are intended for the entire network of healthcare providers, plays an important role in the quality of treatment processes and the sophistication of medical technology. Worldwide, the historical development of scientific and technical progress and the rate of implementation of research into practice is diverse. The Slovak Republic lacks the ability for long-term monitoring of the status of medical equipment in health facilities. Some issues influence healthcare and associated treatment.

The aim of this study is to examine the localisation of selected parameters in use of medical equipment in the Slovak Republic and subsequently to discover potential regional disparities. This aim was partially fulfilled by the finding of unproportional localisation of the medical equipment, although there is to note that further research is needed in this field. The results demonstrate regional disparities in the use of medical equipment throughout the whole analysed period. There are also the regions where medical equipment is not present or is present in considerable low numbers, which creates an inefficient situation. The substantial meaning of the study is to reveal the potential regional disparities throughout the various types of the analyses.

There is a lot of possibilities how to conduct this research in future. The most important point is not created by the obtained results from the conducted analysis. These findings should serve as a monitoring platform to evaluate the accessibility and quality of healthcare technologies for use in this country. It is necessary to obtain more detailed data to obtain more valuable conclusions from this analysis. The results can serve to policymakers and they can create a substantial part of the potential future support systems. We will continue our current research activities and cooperate with the related institutions of the Slovak health system.

Funding

The Scientific Grant Agency of the Ministry of Education, Science, Research and Sport of the Slovak Republic and the Slovak Academy of Sciences project 1/0945/17 Research of the economic quantification of marketing processes aimed at increasing the value for the patient, multi-dimensional analyses of the marketing mix of health facilities and quantification of their importance in the process of establishing a system to measure the quality and effectiveness of health system in the Slovak Republic.

Authors' contributions

BG: Introduction, Discussion, Conclusion; VK: Materials and Methods, Results, Conclusion; JF: Discussion, Conclusion. All authors read and approved the final manuscript.

Competing interests

The authors declare that they have no competing interests.

Author details

[1]Department of Banking and Investment, Faculty of Economics, Technical University of Košice, Němcovej 32, 04001 Košice, Slovak Republic. [2]Department of Finance, Faculty of Economics, Technical University of Košice, Němcovej 32, 04001 Košice, Slovak Republic. [3]1st Department of Internal Medicine, Louis Pasteur University Hospital in Košice, Trieda Slovenského národného povstania 1, 04011 Košice, Slovak Republic. [4]Centre of Excellence in Atherosclerosis Research, Pavol Jozef Šafárik University in Košice, Trieda Slovenského národného povstania 1, 04011 Košice, Slovak Republic.

References

1. Rogalewicz V. Health technology assessment as a tool for medical devices management in hospitals. In: EHB 2015. Proceedings of the 5th IEEE international conference on E-health and. Bioengineering. 2015; doi: 10.1109/ehb.2015.7391561.

2. Zavadil M, Rogalewicz V, Kubátová L, Matloňová V, Salačová K. Hospital-based health technology assessment. Cas Lek Cesk. 2016;155(5):254–9.

3. Ivlev I, Jablonsky J, Kneppo P. Multiple-criteria comparative analysis of magnetic resonance imaging systems. Int J Med Eng Inform. 2016;8(2):124–41. doi: 10.1504/ijmei.2016.075757.

4. Pharr JR. Accessible medical equipment for patients with disabilities in primary care clinics: why is it lacking? Disabil Health J. 2013;6(2):124–32. https://doi.org/10.1016/j.dhjo.2012.11.002.

5. Bem A, Prędkiewicz P, Ucieklak-Jeż P, Siedleck R. Profitability versus debt in hospital industry. In: European financial systems 2015 – proceedings of the 12th international scientific conference; 18–19 June 2015; Brno, Czech Republic. Brno: Masaryk University; 2015. p. 20–7.

6. Bem A, Prędkiewicz P, Ucieklak-Jeż P, Siedleck R. Impact of hospital's profitability on structure of its liabilities. In: Strategica. Local versus global. Proceedings of the third Strategica international conference; 29–30 October, vol. 2015. Bucharest: Romania. Tritonic; 2015. p. 657–65.

7. Bojnický M. Hodnotenie zdravotníckych technológií HTA. In: Verejné zdravotníctvo. 2010;7(2):1–10. http://verejnezdravotnictvo.szu.sk/SK/2010/2/Bojnicky.pdf. Accessed 23 Sept 2017

8. Soltes M, Gavurova B. Quantification and comparison of avoidable mortality – causal relations and modification of concepts. Technol Econ Dev Econ. 2015;21(6):917–38. doi: 10.3846/20294913.2015.1106421.

9. Barták M, Rogalewicz V, Jílková J, Jeřábková S. Cross-border healthcare in European Union and Czech Republic. Cas Lek Cesk. 2016;155(5):247–53.

10. Gavurová B, Vagašová T. Regional differences of standardised mortality rates for ischemic heart diseases in the Slovak Republic for the period 1996–2013 in the context of income inequality. Health Econ Rev. 2016;6(1):1–12. doi: 10.1186/s13561-016-0099-1.

11. Beyer D, Flanagan A, Heinemann A, Poengsen A. Health Care Regulation Across Europe. The Boston Consulting Group. 2007. https://www.bcg.com/documents/file15096.pdf. Accessed 23 Sept 2017.

12. Šoltés V, Gavurová B. The Functionality Comparison of the Health Care Systems by the Analytical Hierarchy Process Method. E+M Ekonomie a Management. 2014;17(3):100–18. 10.15240/tul/001/2014-3-009.

13. Zelený T, Bencko V. Healthcare system financing and profits: all that glitters is not gold. Cent Eur J Public Health. 2015;23(1):3–7. 10.21101/cejph.a4027.

14. Szczygieł N, Rutkowska-Podolska M, Michalski G. Information and Communication Technologies in Healthcare: Still innovation or reality? Innovative and entrepreneurial value-creating approach in healthcare management. Proceedings of the 5th central European conference in regional science; 5–8 October 2014; Košice, Slovak Republic. Košice: Technical University of Košice; 2015: 1020–1029.

15. Smatana M, Pažitný P, Kandilaki D, Laktišová M, Sedláková D, Palušková M, von Ginneken E, Spranger A. Slovakia: health system review. Health Systems in Transition. 2016;18(6):1–243. http://www.euro.who.int/__data/assets/pdf_file/0011/325784/HiT-Slovakia.pdf?ua=1. Accessed 23 Sept 2017

16. Pol LG, Thomas RK. The demography of health and healthcare. London: Springer; 2013.

17. Population Projections 2008–2060. 2014. europa.eu/rapid/press-release_STAT-08-119_en.pdf. Accessed 25 Feb 2017.

18. Meszaros J, Burcin B. Vývoj odvrátiteľnej úmrtnosti na Slovensku. Slovenská štatistika a. demografia. 2008;18(2–3):24–39.

19. Newey C, Nolte M, McKee M, Mossialos E. Avoidable mortality in the enlarged European Union. 2003.

20. Nolte E, McKee M. Measuring the health of nations: updating an earlier analysis. Health Aff. 2008;27(1):58–71. doi: 10.1377/hlthaff.27.1.58.

21. Rutstein DD, Berenberg W, Chalmers TC, Child CG 3rd, Fishman AP, Perrin EB, Feldman JJ, Leaverton PE, Lane M, Sencer DJ, Evans CC. Measuring the quality of medical care – a clinical method. N Engl J Med. 1976;294(11):582–8. doi: 10.1056/NEJM197603112941104.

22. Westerling R. Commentary: evaluating avoidable mortality in developing countries – an important issue for public health. Int J Epidemiol. 2001;30(5):973–5. doi: 10.1093/ije/30.5.973.

23. Tobias M, Yeh L. How much does health care contribute to health gain and to health inequality? Trends in amenable mortality in New Zealand 1981–2004. J Public Health Policy. 2009;33(1):70–8. doi: 10.1111/j.1753-6405.2009.00342.x.

24. Bendixen MA. Practical guide to the use of correspondence analysis in marketing research. The. Mark Bull. 2003;14(2):1–15. http://marketing-bulletin.massey.ac.nz/V14/MB_V14_T2_Bendixen.pdf. Accessed 23 Sept 2017

25. Yelland PM. An introduction to correspondence analysis. Math J. 2010;12(1):1–23. doi: 10.3888/tmj.12-4.

26. Hartigan JA, Kleiner B. Mosaics for contingency tables. Computer science and statistics: proceedings of the 13th symposium on the. Interface. 1981:268–73.

27. Friendly M. Mosaic displays for multi-way contingency tables. J Am Stat Assoc. 1994;89(425):190–200.

28. Cohen A. On the graphical display of the significant components in a two-way contingency table. Commun Stat Theory Methods. 1980;9(10):1025–41.

29. Friendly M. Graphical methods for categorical data. Statistical Analysis System Global Forum Proceedings. April 1992:1367–73. http://www.sascommunity.org/sugi/SUGI92/Sugi-92-233%20Friendly.pdf. Accessed 23 Sept 2017

30. Caglayan G. Making sense of eigenvalue–eigenvector relationships: math majors' linear algebra – geometry connections in a dynamic environment. J Math Behav. 2015;40(B):131–53. doi: 10.1016/j.jmathb.2015.08.003.

31. Cardoso DM, Lozin VV, Luz CJ, Pacheco MF. Efficient domination through eigenvalues. Discret Appl Math. 2016;214:54–62. doi: 10.1016/j.dam.2016.06.014.

32. Cook L. Constraints on universal health Care in the Russian Federation: inequality, informality and the failures of mandatory health insurance reforms. United Nations research institute for. Soc Dev. 2015;

33. Chevreul K, Brigham KB, Durand-Zaleski I, Hernández-Quevedo C. France: health system review. Health Syst Transit. 2015;17(3):1–218.

34. O'Neill JE, O'Neill DM. Health Status, Health Care and Inequality: Canada vs. the U.S. National Bureau of Economic Research Working Paper Series 13429. 2007; doi: 10.3386/w13429.

35. Tragakes E, Lessof S. Health Care Systems in Transition: Russian Federation. Copenhagen: European Observatory on Health Systems and Policies. 2003; 5 (3). http://www.euro.who.int/__data/assets/pdf_file/0005/95936/e81966.pdf. Accessed 23 Sept 2017.

36. Dragomiristeanu A. Reducing inequities in healthcare: a priority for European policies and measures. Manag Health. 2010;14(3):14–9. doi: 10.5233/mih.2010.0019.

37. Ruggieri-Pignon S, Pignon T, Marty M, Rodde-Dunet MH, Destembert B, Fritsch B. Infrastructure of radiation oncology in France: a large survey of evolution of external beam radiotherapy practice. Int J Radiat Oncol Biol Phys. 2005;61(2):507–16. doi: 10.1016/j.ijrobp.2004.06.009.

38. Ventola CL. Challenges in evaluating and standardizing medical devices in health care facilities. PT. 2008;33(6):349–59. http://citeseerx.ist.psu.edu/viewdoc/download?doi=10.1.1.567.4456&rep=rep1&type=pdf. Accessed 23 Sept 2017

39. Miao CX, Zhuo L, YM G, Qin ZH. Study of large medical equipment allocation in Xuzhou. J Zhejiang Univ Sci B. 2007;8(12):881–4. doi: 10.1631/jzus.2007.b0881.

3

Identification determinant factors on willingness to pay for health services in Iran

Javad Javan-Noughabi[1,2], Zahra Kavosi[3], Ahmad Faramarzi[4] and Mohammad Khammarnia[5*]

Abstract

Background: A common method used to examine the relationship between internal preferences and caring externalities is willingness to pay (WTP) approach. We aimed to estimate WTP for health status with different severity level and identify determinant factors on WTP.

Methods: For determining main factors in WTP, a cross-sectional study was conducted in Shiraz in the southeast of Iran, in March to April 2015. The open-ended method was used to estimate monthly WTP in private and altruistic section. Multivariate regression analyses using ordinary least squares were applied to examine the effect of Scio–demographic factors on WTP using SPSS software 21.

Results: Participants were willing to pay an average amount of $ 295 in health status 1 and an average amount of $ 596 in health status 6 (worst status) for internal preferences. Altruistic WTP for health status 1 was $ 294 and participants were willing to pay an average amount of $ 416 in health status 6. Multiple regression analysis identified monthly income as the key determinant of WTP for internal preferences and caring externalities ($P < 0.01$). With an increase of 1% in income, private WTP increase 1.38% in health status 1.

Conclusions: The finding indicates that the mean of WTP increases at severe health status; therefore, health policy maker should allocate resources toward severe health status.

Keywords: Willingness to pay, Altruistic, Private, Iran

Background

Many economists believe that healthcare is different in ways that generate market failure, therefore it is important for formulating public policy in the health sector [1–3]. externalities is one of the most discussed in health market failure, an external effect is existed when benefits and costs of an activity by some agent accrue to someone not directly involved in the activity, and this effect is not prized by the market [4].

In the economic evaluation are existed some procedures for measuring of caring externalities that one approach is altruistic willingness to pay (WTP). Auguste Comte first time used the concept of altruism and believed that there are two separate forces or motivation in every human, one of them focused on their own interests that are selfishness and other force focused on others and the interests of others that is altruism [5].

WTP is the maximum amount of income an individual is willing to give up to ensure that a proposed service or good is available [6].

In the health sector, various studies have been estimated WTP with different methods for health services. For instance, Wang et al. (2015) done study on the Impacts of Healthy Eating and Anti-Obesity Advertising on Willingness-to-Pay by Consumer Body Mass Index [7, 8]. X Yu et al. (2014) estimated WTP for the "Green Food" in China [9] Dror found that using bidding game among 3024 households at the rural location in India, about two-third of sample agree to WTP for health insurance [10]. Basu (2013) applied contingent valuation approach to estimate willingness to pay for prevent Alzheimer's disease and demonstrated the mean of WTP is $155 per month [11].

Open – ended is an approach which is used for the measurement of WTP, in this approach as respondent is asked, "How much would you be willing to pay to be cured?" [12] this approach has been frequently used in

* Correspondence: m_khammar1985@yahoo.com
[5]Health Promotion Research Center, Zahedan University of Medical Sciences, Zahedan, Iran

the economic evaluation [13–17]. For example, Li et al. (2017) used open-ended format to estimate to WTP for newborn screening test for spinal muscular atrophy which their study showed that People expressed a willingness to pay for spinal muscular atrophy screening even without an available therapy (median: \$142; mean: \$253). Willingness to pay increased with treatment availability and respondent income [18, 19].

The relationship between caring externalities and internal preferences (altruistic WTP and private WTP) for health status with different severity levels and determinant factors on WTP were studied as the purpose of the current research. The results of the study could be helpful for health policy makers and mangers in accurate planning in health system.

Methods

Setting and sample

A cross-sectional study was conducted among adults that have income from the general population in Shiraz, Iran, in March to April 2015. Shiraz is the center of health care and medical tourism in Iran and is located in the southeast of Iran [20]. The design of the study was explorative; therefore, it was important to obtain the views of different social groups. By that, the participants were selected from different settings. The sample size was determined using the following equation in which $p = 0.8$, and $d = 0.055$ [21].

$$N = \frac{Z_{1-\frac{\alpha}{2}p(1-p)}}{d^2} = 200$$

For sampling, the population was divided into 9 areas then on average 25 participants was randomly selected of each region.

The used scenarios in the study was based on that participants do not have insurance to pay for different status or services are not free, in addition health status were independent from each other. Data collection was conducted by open-ended questionnaire in a face-to-face interview. To recognize of external factors that might influence on WTP in this study, the participants were asked to provide their sex, educational background, employment status, and income per month. In other parts of the questionnaire, it was possible to compare private WTP and altruistic WTP.

Data collection tool

Data was collected by questionnaire, which had included two parts; the first part was included demographic variable (sex, educational background, employment status and income per month). In other part, the questionnaire asked from participants to declare private WTP and altruistic WTP in six level of health status. Six levels

regarding mobility(physical activity) were used from a scale constructed by Nord [22]; which included: first, can move about without difficulty anywhere, but has difficulties with walking more than a kilometre. Second, can move about with difficulty at home, but has difficulties in stairs and outdoors. Third, moves about with difficulty at home, needs assistance in stairs and outdoors. Fourth, can sit, needs assistance to move about - both at home and outdoors. Fifth, to some degree bedridden can sit on a chair in part of the day if helped up by others and sixth, completely bedridden.

WTP measurement

There are four ways to measure WTP in economic evaluation: open-ended, take-it-or-leave-it (or alternatively discrete choice), payment card, and bidding games types of questions [23, 24]. We chose the open-ended method for this study, this method has previously been used in many studies, in addition there is little information for altruistic and private willingness to pay in health care and the open-ended technique is a good method for obtaining first estimates [25, 26].

We applied private WTP and altruistic WTP for evaluation internal preferences and caring externalities. To estimate private WTP, the question dealt with the health status of participants and was asked as respondent in current way: "If you are suffering from the different health status. How much are you willing to pay to be cured from each health state?"

The scenarios were used to estimate the altruistic WTP the same as in private WTP, but the question relates to others health status and was asked as participants in following way: "suppose a stranger person suffers as described health status and you don't know exactly who she/he is, but he/she cannot be treated due to inability to pay medical expenses. How much are you willing to pay for her/him treatment of any health status?"

Data analysis

Data was analysed on STATA 13 version. The data analysis was started with descriptive analysis (frequency and mean) which would allow us to explore the data and identify specific trend of the study's variables. In the descriptive phase of the study, private WTP compared to altruistic WTP. In addition, since data in private WTP had non-normal distribution; therefore, logarithm was used for analysis while there was no need to get Logs for altruistic WTP data. Moreover, to test the effect of explanatory variables on private WTP and altruistic WTP was applied of OLS regression in each health status.

The below model was performed in analysis:

$$Y_i = \alpha + \beta_1 X_{1i} + \beta_2 X_{2i} + \ldots + e_i \qquad i = 1\ldots\ldots n$$

Where Y_i denotes natural logged private WTP; however, for altruistic WTP is dollar (\$), α is a constant, X_i denotes the control variables, β represents the coefficient and e is an error term.

- Ethics approval and consent to participate:

This study was approved by Ethic Committee of Shiraz University of Medical Sciences.

Results

Scio-demographic characteristics of the study population

A total of 200 participants take part in this study. More than 60% of them have academics education. Furthermore, more than of 50% of participants were male. (See Table 1).

According to the results, about 88.8% of the participants were willing to pay for health status. The study results showed that the mean of participants' income was US\$ 707. They were willing to pay an average amount of \$ 295 in health status 1 and an average amount of \$ 596 in health status 6 (worst status) for internal preferences. Moreover, altruistic WTP for health status 1 was \$ 294 and participants were willing to pay an average amount of \$ 416 in health status 6.

According to Table 1, the mean of monthly income was significant for gender and education ($P = 0.001$ and $P = 0.001$, respectively.). So male participants had higher income rather than females and persons with academic education had higher income rather than others. Table 1 shows monthly income for participant regarding to demographic variables.

Private WTP compare to altruistic WTP for different health status are shown in Fig. 1. Based on the Figure, the mean value of private WTP is higher than the mean value of the altruistic WTP in all health status and difference in the WTP is higher in the sever status. This means that, the mean value of private WTP for owns improvement from first and last health status were \$ 295 and \$ 596 respectively. But, Altruistic WTP for

Table 1 The average monthly income of participants regarding to demographics variables

Variables		Frequency (%)	Month mean (USA \$)	P value
Sex	Male	111 (55.5)	866	0.001
	Female	89 (44.5)	508.5	
Age	<35	112 (56.0)	667	0.112
	≥35	88 (44.0)	759	
Marital Status	Single	93 (46.5)	748	0.201
	Married	107 (53.5)	670.5	
Education	non-academics	66 (33.0)	519.5	0.001
	academics	134 (67.0)	799.5	

others health improvement from first and sixth health status were \$ 294 and \$ 416 respectively. This demonstrates that the respondents had understood the different scenarios.

Table 2 shows determinant factors on private WTP in different status of health. For example, model 1 shows the effect of studied variables on the private WTP for first health status that explanted in the method. Regression analysis showed that among the studied variables only monthly income of participant had significantly influenced on private WTP in all different status of health in significant level of 0.01. For instance, in first health status, the increase of 1% of the monthly income results in 1.3% increase in the private WTP. Moreover, in significant level of 0.01, sex had significant effect on private WTP for first and second health status (Model one and two).According to Table 2, in significant level of 0.05, only education status had significant effect on private WTP for fourth health status (Model four).

Table 3 shows determinants factors that effect on the person's WTP who tendency to pay for other's health improvement (altruistic WTP). Regression analysis in Table 3 showed that monthly income of respondents significantly influenced on altruistic WTP in all different status of health ($P < 0.01$). For example, in first health status (Model one), the increase of 1% of the monthly income results in \$ 251 increase in the altruistic WTP. Also, in significant level of 0.01, sex in model two, three and four had statistically significant on altruistic WTP. Moreover, in significant level of 0.05, sex had significant effect on altruistic WTP for first and fifth health status (Model one and five).

Discussion

The study was designed to determine important factors which are effective on private and altruistic WTP in Iran. We found that a large proportion of participants had willing to pay for one's own (private WTP) and for others' (altruistic WTP) hypothetical health improvement. Moreover, amount of private WTP and altruistic WTP increases with worsening health status; however, in all of health status the value of private WTP was higher than value of altruistic WTP and the difference becomes further in the severity health status. A similar study conducted by Jacobsson in Sweden found that the mean value of private WTP and altruistic WTP for sixth health status were \$1000 and \$8000 respectively, which were higher than from our study [27]. The difference of WTP in our study compared to Jacobsson could be several reasons. First, the study was conducted in countries that are different as culturally, so the willingness to pay is usually lower in developing countries, for example, the average of WTP for health insurance in the USA in 2008 was 75 to \$ 125; however, this amount was \$ 47 in

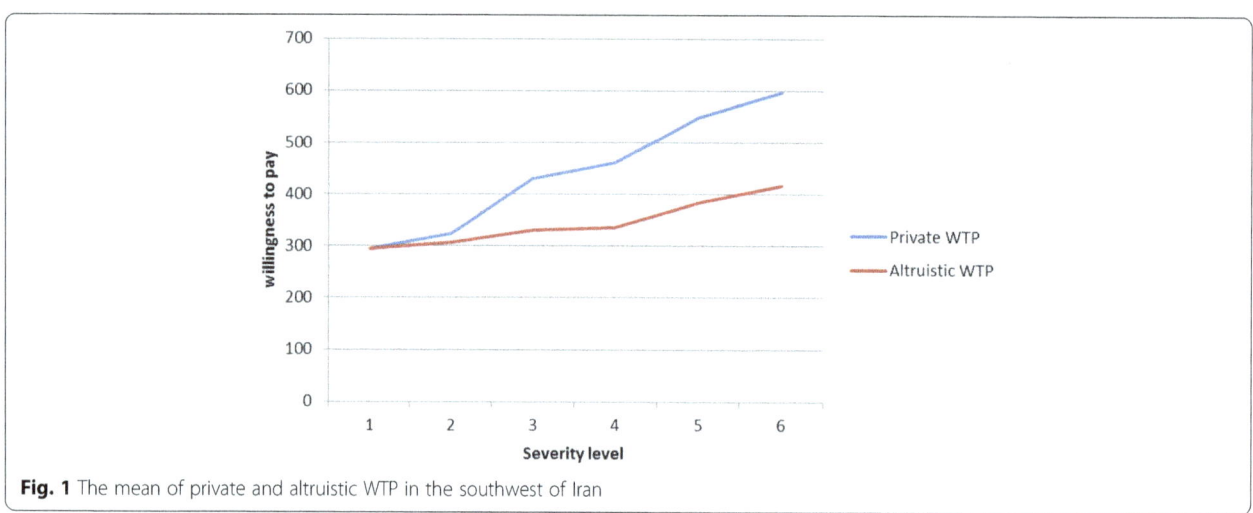

Fig. 1 The mean of private and altruistic WTP in the southwest of Iran

Namibia [28, 29]. Second, Jacobsson's study was conducted in 2001, so it could be discounted the time-value of money. According to the formula of the discount rate, the value of money has been decreased over time [30, 31].

Our results have indicated income is an important predictor for willingness to pay. If income increases 1%, private WTP will be increased 1.38% and 1.02% in health status 1 and 6, respectively. Moreover, with an increase of 1% of income, the altruistic WTP is increased $ 251 and $ 292 in health status 1 and 6, respectively. In line with the study's findings, Ahmed et al. 2015, Wright et al. 2009, Krupnick et al. 2002, also observed significant association between WTP and income [28, 32, 33].

Our analysis was explained that none of demographic variables has significant relationship with WTP for different health status however, gender, for example in the health status 1 the value of private WTP for women is higher than men but the amount of altruistic WTP for men is higher. There are no similar previous studies which confirm our results.

There are some limitations of the present study that need to be considered. One potential limitation of open–ended methods is related to bias that participants express the value of WTP incorrectly. Second, it is possible that respondent don't understand which scenarios are independent from each other, so WTP for each strategy was related to other scenarios. Third, it is

Table 2 Ordinary least square regression for private WTP (Log) in different health status

Variables	Model 1	Model 2	Model 3	Model 4	Model 5	Model 6
	WTP (SE)	WTP (SE)	WTP (SE)	WTP (SE)	WTP (SE)	WTP (SE)
Cons	−8.07[b]	−5.85[b]	−2.59[b]	−1.94[b]	−1.31[b]	−.53
	(0.82)	(0.75)	(0.56)	(0.65)	(0.40)	(0.45)
Sex (ref = male)	0.21[b]	0.16[b]	0.07	0.07	0.01	−0.03
	(0.06)	(0.05)	(0.04)	(0.04)	(0.03)	(0.03)
Age (ref = less than 35 year)	0.04	0.01	−0.007	0.01	−0.03	0.01
	(0.06)	(0.05)	(0.04)	(0.04)	(0.03)	(0.03)
Marital status (ref = single)	0.10	0.09	0.02	0.02	0.004	−.03
	(0.06)	(0.05)	(0.04)	(0.04)	(0.03)	(0.03)
Education (ref = nonacademic)	0.02	0.02	0.05	0.11[a]	0.04	−0.02
	(0.06)	(0.05)	(0.04)	(0.05)	(0.03)	(0.03)
Income	1.38[b]	1.27[b]	1.1[b]	1.06[b]	1.05[b]	1.02[b]
	(0.04)	(0.04)	(0.03)	(0.03)	(0.02)	(0.02)
R square	0.82	0.83	0.87	0.82	0.92	0.90

[a]Significant level at 0.05
[b]Significant level at 0.01

Table 3 Ordinary least square regression for altruistic WTP in different health status

	Model 1 WTP (SE)	Model 2 WTP (SE)	Model 3 WTP (SE)	Model 4 WTP (SE)	Model 4 WTP (SE)	Model 4 WTP (SE)
Cons	−1330.26[b]	−1274.28[b]	-1311[b]	−1245.95[b]	−1341.48[b]	−1314.88[b]
	(115.69)	(112.04)	(106.55)	(111.79)	(210.38)	(337.53)
Sex (ref = male)	−48.12[a]	−58.22[b]	−58.38[b]	−60.29[b]	−85.53[a]	−102.45
	(19.71)	(19.09)	(18.15)	(19.04)	(35.84)	(57.5)
Age (ref = less than 35 year)	27.08	25.9	33.17	26.81	−23.99	1.36
	(20.06)	(19.43)	(18.48)	(19.39)	(36.49)	(58.54)
Marital status (ref = single)	35.17	32.9	28.31	25.98	67.98	−15.53
	(19.49)	(18.88)	(17.95)	(18.83)	(35.45)	(56.87)
Education (ref = nonacademic)	1.93	3.7	4.97	2.91	16.95	23.13
	(20.24)	(19.6)	(18.64)	(19.56)	(36.81)	(59.06)
Income	251.1[b]	246.76[b]	255.65[b]	249.30[b]	274.76[b]	292.54[b]
	(15.41)	(14.92)	(14.19)	(14.89)	(28.02)	(44.95)
R square	0.65	0.66	0.7	0.67	0.42	0.24

[a]Significant level at 0.05
[b]Significant level at 0.01

difficult to disclose the real income of the participants; in particular the study was designed at the individual level and cross sectional.

Conclusions

This current study is provided evidence on WTP for health status and demonstrated that a large proportion of participants had WTP for health status. The value of WTP was difference for internal preference and caring externalities. This study indicates that the mean of WTP increases at severe health status, therefore health policy maker should allocate resources toward severe health status. Among the Scio-economics and demographic factors only income and gender was associated with the WTP significantly.

Acknowledgements
We would to thanks from any participants who contributed in the study. This study was supported by Shiraz University of Medical Science. Also, we would like to thanks from Samin Nobakht who contributed in data collection in the study.

Funding
This study was supported by Shiraz University of Medical Science (grant no. 92–01–21-7009).

Authors' contributions
All authors contributed equally. All authors read and approved the final manuscript.

Competing interests
The authors declare that they have no competing interests.

Author details
[1]Health Management and Economics Research Center, Iran University of Medical Sciences, Tehran, Iran. [2]Department of Health Economics, School of Health Management and Information Sciences, Iran University of Medical Sciences, Tehran, Iran. [3]Health Human Resources Research Center, Shiraz University of Medical Sciences, Shiraz, Iran. [4]Department of Health Management and Economics, School of Public Health, Tehran University of Medical Sciences, Tehran, Iran. [5]Health Promotion Research Center, Zahedan University of Medical Sciences, Zahedan, Iran.

References
1. Wong LY. Development of a holistic internet marketing strategy framework (IMSF) in promoting medical tourism industry (MTI) in Malaysia: Universiti Tun Hussein Onn Malaysia; 2016.
2. Durham J, Blondell SJ. Research protocol: a realist synthesis of cross-border patient mobility from low-income and middle-income countries. BMJ Open. 2014;4(11):e006514.
3. Culyer AJ, Newhouse JP. Handbook of health economics: Elsevier; 2000.
4. Briggs A. Sugar tax could sweeten a market failure: Britain has announced a tax on sugary drinks. Countries should go further and target foods that have large carbon footprints, says Adam Briggs. Nature. 2016;531(7596):551–2.
5. Campbell RL. Reply to Robert H. Bass," egoism versus rights"(spring 2006): altruism in Auguste Comte and Ayn Rand. The Journal of Ayn Rand Studies. 2006;7(2):357–69.
6. Mbachu C, Okoli C, Onwujekwe O, Enabulele F. Willingness to pay for antiretroviral drugs among HIV and AIDS clients in south-east Nigeria. Health Expect. 2017;00:1-9. doi:org/10.1111/hex.12612
7. Wang R, Liaukonyte J, Kaiser HM. Does advertising content matter? Impacts of healthy eating and anti-obesity advertising on willingness-to-pay by consumer body mass index. J Agric Resour Econ. 2015;8:1–41.
8. Green CH, Tunstall SM. The evaluation of river water quality improvements by the contingent valuation method. Appl Econ. 1991;23(7):1135–46.
9. Yu X, Gao Z, Zeng Y. Willingness to pay for the "green food" in China. Food Policy. 2014;45:80–7.
10. Dror DM, Radermacher R, Koren R. Willingness to pay for health insurance among rural and poor persons: field evidence from seven micro health insurance units in India. Health policy. 2007;82(1):12–27.
11. Basu R. Willingness-to-pay to prevent Alzheimer's disease: a contingent valuation approach. Int J Health Care Finance Econ. 2013;13(3–4):233–45.
12. Damschroder LJ, Ubel PA, Riis J, Smith DM. An alternative approach for eliciting willingness-to-pay: a randomized internet trial. Judgm Decis Mak. 2007;2(2):96.

13. Shi L, Gao Z, Chen X. The cross-price effect on willingness-to-pay estimates in open-ended contingent valuation. Food Policy. 2014;46:13–21.
14. Tussupova K, Berndtsson R, Bramryd T, Beisenova R. Investigating willingness to pay to improve water supply services: application of contingent valuation method. Water. 2015;7(6):3024–39.
15. Sousa N, Costa T, Monteiro-Soares M, Rocha Gonçalves F, Azevedo LF. Bias in valuation of health care benefits in metastatic prostate cancer: a contingent valuation of willingness to pay. ASCO Annual Meeting. 2017.
16. Botelho A, Pinto LC. Hypothetical, real, and predicted real willingness to pay in open-ended surveys: experimental results. Appl Econ Lett. 2002;9(15):993–6.
17. Veisten K. Willingness to pay for eco-labelled wood furniture: choice-based conjoint analysis versus open-ended contingent valuation. J For Econ. 2007; 13(1):29–48.
18. Frew EJ, Wolstenholme JL, Whynes DK. Comparing willingness-to-pay: bidding game format versus open-ended and payment scale formats. Health Policy. 2004;68(3):289–98.
19. Lin P-J, Yeh W-S, Neumann PJ. Willingness to pay for a newborn screening test for spinal muscular atrophy. Pediatr Neurol. 2017;66:69–75.
20. Asadi H, Garavand A, Khammarnia M, Abdollahi MB. TheThe sources of work stress among nurses in private hospitals in shiraz, 2016 sources of work stress among nurses in private hospitals in shiraz, 2016. Journal of Health Management and Informatics. 2017;4(3):71–5.
21. Ryan TP. Sample size determination and power: John Wiley & Sons; 2013.
22. Nord E. The trade-off between severity of illness and treatment effect in cost-value analysis of health care. Health Policy. 1993;24(3):227–38.
23. Breidert C, Hahsler M, Reutterer T. A review of methods for measuring willingness-to-pay. Innovative Marketing. 2006;2(4):8–32.
24. Florax RJ, Travisi CM, Nijkamp P. A meta-analysis of the willingness to pay for reductions in pesticide risk exposure. Eur Rev Agric Econ. 2005;32(4):441–67.
25. Asenso-Okyere WK, Osei-Akoto I, Anum A, Appiah EN. Willingness to pay for health insurance in a developing economy. A pilot study of the informal sector of Ghana using contingent valuation. Health policy. 1997;42(3):223–37.
26. Bärnighausen T, Liu Y, Zhang X, Sauerborn R. Willingness to pay for social health insurance among informal sector workers in Wuhan, China: a contingent valuation study. BMC Health Serv Res. 2007;7(1):1.
27. Jacobsson F, Carstensen J, Borgquist L. Caring externalities in health economic evaluation: how are they related to severity of illness? Health Policy. 2005;73(2):172–82.
28. Gustafsson-Wright E, Asfaw A, van der Gaag J. Willingness to pay for health insurance: an analysis of the potential market for new low-cost health insurance products in Namibia. Soc Sci Med. 2009;69(9):1351–9.
29. Bustamante AV, Ojeda G, Castañeda X. Willingness to pay for cross-border health insurance between the United States and Mexico. Health Aff. 2008; 27(1):169–78.
30. Hirth RA, Chernew ME, Miller E, Fendrick AM, Weissert WG. Willingness to pay for a quality-adjusted life year in search of a standard. Med Decis Mak. 2000;20(3):332–42.
31. Brouwer WB, Niessen LW, Postma MJ, Rutten FF. Need for differential discounting of costs and health effects in cost effectiveness analyses. BMJ. 2005;331(7514):446–8.
32. Ahmed S, Hoque ME, Sarker AR, Sultana M, Islam Z, Gazi R, et al. Willingness-to-pay for community-based health insurance among informal Workers in Urban Bangladesh. PLoS One. 2016;11(2):e0148211.
33. Krupnick A, Alberini A, Cropper M, Simon N, O'Brien B, Goeree R, et al. Age, health and the willingness to pay for mortality risk reductions: a contingent valuation survey of Ontario residents. J Risk Uncertain. 2002;24(2):161–86.

4

Health care utilisation amongst older adults with sensory and cognitive impairments in Europe

David G. Lugo-Palacios[1][*] [iD] and Brenda Gannon[2]

Abstract

Worldwide, the high prevalence of multiple chronic conditions amongst older population has led to increased utilisation of health care and rising associated costs, becoming a major public health concern. Hearing, vision and cognitive disorders are common chronic conditions amongst older Europeans and recent studies have documented its high co-occurrence. While it has been shown separately that suffering either mental disorders or sensory (hearing and vision) impairments is associated with higher health care utilisation, the association between health care utilisation and the interaction of these conditions has received little attention in the literature. Therefore, using four waves of the Survey of Health, Ageing and Retirement in Europe (SHARE), this study applies the correlated random effects method to the negative binomial and finite mixture models to analyse the extent to which the interaction of cognitive and sensory impairments is associated with health care use. We found that individuals with cognitive impairment tend to have more hospitalisations. The finite mixture approach indicates a positive association between sensory impairment and the number of hospitalisations amongst low users of health care. Additionally, our findings suggest a positive association between suffering both impairments at the same time and the number of doctor and GP visits.

Keywords: Ageing, cognitive impairment, Sensory impairment, Health care utilisation, Correlated random effects, SHARE

Jel classification: I110, I120, I140

Background

The high prevalence of multiple chronic conditions amongst older population has led to decreased quality of life, to increased utilisation of health care services and rising associated costs across the world; thus, becoming a major public health concern [1, 2]. Even in the coexistence of chronic conditions, individual diseases dominate health care delivery. However, the use of many services to manage individual diseases can become duplicative, inefficient and, in some cases, unsafe for patients [3]. Hearing, vision and cognitive disorders are common chronic conditions amongst older Europeans and recent studies have documented its high co-occurrence [4–6]. Moreover, significant statistical associations between sensory impairment and cognitive decline have been found in previous research and several hypothesis have been proposed to account for the relationship between them [7, 8]. While it has been shown separately that suffering either mental disorders or sensory impairments is associated with higher utilisation of health care resources, the association between health care utilisation and the interaction of these conditions has received little attention in the literature [9–11]. Therefore, in an effort to better understand health care utilisation amongst older population suffering sensory and cognitive impairments, this study examines the extent to which older Europeans with both impairments visit any medical doctor, a general practitioner (GP) and a hospital in comparison with individuals with only sensory impairment, with only cognitive impairment or with none of these conditions.

Grossman considers that an individual, seen both as consumer and producer of its own health, inherit an

* Correspondence: david.lugopalacios@manchester.ac.uk
[1]Centre for Health Economics, University of Manchester, 4.306 Jean McFarlane Building, Oxford Road, M13 9PL, Manchester, UK

initial stock of health that depreciates with age and can be increased by investment [12, 13]. Time and other inputs, such as health care and regular physical activity, are used to produce healthy time. Hence, the net investment in the stock of health equals gross investment minus depreciation. In the original Grossman model, while the rates of depreciation are exogenous, they depend on age. As the depreciation rate increases, the marginal cost of healthy days increases as well and, thus, a utility-maximiser individual will choose a lower stock of health. An increase in the shadow price of capital, caused by a higher depreciation rate, reduces not only the demand for health capital, but also the amount of health capital supply to the individual by a given amount of gross investment [14, 15]. Nevertheless, assuming that the demand for health is inelastic, the demand for health inputs (i.e. health care) will increase with age to compensate part of the reduction in health capital. The negative relationship between the demand for health and the one for health care predicts that people who are older and less healthy will increase their consumption of health care [14].

Previous studies have shown that hearing, vision and cognitive impairments amongst older adults impact negatively on functional independence, mental health and reduce quality of life, increasing the need for support services [11, 16]. Furthermore, it has been postulated that sensory impairment and cognitive decline may both be the result of age-related changes in a shared factor, such as degeneration of central nervous structures [7]. In addition, Kumagai and Ogura (2014) found that increasing the intensity of regular physical activity has positive effects on health stock suggesting that health enhancement behaviours may reduce the need and use of health care [17]. Therefore, holding the rest constant, it is expected that older population with sensory and cognitive impairments with no regular physical activity (higher depreciation rate and lower stock of health capital) use more health services than older population with only one or none of these impairments.[1] The objective of this paper is to test the validity of this hypothesis amongst older Europeans.

Data

The analysis uses data from waves 1, 2, 4 and 5 of the Survey of Health, Ageing and Retirement in Europe (SHARE), Release 5.0.0 collected between 2004 and 2013 [18]. SHARE is a multidisciplinary cross-national panel survey representative at the national level that collects data on health, socio-economic status and family networks of more than 123,000 non-institutionalised individuals aged 50 or over (and their spouses) from 20 European countries. Data from the third wave are excluded in this analysis since it only collects the retrospective histories of the respondents and does not contain data on recent health conditions and health care utilisation. The present study only uses data from nine countries present in all the available waves (Austria, Belgium, Denmark, France, Germany, Italy, the Netherlands, Spain, and Switzerland).

Health care utilisation within the last 12 months is examined separately with three different variables: number of times the respondent has seen a medical doctor, the number of these contacts that were visits to a GP, and the number of times that the respondent was a patient in a hospital overnight. Unfortunately, in wave 5 the number of times that a person visited the GP was not separated from the overall visits to a medical doctor. For this reason, wave 5 was excluded from the analysis that takes visits to the GP as the dependent variable.

This paper uses measures of episodic memory and verbal fluency as indicators of cognitive function [19]. The episodic memory test in SHARE consists of a verbal recall of a list of ten words (in waves 1 and 2 the same list was used whereas in waves 4 and 5 respondents were assigned randomly to one of four sets of ten words). This test is implemented two times: immediately after the respondent hears the complete list (immediate recall) and at the end of the cognitive function module (delayed recall).

The number of words remembered correctly from both the immediate and the delayed recall are added generating a new episodic memory variable that ranges between 0 and 20 [20]. In the literature on cognitive decline, a memory score of 1.5 standard deviations below the age-specific mean has been considered an indicator of mild cognitive impairment [21, 22]. Therefore, this method is applied within each country using the statistics of the episodic memory variable to generate a binary variable that identifies individuals with mild cognitive impairment. Due to a very low cut-off point for individuals aged 75 or older (due to a relatively low number of observations), a different cut-off was defined for these individuals. For this age group the mean and standard deviation taken into consideration are not age specific and the age group (75 and older) statistics are used instead. Moreover, instead of taking a 1.5 standard deviation below the average as the cut-off point to indicate mild cognitive impairment, only one standard deviation from the age group mean is considered.

In the verbal fluency test, respondents were asked to name as many animals as possible in 60 s. Since naming less than 15 different animals (excluding repetitions) is suggestive of dementia and naming 15 or more are considered normal, a variable indicating if the respondent has a verbal fluency problem was created if respondents failed to name at least 15 correct words [23].

A third dummy variable classifies an individual as cognitive impaired if he/she has either an episodic memory problem or a verbal fluency problem, as defined above.

Sensory impairment is measured using self-reported vision and hearing quality. In the case of vision quality, two self-reported measures were used to identify impairment: distance eyesight and reading eyesight (using glasses or contact lenses as usual). Individuals who responded their eyesight was fair or poor (as opposed to excellent, very good or good) are categorised as visually impaired [24]. In the same line, participants that answered that their hearing was fair or poor (using hearing aid as usual) are classified as having a hearing impairment. Individuals with either vision or hearing impairment are then considered to be sensory impaired.

Along with the sensory and cognitive impairment indicator variables, the interaction term between these two variables are the main covariates of interest in this study as they will allow the investigation of the extent to which individuals with these impairments are using health care services. The choice of additional regressors follows the Andersen model that considers that health care utilisation is a function of an individual's predisposing, enabling and need characteristics, as well as of his/her health behaviours [25]. The predisposing characteristics considered are age and age squared treated as continuous variables, a dummy variable indicating if the individual is married, as well as the person's sex, immigration status and education level. The latter was categorised into three levels (none/primary, secondary, and tertiary) using the International Standard Classification of Education codes reported in SHARE [26]. Household income in its logarithmic form, adjusted for purchase power, and employment status (employed or not employed) are used as enabling characteristics.[2] Apart from the variables indicating sensory and cognitive impairments, the need factors included are the number of chronic diseases reported and the Activity Daily Living (ADL) scale that measures the individual functional status. The ADL scale is treated as a continuous variable ranging between 0 (no impediment) and 6 (total dependence). To account for health behaviours, both risky and health enhancement activities were considered in this study: two variables are introduced to indicate whether the individual smokes at the moment of the interview and whether the individual drinks alcohol more than three days a week; it was considered that an individual undertook health enhancement activities if he/she engaged more than once a week in vigorous physical activity. Finally, SHARE wave dummy variables are also considered.

The observations with missing values for at least one of the variables mentioned are dropped. Likewise, as described below, only individuals with two or more observations in the panel are included in the analysis. The resulting data set is an unbalanced panel with 85,473 observations from 32,229 individuals. Table 1 shows the descriptive statistics of the data set analysed. SHARE respondents had on average 7 visits to the doctor, 4.7 visits to the GP and 0.24 hospitalisations during the whole period of study. Pooling the four SHARE waves, 28% interviews identified individuals with cognitive impairment, 38% with sensory impairment, and 14% with both impairments at the same time. Furthermore, 57.9% of the 32,229 individuals were considered sensory impaired at least once in the study period; the percentages for individuals with at least one report of being cognitively impaired and at least one report of having both impairments at the same time are 42.7% and 24.2%, respectively (not shown).

Table 1 also displays the zero counts in the variables measuring the use of health care. The percentage of zeros is 10.3% for doctor visits, 15.8% for GP visits, and 85.2% for hospitalisations.

Methods

This paper analyses health care utilisation amongst SHARE population over time. A key decision when analysing panel data is to choose how to handle the panel heterogeneity caused by the time-invariant individual-specific components. One option is to treat individual heterogeneity as an unobserved random variable uncorrelated with the regressors (random effects, RE). The problem with this approach is that if the no-correlation assumption between the individual effects and the covariates is violated, then estimates obtained from a RE model will not be consistent. A popular alternative in the applied micro-econometrics literature is the use of fixed effects (FE) models as they allow the individual-specific effects and the regressors to be correlated [27]. In a FE model, individual effects are eliminated by either first differencing or applying the deviations-from-mean transformation, but time-invariant regressors are also swept out with this transformation [28]. This can be problematic if time-invariant covariates or with little variance across the panel are of special interest. There is, however, an alternative to FE models that can yield consistent estimates while allowing the inclusion of time-invariant regressors: conditionally correlated random effects (CCRE) [29, 30]. This approach was originally proposed for linear regression, but has been adapted for count data models [31].

This paper follows the CCRE approach by estimating two different models. The first is a conditionally correlated random effects negative binomial (CCRENB) model and the second is a latent class negative binomial model for panel data with correlated random effects (LCNB_CRE).

The CCRENB model

Table 1 suggests that the three health care variables used in this paper are overdispersed (conditional variance significantly higher than the conditional mean). Negative binomial models are often used in this case as they can accommodate overdispersed data and may improve efficiency in estimation compared to Poisson models [27].

Table 1 Descriptive statistics

Variable	Observations	Mean	Std. Dev.	Min	Max
Health care utilisation					
Doctor visits	85,147	7.00	9.59	0	98
GP visits	59,965	4.73	7.01	0	98
Hospitalisations	85,473	0.24	0.80	0	10
Predisposing factors					
Age	85,473	65.69	9.73	50	104
Male	85,473	0.45	0.50	0	1
Married	85,473	0.72	0.45	0	1
Immigrant	85,473	0.08	0.27	0	1
Primary education	85,473	0.27	0.44	0	1
Secondary education	85,473	0.51	0.50	0	1
Tertiary education	85,473	0.22	0.41	0	1
Enabling factors					
Employed	85,473	0.26	0.44	0	1
ln(income_ppp)	85,473	10.03	1.40	−5.62	15.99
Health behaviours					
Present smoker	85,473	0.18	0.38	0	1
Regular alcohol consumption	85,473	0.37	0.48	0	1
Regular physical activity	85,473	0.34	0.47	0	1
Need factors					
ADL scale	85,473	0.19	0.72	0	6
No. of chronic diseases	85,473	1.40	1.31	0	11
Cognitive impairment	85,473	0.28	0.45	0	1
Sensory impairment	85,473	0.38	0.48	0	1
Sense_Cog impairment	85,473	0.14	0.34	0	1
Country dummies					
Austria	85,473	0.12	0.32	0	1
Germany	85,473	0.07	0.26	0	1
Netherlands	85,473	0.10	0.30	0	1
Spain	85,473	0.11	0.31	0	1
Italy	85,473	0.11	0.32	0	1
France	85,473	0.15	0.36	0	1
Switzerland	85,473	0.09	0.28	0	1
Belgium	85,473	0.16	0.37	0	1
Denmark	85,473	0.09	0.28	0	1
Wave dummies					
SHARE Wave 1	85,473	0.18	0.38	0	1
SHARE Wave 2	85,473	0.21	0.41	0	1
SHARE Wave 4	85,473	0.31	0.46	0	1
SHARE Wave 5	85,473	0.30	0.46	0	1

Table 1 Descriptive statistics *(Continued)*

Variable	Observations	Mean	Std. Dev.	Min	Max
Number of waves	85,473	2.91	0.87	2	4
Number of zero counts					

	Observations	Zeros	Percentage of zeros
Doctor visits	85,147	8784	10.32%
GP visits	59,965	9485	15.82%
Hospitalisations	85,473	72,796	85.17%

The negative binomial random effects (RE) model was first proposed in [32] by supposing that y_{it} is independent and identically distributed negative binomial with quadratic variance function with parameters $\alpha_i \lambda_{it}$ and ϕ_i, where α_i is a time-invariant individual-specific random effect, $\lambda_{it} = \exp(x'_{it}\beta)$, ϕ_i is a dispersion factor, x_{it} are the exogenous covariates, and β is the vector of regression parameters. This implies that y_{it} has mean $\alpha_i \lambda_{it}/\phi_i$ and variance $(\alpha_i \lambda_{it}/\phi_i) \times (1 + \alpha_i/\phi_i)$ [27]. If $(1 + \alpha_i/\phi_i)$-1 is a beta-distributed random variable with parameters (a, b), then the joint density of individual i's health care utilisation is

$$f(y_{it}|X_{it},\beta,a,b) = \prod_{t=1}^{T}\left(\frac{\Gamma(\lambda_{it}+y_{it})!}{\Gamma(\lambda_{it})!\Gamma(y_{it}+1)!}\right)$$
$$\times \frac{\Gamma(a+b)\Gamma(a+\sum_t\lambda_{it})\Gamma(b+\sum_t y_{it})}{\Gamma(a)\Gamma(b)\Gamma(a+b+\sum_t\lambda_{it}+\sum_t y_{it})} \quad (1)$$

where y_{it} is the count of doctor visits (or hospitalisations) and $\Gamma(.)$ is the gamma function. Eq. (1) is the basis for maximum likelihood estimation of β, a and b. As any other RE model, the estimated coefficients are only consistent if the RE are uncorrelated with the covariates. The no-correlation assumption between the individual effects and the covariates can be relaxed in a RE framework by applying the Mundlak-Chamberlain method to the count data case. This is done by allowing the time-invariant individual effect to depend on the average of individual effects:

$$\alpha_i = \exp(\overline{x}'_i \varphi + \varepsilon_i) \quad (2)$$

where $\overline{x}_i$ is the time-average of the covariates and ε_i may be interpreted as unobserved heterogeneity that is uncorrelated with the regressors [31]. The conditional mean of y_{it} can then be expressed by

$$E[(y_{it}|X_{it},\alpha_i) = \exp(x'_{it}\beta + \overline{x}'_i\varphi + \varepsilon_i)] \quad (3)$$

Equation (3) can be estimated as an RE model, with $\overline{x}'_i$ as an additional regressor [31]. Only individuals observed at least in two different waves are included in the analysis as changes over time are unobserved for individuals with only one observation [33].

Although the negative binomial model is superior to the Poisson in that it allows for overdispersion, its use might be inadequate in analysing data with excess zeros [34]. While on this paper excess zeros is not a concern in the case of doctor and GP visits, it is in the case of hospitalisations. Therefore, in addition to the CCRENB model, this paper also considers a methodology that takes this excess of zeros into account.

The LCNB_CRE model

An alternative approach to handle heterogeneity in a count data framework is to use latent class (or finite mixture) models. These models can provide an effective way of handling both excess zeros and overdispersion in count models [31, 35, 36]. This method assumes that the sample of individuals is drawn from a population divided in C different latent classes with a probability π_j of belonging to the jth latent class, where $\sum_{j=1}^{C}\pi_{ij} = 1$, $0 \leq \pi_{ij} \leq 1$, $j = 1, ..., C$. It is also assumed that the variable of interest (y_{it}) follows a different underlying distribution within each latent class. Here, the latent classes are assumed to be based on the individual's latent long-term health status which may not be well captured by proxy variables. In this sense, the latent class framework represents unobserved time-invariant heterogeneity [37].

Following Jones et al. (2013), the panel structure is accounted for in the formulation of the mixture of probabilities and densities [38]. Let y_{it} represent the number of doctor visits (or hospitalisations) in year t. Conditional on the class that individual i belongs to, y_{it} has density $f_j(y_{it}| x_{it}; \theta_j)$ with θ_j vectors of parameters specific to each class. Given class j, the joint density of y_{it} over the observed periods (T_i) is a product of T_i independent densities $f_j(y_{it}| x_{it}; \theta_j)$. Unconditionally on the latent class, the joint density of $y_i = [y_{i1}, ..., y_{iT_i}]$ is given by

$$g(y_i|x_i; \pi_{i1}, ..., \pi_{iC}; \theta_1, ..., \theta_C) = \sum_{j=1}^{C}\pi_{ij}\prod_{t=1}^{T_i}f_j(y_{it}|x_{it}; \theta_j) \quad (4)$$

Class membership probabilities are commonly taken in the literature as fixed parameters to be estimated along with θ_j [37]. This is analogous to a RE specification that assumes no correlation between individual heterogeneity and the regressors [38]. To relax this assumption, the Mundlak-Chamberlain approach is followed again, but now modelling class membership as a function of time-invariant individual characteristics using a multinomial logit [37]:

$$\pi_{ij} = \frac{\exp\left(\overline{x_i}\gamma_j\right)}{\sum_{g=1}^{C}\exp\left(\overline{x_i}\gamma_g\right)}, \quad j = 1, ..., C \quad (5)$$

with $\gamma_C = 0$, $\overline{x_i}$ defined as in eq. (2), and defining each of the j density functions in [4] in the same way as eq. (1). The vectors of parameters θ_j and γ_j are estimated jointly by maximum likelihood using the Broyden-Fletcher-Goldfarb-Shanno quasi-Newton algorithm. Following most applications of the latent class approach in health care, this paper defines C = 2 and based on the predicted number of counts these classes are referred as "low users" and "high users" of health care. STATA 14 is used in all estimations [39].

Results

Regression results of the CCRENB model

Results of the CCRENB model are presented in the form of incidence-rate-ratios (IRR) in Table 2. IRRs significantly lower than one for a given covariate are interpreted as indicative of a negative association between the covariate in question and the type of care analysed; IRRs significantly higher than one suggest a positive relationship. Results in this paper are reported as IRRs instead of marginal effects, as estimation of the latter would require assumptions that would undermine the existence of heterogeneity across individuals; specifically, marginal effects would be estimated by assuming that all the random effects are zero [40].

Two separate regressions are carried out for each type of health care: one including the interaction term of sensitive and cognitive impairments (even columns) and other without this interaction (odd columns). Bayesian Information Criteria (BIC) is reported as measures of goodness of fit, models with smaller values of BIC are preferred.

The models that include the Sense-Cog interaction show that having a cognitive but no sensory impairment is associated with 1.9% fewer doctor visits and 7.5% more hospitalisations at the 10% significance level. Column [4] indicates that individuals with both cognitive and sensory impairments tend to have 4.9% more GP visits than individuals with none of these impairments at the 5% significance level.

When the Sense-Cog interaction is not included in the model, the estimates of cognitive and sensory impairment are interpreted considering the rest of the other factors constant. Hence, ceteris paribus, having a cognitive impairment is not significantly associated with doctor and GP visits, but individuals with this impairment tend to have 8.1% more hospitalisations than individuals without this impairment. Columns [1] and [5] show that sensory impairment is significantly associated at the 5% level with 1.7% more doctor visits and at the 10% significance level with 4.7% more hospitalisations.

The associations found for the rest of the covariates are robust to the inclusion of the Sense-Cog interaction term. The number of chronic diseases is strongly associated with the use of health care; suffering an additional chronic disease is associated with 12% more doctor visits, 9% more GP visits and 19% more hospitalisations. The ADL scale is also positively associated with health care utilisation. Unhealthy behaviours are negatively associated with the use of health care: present smokers tend to have 12% fewer visits to the doctor and 41% fewer hospitalisations. A health enhancement behaviour is also negatively associated with the use of health care: being physically active more than one day a week

Table 2 Health care utilisation in SHARE: negative binomial conditionally correlated random effects model

	Doctor Visits		GP visits		Hospitalisations	
	[1]	[2]	[3]	[4]	[5]	[6]
Predisposing factors						
Age	0.970***	0.969***	0.951***	0.950***	0.987	0.986
	[0.009]	[0.009]	[0.011]	[0.011]	[0.033]	[0.033]
Age squared	1.000	1.000	1.000	1.000	1.000	1.000
	[0.000]	[0.000]	[0.000]	[0.000]	[0.000]	[0.000]
Male	0.928***	0.927***	0.963***	0.963***	1.198***	1.197***
	[0.008]	[0.008]	[0.009]	[0.009]	[0.026]	[0.026]
Married	1.009	1.008	1.006	1.005	1.089	1.089
	[0.024]	[0.024]	[0.033]	[0.033]	[0.092]	[0.092]
Immigrant	1.045***	1.045***	1.029*	1.028	1.021	1.020
	[0.015]	[0.015]	[0.017]	[0.017]	[0.038]	[0.038]
Secondary education	0.993	0.992	0.956***	0.955***	1.035	1.032
	[0.010]	[0.010]	[0.012]	[0.012]	[0.028]	[0.028]
Tertiary education	1.043***	1.043***	0.903***	0.903***	1.022	1.022
	[0.013]	[0.013]	[0.014]	[0.014]	[0.036]	[0.036]
Enabling factors						
Employed	0.904***	0.904***	0.936***	0.936***	0.865***	0.864***
	[0.013]	[0.013]	[0.018]	[0.018]	[0.048]	[0.048]
ln(Income_ppp)	1.014***	1.014***	1.011***	1.011***	0.999	0.999
	[0.003]	[0.003]	[0.003]	[0.003]	[0.010]	[0.010]
Health behaviours						
Present smoker	0.877***	0.877***	0.914***	0.914***	0.587***	0.587***
	[0.015]	[0.015]	[0.020]	[0.020]	[0.034]	[0.034]
Regular alcohol consumption	0.956***	0.956***	0.952***	0.952***	0.844***	0.844***
	[0.010]	[0.010]	[0.012]	[0.012]	[0.031]	[0.031]
Regular physical activity	0.937***	0.937***	0.951***	0.951***	0.832***	0.832***
	[0.008]	[0.008]	[0.011]	[0.011]	[0.026]	[0.026]
Need factors						
ADL scale	1.033***	1.033***	1.032***	1.032***	1.156***	1.156***
	[0.005]	[0.005]	[0.006]	[0.006]	[0.017]	[0.017]
Number of chronic diseases	1.117***	1.117***	1.093***	1.093***	1.185***	1.185***
	[0.004]	[0.004]	[0.005]	[0.005]	[0.013]	[0.013]
Cognitive impairment	0.991	0.981*	1.001	0.98	1.081**	1.075*
	[0.009]	[0.011]	[0.012]	[0.014]	[0.035]	[0.044]
Sensory impairment	1.017**	1.009	1.007	0.989	1.047*	1.042
	[0.008]	[0.009]	[0.010]	[0.012]	[0.029]	[0.034]
Sense_cog impairment		1.023		1.049**		1.014
		[0.015]		[0.020]		[0.053]
Austria	1.311***	1.310***	1.146***	1.145***	1.877***	1.876***
	[0.024]	[0.024]	[0.025]	[0.025]	[0.088]	[0.088]
Germany	1.567***	1.566***	1.263***	1.262***	1.419***	1.417***
	[0.031]	[0.031]	[0.029]	[0.029]	[0.074]	[0.074]
Netherlands	1.085***	1.084***	0.905***	0.904***	0.921	0.92

Table 2 Health care utilisation in SHARE: negative binomial conditionally correlated random effects model *(Continued)*

	Doctor Visits		GP visits		Hospitalisations	
	[1]	[2]	[3]	[4]	[5]	[6]
	[0.020]	[0.020]	[0.020]	[0.020]	[0.049]	[0.049]
Spain	1.252***	1.252***	1.132***	1.132***	0.755***	0.757***
	[0.024]	[0.024]	[0.026]	[0.026]	[0.041]	[0.041]
Italy	1.375***	1.375***	1.314***	1.314***	0.836***	0.837***
	[0.026]	[0.026]	[0.029]	[0.029]	[0.044]	[0.044]
France	1.540***	1.539***	1.467***	1.465***	1.178***	1.176***
	[0.026]	[0.026]	[0.030]	[0.030]	[0.056]	[0.056]
Switzerland	1.131***	1.131***	0.966	0.966	1.350***	1.349***
	[0.022]	[0.022]	[0.023]	[0.023]	[0.072]	[0.072]
Belgium	1.564***	1.563***	1.497***	1.495***	1.175***	1.173***
	[0.026]	[0.026]	[0.030]	[0.030]	[0.054]	[0.054]
SHARE Wave 2	1.109***	1.109***	1.108***	1.108***	1.141*	1.142*
	[0.023]	[0.023]	[0.027]	[0.027]	[0.085]	[0.085]
SHARE Wave 4	1.243***	1.245***	1.311***	1.315***	1.139	1.140
	[0.069]	[0.069]	[0.089]	[0.089]	[0.227]	[0.228]
SHARE Wave 5	1.406***	1.408***	.	.	1.227	1.229
	[0.101]	[0.101]	.	.	[0.316]	[0.317]
N	85,147	85,147	59,965	59,965	85,473	85,473
ll	−239,098.39	−239,094.79	−146,884.11	−146,879.70	−45,976.20	−45,974.52
AIC	478,284.78	478,281.57	293,854.22	293,849.40	92,040.40	92,041.05
BIC	478,696.28	478,711.77	294,241.29	294,254.47	92,452.06	92,471.42

IRR Incidence-rate ratios. * $p < 0.10$, ** $p < 0.05$, *** $p < 0.01$. IRR of time-averaged covariates are not shown. Standard errors in brackets

is associated with 6% fewer doctor visits, 5% fewer GP visits and nearly 17% fewer hospitalisations. The direction and the magnitude of the association of health care utilisation with other factors depend on the type of care analysed. For example, males tend to have fewer visits to the doctor and to the GP, but more hospitalisations; and higher income level is only positively associated with more visits to the doctor and to the GP, but it is not significantly associated with the number of hospitalisations.

For presentation purposes the IRRs of the average across the panel of the time-varying covariates were not reported in Table 2, but they are available in the Appendix. The estimated coefficients can be interpreted as long-term associations with the use of health care. In this sense, the long-term association of being cognitively impaired is positive and significantly associated with doctor and GP visits. In the same line, smoking is positively associated in the long term with hospitalisations. The strongest long-term association displayed in Table 5 in Appendix is the one between the number of chronic conditions and GP visits.

Regression results of the LCNB_CRE model

Table 3 shows the estimation results of the LCNB_CRE model. By design, these models are estimated using balanced

panels [38]. Consequently, a significant amount of observations are lost with the implementation of this method. Given that the BIC in the CCRENB model favours the specification without the Sense-Cog interaction, only this is considered in Table 3 but the unrestricted alternative is reported in the Appendix.

Having a cognitive impairment is associated with 6% fewer doctor visits amongst low users, but has no significant association with high users. Contrary to this finding, but in the same direction to what was found in the CCRENB model, this impairment is associated with more hospitalisations amongst high users; however, amongst low users this association is negative. The insignificant association between GP visits and being cognitively impaired found in the CCRENB still holds amongst low users, but not for frequent users of GP services as having this impairment is associated with 6% more visits.

Column [5] shows that there is strong evidence supporting that sensory impairment is associated with 17% more hospitalisations amongst infrequent users of hospital services. The positive association amongst individuals with this impairment and visits to the doctor found in Table 2 is not supported anymore in the LCNB_CRE model.

With the only exception of the ADL scale amongst infrequent users of GP services, the strong, positive and

Table 3 Health Care utilisation in SHARE: latent class negative binomial conditionally correlated random effects model

	Doctor Visits		GP visits		Hospitalisations	
	[1]	[2]	[3]	[4]	[5]	[6]
	Low users	High users	Low users	High users	Low users	High users
Predisposing factors						
Age	1.012	1.021	1.016	0.989	1.055	1.000
	[0.013]	[0.014]	[0.015]	[0.013]	[0.048]	[0.056]
Age squared	1.000	1.000	1.000	1.000	1.000	1.000
	[0.000]	[0.000]	[0.000]	[0.000]	[0.000]	[0.000]
Male	0.909***	0.99	0.967*	1.013	1.239***	1.186**
	[0.016]	[0.019]	[0.019]	[0.020]	[0.069]	[0.089]
Married	1.057**	1.000	1.032	0.983	1.045	1.155
	[0.025]	[0.023]	[0.027]	[0.023]	[0.081]	[0.132]
Immigrant	1.042	0.978	0.977	0.996	1.212*	0.738*
	[0.037]	[0.038]	[0.035]	[0.037]	[0.123]	[0.125]
Secondary education	1.029	1.008	0.989	0.917***	1.048	1.062
	[0.023]	[0.023]	[0.025]	[0.021]	[0.072]	[0.097]
Tertiary education	1.077***	1.082**	0.921***	0.857***	0.964	1.154
	[0.029]	[0.034]	[0.028]	[0.028]	[0.082]	[0.137]
Enabling factors						
Employed	0.922***	0.859***	0.951*	0.845***	0.872	0.818
	[0.024]	[0.025]	[0.026]	[0.027]	[0.103]	[0.105]
ln(income_ppp)	1.025***	0.995	1.014*	0.993	1.001	0.98
	[0.008]	[0.006]	[0.008]	[0.006]	[0.024]	[0.025]
Health behaviours						
Present smoker	0.833***	0.938**	0.835***	0.966	0.911	0.744***
	[0.023]	[0.024]	[0.024]	[0.026]	[0.098]	[0.082]
Regular alcohol consumption	0.964**	0.876***	0.962**	0.913***	0.858**	0.837**
	[0.018]	[0.017]	[0.019]	[0.019]	[0.053]	[0.074]
Regular physical activity	0.883***	0.920***	0.907***	0.908***	0.842***	0.761***
	[0.015]	[0.018]	[0.017]	[0.019]	[0.054]	[0.065]
Need factors						
ADL scale	1.042**	1.129***	1.012	1.101***	1.272***	1.120**
	[0.017]	[0.015]	[0.023]	[0.012]	[0.040]	[0.060]
Number of chronic diseases	1.339***	1.144***	1.338***	1.116***	1.329***	1.090***
	[0.010]	[0.008]	[0.012]	[0.008]	[0.028]	[0.034]
Cognitive impairment	0.942***	1.019	0.978	1.063***	0.890*	1.164*
	[0.020]	[0.021]	[0.024]	[0.022]	[0.062]	[0.102]
Sensory impairment	0.989	0.992	0.988	1.01	1.167***	0.946
	[0.017]	[0.017]	[0.019]	[0.019]	[0.066]	[0.072]
Country dummies						
Austria	1.345***	1.224***	1.112**	1.338***	2.069***	1.073
	[0.069]	[0.059]	[0.055]	[0.068]	[0.260]	[0.196]
Germany	1.984***	1.652***	1.346***	1.496***	1.924***	0.908
	[0.071]	[0.080]	[0.054]	[0.074]	[0.234]	[0.159]
Netherlands	1.133***	1.135***	0.948	0.867***	0.894	0.781

Table 3 Health Care utilisation in SHARE: latent class negative binomial conditionally correlated random effects model *(Continued)*

	Doctor Visits		GP visits		Hospitalisations	
	[1]	[2]	[3]	[4]	[5]	[6]
	[0.040]	[0.051]	[0.040]	[0.042]	[0.115]	[0.121]
Spain	1.419***	1.158***	1.182***	1.337***	0.704**	0.616***
	[0.057]	[0.053]	[0.058]	[0.064]	[0.097]	[0.102]
Italy	1.529***	1.491***	1.156***	1.853***	0.837	0.629***
	[0.060]	[0.065]	[0.050]	[0.086]	[0.109]	[0.100]
France	1.673***	1.271***	1.610***	1.333***	1.276**	0.954
	[0.057]	[0.057]	[0.060]	[0.062]	[0.151]	[0.143]
Switzerland	1.124***	1.151**	0.921*	1.100	1.458***	1.396
	[0.049]	[0.068]	[0.045]	[0.070]	[0.198]	[0.290]
Belgium	1.649***	1.426***	1.504***	1.569***	1.291**	0.734**
	[0.052]	[0.057]	[0.053]	[0.067]	[0.014]	[0.014]
N	28,328		26,571		28,736	
ll	−79,603.25		−65,226.65		−14,502.19	
AIC	159,334.50		130,581.31		29,132.39	
BIC	159,773.88		131,035.00		29,572.68	

IRR Incidence-rate ratios. * $p < 0.10$, ** $p < 0.05$, *** $p < 0.01$. IRR of time-averaged covariates are not shown. Standard errors in brackets

significant association between health care utilisation and the rest of the need factors found in the CCRENB is still present in the latent class approach. Also consistent with the findings of the previous model, being employed and both unhealthy and health enhancement behaviours are negatively associated with all types of health care utilisation. In the CCRENB model income was positively associated with doctor and GP visits, now this association is only present amongst low users of health care.

Interestingly, the association found between immigration status and the number of hospitalisations depends on whether the individual is a frequent or an infrequent user. Being an immigrant is associated with 21% more hospitalisations amongst lower users but with 26% fewer hospitalisations amongst high users.

Table 4 reports the sample average of predicted probability of belonging to the high user class for each type of health care as well as the expected number of visits for each class and type of care.

Table 4 Predicted probability and expected number of visits by class

	Prob. High user	E[visits] if low user	E[visits] if high user
Doctor Visits	0.43	4.07	10.54
		[2.77]	[4.19]
GP visits	0.45	2.62	7.03
		[1.75]	[2.86]
Hospitalisations	0.18	0.14	0.70
		[0.17]	[0.41]

Standard errors in brackets

The results of the analysis of the determinants of latent class membership are shown in Table 7 in Appendix. It is worth noting that having a cognitive impairment is associated with a higher probability of being a frequent user of doctor and GP visits. In the same direction, sensory impaired individuals are associated with a higher probability of visiting a doctor frequently.

Discussion

This paper analyses the utilisation of health care services by older Europeans with cognitive and sensory impairments. This is carried out by using two different applications of the correlated random effects (CRE) method to describe the variation in the number of visits to any doctor, to the GP, and to the hospital amongst respondents of the SHARE survey. These econometric techniques test the hypothesis that individuals with cognitive and sensory impairments with no regular physical activity will tend to use more health care than people with only one or with none of these impairments in order to partly compensate for the higher depreciation of their health stock. This analysis provides evidence suggesting that, in some cases, cognitive and sensory impairments are associated with higher utilisation of health care services, even after conditioning for other major health conditions. Specifically, the correlated random effects negative binomial model (CCRENB) shows that cognitive impairment is associated with more hospitalisations. Likewise, the latent class approach (LCNB_CRE) finds that amongst high users of health care those with cognitive impairment are significantly associated with more hospitalisations and more GP visits. Additionally, estimates from the LCNB_CRE model indicate a strong, positive and significant association between sensory impairment and the number of hospitalisations amongst low users. Furthermore, the unrestricted models suggest a positive association between suffering both impairments at the same time and the number of doctor and GP visits. Although in some specifications the estimates of the interaction term were statistically significant, the models from which they were obtained are outperformed by the restricted models that omit the Sense-Cog interaction.

On the other hand, the CCRENB shows that individuals with cognitive but no sensory impairment have a negative association with doctor visits. The LCNB_CRE also finds a negative association between cognitive impairment and this type of care amongst low users. These results are not necessarily contrary to the hypothesis tested here as they may be reflecting barriers to outpatient health care access amongst cognitively impaired individuals. Walsh and colleagues suggested that individuals with cognitive impairment may not recognise or be able to communicate health problems requiring outpatient care [41]. One may argue that this lack of outpatient care could lead to more severe illnesses requiring hospitalisations; thus, suggesting that the observed negative association with doctor visits and the positive association with hospitalisations amongst high users of health care could be potentially related. However, testing the existence of substitution and/or complementary behaviours in the use of the different types of health care requires the estimation of a structural demand model which is beyond the scope of this paper.

Regarding the rest of the factors that condition for health need, the results of both econometric models are as predicted by the Grossman theory. Individuals in major health need (higher number of chronic diseases and of daily life limitations) are associated with higher utilisation of health care while individuals with alternative ways of health investment, i.e. regular physical activity, tend to use fewer health care services. Recent studies analysing health care utilisation amongst older Europeans using either SHARE or other surveys have also found these associations [42–45].

In a cross-sectional study using SHARE, Solé-Auro et al. found in their pooled (11 country sample) model a positive association between being an immigrant and visiting the doctor, the GP and the hospital [45]. Interestingly, while the CCRENB model in the present analysis also finds a positive association for the first two types of care, the results of the LCNB_CRE model show that the direction of the association for hospital visits depends on its intensity: the association is positive for low users, but negative for high users.

This paper is subject to three main limitations. First, as with any other study using panel surveys, the results presented here are subject to non-response and attrition bias. However, a recent study using SHARE rejected the hypothesis of significant correlation patterns of missing values and health care utilisation variables [43]. This, nevertheless, does not necessarily apply to the results of the LCNB_CRE model as it was estimated using the balanced panel. Long-term survivors who remain in a panel are likely to be healthier on average than the original sample at the beginning of the panel; this is the source of potential bias in the estimated associations [38]. Second, health care use based on recall of respondents' past utilisation in the last year may be subject to be underreported. Recall bias may be a particularly important issue amongst cognitively impaired individuals [41]. Unfortunately, without an effective linkage between population surveys and administrative records similar studies will continue to face the same limitation. Third, the models estimated here are not demand functions and treating the three types of health care as independent is a strong assumption. However, the methodology followed in this paper allows the identification of associations between suffering sensory and/or cognitive impairments and using these types of care over and above other individual characteristics. This initial analysis can be complemented with the further estimation of demand functions using structural models that apart from identifying factors associated with the use of health care could also identify price elasticities as well as substitution and complimentary behaviours amongst the types of care studied here. This is, however, beyond the scope of this paper.

Conclusions

While some evidence suggests that individuals with both sensory and cognitive impairments tend to have more doctor and GP visits that individuals with only one and with none of these impairments, the models that better fit the data did not include the interaction of these impairments. Nevertheless, this analysis shows the existence of a positive association between health care utilisation and cognitive and sensory impairments over and above the existing association of health care utilisation with other major chronic conditions. Given that 24% of the individuals in the sample studied were classified as having both sensory and cognitive impairments, a potential improvement in the efficiency of health care delivery may come from taking a systematic integrated care approach in the treatment of these conditions.

Endnotes

[1]We thank an anonymous reviewer for stressing the importance of emphasising the role of regular physical activity in this hypothesis.

[2]Due to a relatively high rate of non-response, the imputed values provided in SHARE were used. For simplicity, the average of the imputations provided was used. This simplification does not affect the main results of this paper.

Appendix

Table 5 IRR of time average of covariates in CCRENB

Age	Doctor Visits		GP visits		Hospitalisations	
	1.016*	1.017*	1.029***	1.029***	0.981	0.982
	[0.009]	[0.009]	[0.011]	[0.011]	[0.030]	[0.030]
Married	1.002	1.003	1.003	1.004	0.873	0.873
	[0.025]	[0.025]	[0.035]	[0.035]	[0.077]	[0.077]
Employed	0.945***	0.946***	0.903***	0.904***	0.817***	0.820***
	[0.019]	[0.019]	[0.023]	[0.023]	[0.054]	[0.054]
ln(Income_ppp)	1.005	1.005	0.982***	0.982***	1.000	1.000
	[0.005]	[0.005]	[0.006]	[0.006]	[0.015]	[0.015]
Present smoker	1.011	1.011	0.977	0.977	1.744***	1.744***
	[0.020]	[0.020]	[0.025]	[0.025]	[0.112]	[0.112]
Regular alcohol consumption	0.992	0.992	0.975	0.975	1.076	1.075
	[0.014]	[0.014]	[0.017]	[0.017]	[0.048]	[0.048]
Regular physical activity	0.919***	0.919***	0.896***	0.896***	0.963	0.963
	[0.013]	[0.013]	[0.016]	[0.016]	[0.042]	[0.042]
ADL scale	1.000	1.001	1.019**	1.021**	1.050**	1.053**
	[0.008]	[0.008]	[0.010]	[0.010]	[0.023]	[0.023]
No. of chronic diseases	1.210***	1.210***	1.219***	1.219***	1.181***	1.182***
	[0.006]	[0.006]	[0.007]	[0.007]	[0.017]	[0.017]
Cognitive impairment	1.020	1.055***	1.117***	1.163***	0.974	1.035
	[0.016]	[0.021]	[0.021]	[0.028]	[0.045]	[0.062]
Sensory impairment	1.015	1.038**	1.007	1.039*	1.048	1.091*
	[0.013]	[0.016]	[0.016]	[0.021]	[0.041]	[0.052]
Sense_Cog impairment		0.927***		0.913***		0.879
		[0.026]		[0.031]		[0.072]
SHARE Wave 2	0.976	0.975	0.947	0.946	1.012	1.011
	[0.049]	[0.049]	[0.057]	[0.057]	[0.150]	[0.150]
SHARE Wave 4	0.826***	0.824***	0.733***	0.731***	1.023	1.019
	[0.054]	[0.054]	[0.057]	[0.057]	[0.227]	[0.226]
SHARE Wave 5	0.749***	0.747***	0.703***	0.701***	0.812	0.81
	[0.060]	[0.060]	[0.068]	[0.068]	[0.225]	[0.224]

IRR Variables are individual averages over the observed panel. Estimates are reported as incidence-rate ratios. * $p < 0.10$, ** $p < 0.05$, *** $p < 0.01$. Standard errors in brackets

Table 6 Health Care utilisation in SHARE: LCNB_CRE with Sense-Cog impairment

	Doctor Visits		GP visits		Hospitalisations	
	[1]	[2]	[3]	[4]	[5]	[6]
Predisposing factors	*Low users*	*High users*	*Low users*	*High users*	*Low users*	*High users*
Age	1.012	1.021	1.015	0.99	1.056	0.998
	[0.013]	[0.014]	[0.015]	[0.013]	[0.048]	[0.056]
Age squared	1.000	1.000	1.000	1.000	1.000	1.000
	[0.000]	[0.000]	[0.000]	[0.000]	[0.000]	[0.000]
Male	0.909***	0.991	0.967*	1.013	1.240***	1.182**
	[0.016]	[0.019]	[0.019]	[0.020]	[0.070]	[0.089]
Married	1.057**	1.000	1.032	0.984	1.048	1.157
	[0.025]	[0.023]	[0.027]	[0.023]	[0.081]	[0.132]
Immigrant	1.041	0.978	0.976	0.995	1.213*	0.737*
	[0.037]	[0.038]	[0.035]	[0.037]	[0.123]	[0.124]
Secondary education	1.029	1.011	0.988	0.917***	1.051	1.061
	[0.023]	[0.023]	[0.025]	[0.021]	[0.073]	[0.096]
Tertiary education	1.077***	1.083**	0.920***	0.855***	0.964	1.153
	[0.029]	[0.034]	[0.028]	[0.028]	[0.082]	[0.137]
Enabling factors						
Employed	0.923***	0.859***	0.952*	0.846***	0.874	0.816
	[0.024]	[0.025]	[0.026]	[0.027]	[0.103]	[0.104]
In(income_ppp)	1.025***	0.996	1.015*	0.994	1.001	0.984
	[0.008]	[0.006]	[0.008]	[0.006]	[0.024]	[0.025]
Health behaviours						
Present smoker	0.832***	0.936**	0.836***	0.966	0.912	0.748***
	[0.023]	[0.024]	[0.024]	[0.026]	[0.098]	[0.083]
Regular alcohol consumption	0.964**	0.876***	0.961**	0.915***	0.858**	0.837**
	[0.017]	[0.017]	[0.019]	[0.019]	[0.054]	[0.074]
Regular physical activity	0.883***	0.919***	0.907***	0.908***	0.843***	0.761***
	[0.015]	[0.018]	[0.017]	[0.019]	[0.054]	[0.065]
Need factors						
ADL scale	1.042**	1.128***	1.011	1.099***	1.271***	1.120**
	[0.017]	[0.015]	[0.023]	[0.012]	[0.040]	[0.060]
Number of chronic diseases	1.338***	1.143***	1.339***	1.114***	1.329***	1.088***
	[0.010]	[0.008]	[0.012]	[0.008]	[0.028]	[0.034]
Cognitive impairment	0.946**	0.975	0.986	1.018	0.865	1.061
	[0.025]	[0.026]	[0.029]	[0.027]	[0.078]	[0.118]
Sensory impairment	0.992	0.960*	0.992	0.973	1.151**	0.885
	[0.019]	[0.021]	[0.021]	[0.023]	[0.075]	[0.081]
Sense_Cog impairment	0.988	1.098***	0.979	1.096***	1.061	1.214
	[0.038]	[0.039]	[0.044]	[0.039]	[0.130]	[0.183]
Country dummies						
Austria	1.348***	1.229***	1.114**	1.342***	2.063***	1.074
	[0.069]	[0.060]	[0.055]	[0.068]	[0.259]	[0.197]
Germany	1.982***	1.660***	1.345***	1.502***	1.916***	0.912
	[0.071]	[0.080]	[0.054]	[0.074]	[0.233]	[0.160]

Table 6 Health Care utilisation in SHARE: LCNB_CRE with Sense-Cog impairment *(Continued)*

	Doctor Visits		GP visits		Hospitalisations	
	[1]	[2]	[3]	[4]	[5]	[6]
Netherlands	1.132***	1.139***	0.948	0.868***	0.893	0.781
	[0.040]	[0.051]	[0.040]	[0.042]	[0.114]	[0.122]
Spain	1.417***	1.164***	1.181***	1.341***	0.699***	0.619***
	[0.057]	[0.053]	[0.058]	[0.064]	[0.097]	[0.103]
Italy	1.528***	1.495***	1.153***	1.855***	0.832	0.625***
	[0.060]	[0.066]	[0.050]	[0.086]	[0.108]	[0.099]
France	1.673***	1.274***	1.608***	1.335***	1.270**	0.953
	[0.057]	[0.057]	[0.060]	[0.062]	[0.150]	[0.143]
Switzerland	1.124***	1.154**	0.920*	1.102	1.451***	1.395
	[0.049]	[0.068]	[0.045]	[0.070]	[0.197]	[0.290]
Belgium	1.648***	1.434***	1.502***	1.578***	1.286**	0.738**
	[0.052]	[0.058]	[0.053]	[0.068]	[0.140]	[0.107]
N	28,328		26,571		28,736	
ll	−79,599.46		−65,222.37		−14,501.18	
AIC	159,332.92		130,578.75		29,136.36	
BIC	159,792.90		131,053.71		29,597.29	

IRR Incidence-rate ratios. * $p < 0.10$, ** $p < 0.05$, *** $p < 0.01$. IRR of time-averaged covariates are not shown. Standard errors in brackets

Table 7 Estimated class membership probability (π)

	Doctor visits	GP visits	Hospitalisations
π=	high users	low users	low users
Age	−0.039***	0.001	0.065***
	[0.006]	[0.006]	[0.017]
Married	−0.104	−0.047	0.229
	[0.103]	[0.099]	[0.252]
Employed	−0.272**	0.083	0.389
	[0.133]	[0.128]	[0.297]
ln(Income_ppp)	−0.105**	0.150***	−0.015
	[0.043]	[0.038]	[0.081]
Present smoker	0.203*	−0.203*	−0.773***
	[0.118]	[0.113]	[0.275]
Regular alcohol consumption	0.042	0.134	−0.131
	[0.095]	[0.091]	[0.213]
Regular physical activity	−0.205*	0.265**	−0.037
	[0.113]	[0.106]	[0.244]
ADL scale	0.273**	−0.263***	−0.188
	[0.110]	[0.101]	[0.182]
No. of chronic diseases	0.569***	−0.651***	−0.509***
	[0.044]	[0.045]	[0.078]
Cognitive impairment	0.664***	−0.851***	−0.356
	[0.120]	[0.108]	[0.241]
Sensory impairment	0.330***	−0.151	−0.224
	[0.107]	[0.100]	[0.225]
Constant	2.313***	−0.128	−1.54
	[0.598]	[0.544]	[1.423]

Variables are individual averages over the observed panel.
$*p < 0.10, **p < 0.05, ***p < 0.01$

Abbreviations
ADL: Activity Daily Living; CCRE: Conditionally Correlated Random Effects; CCRENB: Conditionally Correlated Random Effects Negative Binomial; CRE: Correlated Random Effects; FE: Fixed effects; GP: General Practitioner; IRRs: Incidence-rate ratios; LCNB_CRE: Latent Class Negative Binomial with correlated random effects; RE: Random Effects; SHARE: Survey of Health, Ageing and Retirement in Europe

Acknowledgements
This paper uses data from SHARE Waves 1, 2, 4 and 5 (DOIs: 10.6103/ SHARE.w1.500,https//doi.org/10.6103/SHARE.w2.500, doi:10.6103/SHARE.w4.500, doi:10.6103/SHARE.w5.500,), see Börsch-Supan et al. (2013) for methodological details.The SHARE data collection has been primarily funded by the European Commission through FP5 (QLK6-CT-2001-00360), FP6 (SHARE-I3: RII-CT-2006-062193, COMPARE: CIT5-CT-2005-028857, SHARELIFE: CIT4-CT-2006-028812) and FP7 (SHARE-PREP: N°211909, SHARE-LEAP: N°227822, SHARE M4: N°261982). Additional funding from the German Ministry of Education and Research, the Max Planck Society for the Advancement of Science, the U.S. National Institute on Aging (U01_AG09740-13S2, P01_AG005842, P01_AG08291, P30_AG12815, R21_AG025169, Y1-AG-4553-01, IAG_BSR06-11, OGHA_04-064, HHSN271201300071C) and from various national funding sources is gratefully acknowledged (see www.share-project.org).

Funding
This research is part of the Work Package 4 of the SENSE-Cog project, which has received funding from the European Union's Horizon 2020 research and innovation programme under grant agreement no. 668648. The funding body has no role in the study design, data collection, data analysis, data interpretation or manuscript writing.

Authors' contributions
DLP and BG designed the study. DLP conducted the data management, the data analysis, the results interpretation and drafted the manuscript. BG contributed to the interpretation and edited the manuscript before finalisation. All authors read and approved the final manuscript.

Competing interests
The authors declare that they have no competing interest.

Author details
[1]Centre for Health Economics, University of Manchester, 4.306 Jean McFarlane Building, Oxford Road, M13 9PL, Manchester, UK. [2]Centre for the Business and Economics of Health, The University of Queensland, Faculty of Business, Economics and Law, QLD, St Lucia 4072, Australia.

References
1. Fortin M, Stewart M, Poitras M-E, Almirall J, Maddocks HA. Systematic review of prevalence studies on multimorbidity: toward a more uniform methodology. The. Ann Fam Med. 2012;10(2):142–51.
2. Glynn LG, Valderas JM, Healy P, Burke E, Newell J, Gillespie P, et al. The prevalence of multimorbidity in primary care and its effect on health care utilization and cost. Fam Pract. 2011;28(5):516–23.
3. Barnett K, Mercer SW, Norbury M, Watt G, Wyke S, Guthrie B. Epidemiology of multimorbidity and implications for health care, research, and medical education: a cross-sectional study. Lancet. 2012;380(9836):37–43.
4. Humes LE, Busey TA, Craig J, Kewley-Port D. Are age-related changes in cognitive function driven by age-related changes in sensory processing? Attention, Perception, & Psychophysics. 2013;75(3):508–24.
5. Kiely K, Anstey K, Luszcz M. Dual Sensory Loss and Depressive Symptoms: The Importance of Hearing, Daily Functioning, and Activity Engagement. Front Hum Neurosci. 2013;7(837). https://www.frontiersin.org/articles/10. 3389/fnhum.2013.00837/full.
6. Lin FR, Yaffe K, Xia J, et al. Hearing loss and cognitive decline in older adults. JAMA Intern Med. 2013;173(4):293–9.
7. Valentijn SAM, Van Boxtel MPJ, Van Hooren SAH, Bosma H, Beckers HJM, Ponds RWHM, et al. Change in sensory functioning predicts change in cognitive functioning: results from a 6-year follow-up in the Maastricht aging study. J Am Geriatr Soc. 2005;53(3):374–80.
8. Yamada Y, Denkinger MD, Onder G, Henrard J-C, van der Roest HG, Finne-Soveri H, et al. Dual sensory impairment and cognitive decline: the results from the shelter study. J Gerontol: Series A. 2016;71(1):117–23.
9. Genther DJ, Frick KD, Chen D, Betz J, Lin FR. Association of hearing loss with hospitalization and burden of disease in older adults. JAMA. 2013;309(22):2322–4.
10. Javitt JC, Zhou Z, Willke RJ. Association between Vision Loss and Higher Medical Care Costs in Medicare Beneficiaries: Costs Are Greater for Those with Progressive Vision Loss. Ophthalmology. 2007;114(2):238–45. e1
11. Xiang X, An R. The impact of cognitive impairment and comorbid depression on disability, health care utilization, and costs. Psychiatr Serv. 2015;66(11):1245–8.
12. Grossman M. The demand for health: a theoretical and empirical investigation. New York: Columbia University Press of the National Bureau of Economic Research; 1972.
13. Grossman M. The Human Capital Model. In: Culyer A, Newhouse J, editors. Handbook of Health Economics. 1A. Amsterdam: Elsevier; 2000. p. 347–408.
14. McGuire A, Henderson J, Mooney G. The economics of health care: an introductory text. London/New York: Routledge & Kegan Paul; 1988.
15. Wagstaff A. The demand for health: some new empirical evidence. J Health Econ. 1986;5(3):195–233.
16. Gopinath B, Schneider J, McMahon CM, Burlutsky G, Leeder SR, Mitchell P. Dual sensory impairment in older adults increases the risk of mortality: a population-based study. PLoS One. 2013;8(3):e55054.
17. Kumagai N, Ogura S. Persistence of physical activity in middle age: a nonlinear dynamic panel approach. Eur J Health Econ. 2014;15(7):717–35.
18. Börsch-Supan A, Brandt M, Hunkler C, Kneip T, Korbmacher J, Malter F, et al. Data resource profile: the survey of health, ageing and retirement in Europe (SHARE). Int J Epidemiol. 2013;42(4):992–1001.

19. Dregan A, Gulliford MC. Leisure-time physical activity over the life course and cognitive functioning in late mid-adult years: a cohort-based investigation. Psychol Med. 2013;43(11):2447–58.
20. Tampubolon G. Cognitive ageing in great Britain in the new century: cohort differences in episodic memory. PLoS One. 2015;10(12):e0144907.
21. Bennett IJ, Golob EJ, Parker ES, Starr A. Memory evaluation in mild cognitive impairment using recall and recognition tests. J Clin Exp Neuropsychol. 2006;28(8):1408–22.
22. Petersen RC. Mild cognitive impairment as a diagnostic entity. J Intern Med. 2004;256(3):183–94.
23. Simmons BB, Hartmann B, Dejoseph D. Evaluation of suspected dementia. Am Fam Physician. 2011;1(5):9.
24. Whillans J, Nazroo J. Assessment of visual impairment: the relationship between self-reported vision and 'gold-standard' measured visual acuity. Br J Vis Impair. 2014;32(3):236–48.
25. Andersen RM, Davidson PL. Improving access to care in America. Changing the US health care system: key issues in health services policy and management 3a edición San Francisco: Jossey-Bass. 2007:3–31.
26. UNESCO. International standard classification of education 1997. New York; 1997.
27. Cameron AC, Trivedi PK. Microeconometrics: methods and applications. New York, USA: Cambridge University Press; 2005.
28. Deb P, Trivedi Pravin K. Finite Mixture for Panels with Fixed Effects. J Econometric Methods. 2013:35.
29. Chamberlain G. Multivariate regression models for panel data. J Econ. 1982; 18(1):5–46.
30. Mundlak Y. On the pooling of time series and cross section data. Econometrica. 1978;46(1):69–85.
31. Cameron AC, Trivedi PK. Count panel data. In: Baltagi B, editor. The Oxford handbook of panel data. Oxford, UK: Oxford University Press; 2013.
32. Hausman J, Hall BH, Griliches Z. Econometric models for count data with an application to the Patents-R & D Relationship. Econometrica. 1984;52(4):909–38.
33. Wooldridge JM. Correlated random effects models with unbalanced panels. Manuscript Michigan State University 2010.
34. Gurmu S. Semi-parametric estimation of hurdle regression models with an application to Medicaid utilization. J Appl Econ. 1997;12(3):225–42.
35. Deb P, Trivedi PK. Demand for medical care by the elderly: a finite mixture approach. J Appl Econ. 1997;12(3):313–36.
36. Deb P, Trivedi PK. The structure of demand for health care: latent class versus two-part models. J Health Econ. 2002;21(4):601–25.
37. Bago d'Uva T. Latent class models for use of primary care: evidence from a British panel. Health Econ. 2005;14(9):873–92.
38. Jones AM, Rice N, d'Uva TB, Balia S. Applied health economics. New York, USA: Routledge; 2013.
39. StataCorp. Stata Statistical Software: Release 14. College Station, TX: StataCorp LP; 2014.
40. Karaca-Mandic P, Norton EC, Dowd B. Interaction Terms in Nonlinear Models. Health Services Research. 2012;47(1pt1):255–74.
41. Walsh EG, Wu B, Mitchell JB, Berkmann LF. Cognitive function and acute care utilization. J Gerontol: Series B. 2003;58(1):S38–49.
42. Hudson E, Nolan A. Public healthcare eligibility and the utilisation of GP services by older people in Ireland. J Econ Ageing. 2015;6:24–43.
43. Ilinca S, Calciolari S. The patterns of health care utilization by elderly Europeans: frailty and its implications for health systems. Health Serv Res. 2015;50(1):305–20.
44. Schmitz H. More health care utilization with more insurance coverage? Evidence from a latent class model with German data. Appl Econ. 2012;44(34):4455–68.
45. Solé-Auró A, Guillén M, Crimmins EM. Health care usage among immigrants and native-born elderly populations in eleven European countries: results from SHARE. Eur J Health Econ. 2012;13(6):741–54.

5

The costs of repatriating an ill seafarer: a micro-costing approach

Mads D. Faurby[1,2*], Olaf C. Jensen[1], Lulu Hjarnoe[1] and Despena Andrioti[1]

Abstract

Seafarers sail the high seas around the globe. In case of illness, they are protected by international regulations stating that the employers must pay all expenses in relation to repatriation, but very little is known about the cost of these repatriations. The objective of this study was to estimate the financial burden of repatriations in case of illness. We applied a local approach, a micro-costing method, with an employer perspective using four case vignettes: I) Acute myocardial infarction (AMI), II) Malignant hypertension, III) Appendicitis and IV) Malaria. Direct cost data were derived from the Danish Maritime Authority while for indirect costs estimations were applied using the friction cost approach. The average total costs of repatriation varied for the four case vignettes; AMI (98,823 EUR), Malignant hypertension (47,597 EUR), Appendicitis (58,639 EUR) and Malaria (23,792 EUR) mainly due to large variations in the average direct costs which ranged between 9560 euro in the malaria case and 77,255 in the AMI case. Repatriating an ill seafarer is a costly operation and employers have a financial interest in promoting the health of seafarers by introducing or further strengthen cost-effective prevention programs and hereby reducing the number of repatriations.

Keywords: Local level costing method, Case vignette, Health promotion, Direct cost, Indirect cost, Repatriation

Background

Seafarers are an essential workforce to the global economy with around 1.5 million people working day and night [1], securing transportation of more than 90% of the goods across the globe [2, 3]. The remote character of their working environment defines them as a hard to reach population group [4–6]. This vulnerability of seafarers makes their health and wellbeing a concern and priority in a public health point of view. The current international regulation (Maritime Labour Convention (MLC 2006), states that seafarers must receive equal quality of care as the population on shore [7, 8]. In case of sickness on board, seafarers might find themselves in need of medical evacuation and/or repatriation[1] [9].

Limited epidemiological research on repatriations is available [3, 10, 11], but suggests that around 1.7% of all deployments ends with repatriation [10], and it is the employer who must pay the costs of repatriation [9], which is likely to be highly expensive. Direct and indirect costs should be taken into consideration. The direct costs includes paying for transportation from the ship to the hospital, hospital admission, medicines, plus transportation to the home country, accommodation salary and sickness benefits during repatriation and illness [9]. The direct costs are often reimbursed by a third party payer to which ship owners pay annual fees in order for their coverage [12]. Indirect costs, such as production loss and the cost of time spent managing the repatriation case, are not reimbursed or insured against. These indirect costs are all held entirely by the employer, which could be as much as ten times the amount of direct costs [13]. Henny et al. in 2013 estimated that the annual costs of evacuation and medical treatment for the shipping industry amount to a total of 760 million euro. Knowing the costs of repatriation for seafarers can provide valuable insights for the employers, who strive to cost containment at all times and maximizing revenues [14]. A cost-of-illness analysis may thus be the first step in an economic evaluation of repatriations to establish strong arguments to promote the health and welfare of seafarers. A micro-level cost analysis of repatriation establishes information regarding the costs of different

* Correspondence: mfaurby@outlook.dk
[1]Centre of Maritime Health and Society, Institute of Public Health, Faculty of Health Sciences, University of Southern Denmark, Niels Bohrs vej 9, 6700 Esbjerg, Denmark
[2]Faurby Consulting, Aebleparken 190, 3rd floor, 5270 Odense N, Denmark

illnesses and what the major cost drivers are, when sea-farers are repatriated [15]. This type of study will provide value to maritime stakeholders and decision makers [16] and eventually enable employers to implement cost effective preventive measures and better integrated care and thereby save money.

The cost of repatriation is an unexplored field and careful attention should be paid to the costing methodology as at the moment there is no golden standard. It is crucial that the cost formula represents the relevant costing categories, is reliable, valid, and user friendly in order to provide useful data and be implemented in the shipping industry and at the ship level [17].

The European Union HealthBASKET project proposed a case vignette method to estimate the costs of treatment. The case vignette is an innovative and novel approach developed to explore resource use and costs.

A case vignette describes a typical patient in regards to diagnosis, age, gender and possible comorbidity and is a retrospective episode-specific costing approach. The approach was applied to the vignette cases – diagnoses – in order to compare the costs of ten different treatments under DRG tariffs across nine European Union countries [15, 18].

Even though research on the evaluation of the financial burden of a range of diseases in different countries and public administration levels is widely available, very limited research concerns the shipping sector.

The objective of this study was to estimate the average total costs of repatriating seafarers based on four case vignettes.

Methods

Four case vignettes were used (Table 1) based on published epidemiological research, which represent a major disease burden for the seafarers [3, 10].

Identifying the cases

The primary data source for cost information was the Danish Maritime Authority (DMA). DMA reimburses the ship-owners costs of repatriation and keeps records of the reimbursements made. However, DMA keeps paper archives of all the reimbursement cases, making it highly difficult and time consuming to identify the relevant cases to fit the case vignettes. The identification of the cases to fit the case vignettes were instead derived from Radio Medical Denmark records, which contains information on the date of the call, the expected diagnosis, personal identification number, gender of the seafarer and whether a helicopter emergency medical service or deviation was used to get the seafarer from the ship to shore. For each case vignette, one anonymized match was derived from the Radio Medical Denmark records in the period 2011 to 2013 The survey was approved by the responsible Authority, the Danish Data Protection Agency.

Establishing cost categories and measuring costs

This study estimates the average total costs of repatriation with an employer perspective based on the local approach [17] and follows guidelines for a costing study for each of the four case vignettes listed above [19]. In every case the timeframe is no longer than 18 weeks since this is the maximum time that is reimbursed by DMA [20, 21].

Cost formula

The following cost formula was applied to estimate the average total costs of repatriation capturing both the direct and indirect costs of repatriation: $C_{Total} = C_{Direct} + C_{Indirect}$.

The direct costs of repatriation are related to evacuation via helicopter or ship deviation, further transportation costs such as ambulance and airplane to repatriation country, hospitalization, medication, rehabilitation and sickness benefits, expressed in the formula [22]:

$$C_{Direct} = C_{Transport} + C_{Treatment} + C_{Compensation}$$

The indirect costs are expressed as: $C_{Indirect} = C_{production\ loss} + C_{recruit} + C_{overtime} + C_{insurance\ premium} + C_{manage}$.
Where:

$C_{production\ loss}$: the costs resulting from a slowdown in production.

$C_{recruit}$: the costs of hiring an additional worker to replace to repatriated seafarer.

$C_{overtime}$: the costs related to paying overtime to fellow seafarers in order to avoid a slowdown in production.

$C_{insurance\ premium}$: the costs related to an increase in insurance premium, which occurs after having the costs related to repatriation reimbursed.

C_{manage}: the costs related to managing the repatriation case e.g. the captain of the vessel must spend time compiling the receipts and claiming reimbursement [17].

This formula is flexible enough to accommodate the data from DMA and company level.

Table 1 Overview of case vignettes

WHO ICD-10 code	Description
IX Diseases of the circulatory system: I21	Acute myocardial infarction – A male aged 45–55
IX Diseases of the circulatory system: I10	Malignant Hypertension – A male aged 45–55
XI Diseases of the digestive system: K35	Acute appendicitis – Male/Female aged 20–30
I Certain infectious and parasitic diseases: B54	B54 Malaria – Male/Female, all age-groups

Identification and classification of resource items and units of resources utilized

A detailed description of the resource utilization of each of the four case vignettes were created and the resource utilization for each case vignette was measured using the local approach [13, 17]. The local approach is characterized by acknowledging that there can be differences in the costs of a service in different cases. The approach involves an assessment of the costs more directly by the company [13], and it is characterized as a micro-costing approach. This method is the most accurate, but also the most time consuming [14]. Each case was presented with the average indirect, direct and total costs based on the data from DMA. Indirect costs, such as insurance premiums, costs related to managing the repatriation case, and replacement costs are not captured in the data from DMA and assumptions in this regard had to be made. We used adjusted aggregate published data, when data were not available.

Measuring resource units and placing a monetary value on the resource units

The fourth and final step was to measure resource units and place a monetary value on the consumption, taken into consideration both direct and indirect costs.

Direct costs

The data for estimating the direct costs were retrieved from DMA based on the claims filed by the shipping companies [17]. These claims include fees and charges from hospitals, transportation services, pharmacies, general practitioners and sickness benefits. The costs were all provided in Danish Kroner (DKK). This was converted to euro (EUR) with current exchange rate from the European Central Bank [23]. As the costs occurred in different time periods 2011 to 2013, the figures were adjusted to 2013 prices using the Danish retail price index from Statistics Denmark [24]. The repatriated seafarer was entitled to sickness benefits, which were included as a part of the direct costs. Information about sickness benefits, duration of sick leave and salary was available from DMA. Information about salary used estimations from Marine Insight [25].

Indirect costs

Less information was available to estimate the indirect costs including productivity losses, management of the case and recruitment of a new seafarer. Assumptions were based on the available literature (Table 2). The friction method was applied to estimate these costs. It was assumed that the friction period lasted 18 weeks, which was the maximum duration that sickness benefits were covered by the DMA [26].

Results

The average total costs of the four case vignettes varied between 23,792 euro for the least expensive – the malaria case vignette – up to 98,823 for the most expensive – the AMI case vignette. Table 3 illustrates the average direct, indirect and total costs of the four case vignettes.

More specifically:

Case vignette no. 1

The AMI case vignette was comprised of a male seafarer who was evacuated by helicopter to the port of Bergen, Norway in 2011. The treatment was a percutaneous coronary intervention (PCI) and he was hospitalized for 12 days before returning to his home country, where he received further treatment and hospitalization. The seafarer received sickness benefits for the full period of 18 weeks. The total average cost amounted to 98,823 Euro. The main cost driver for this repatriation case was the treatment costs, which accounted for 44.7% of total costs equaling to 44,174 euro.

Case vignette no. 2

The malignant hypertension case vignette was comprised of a male engineer who was evacuated to the port of Shanghai for medical examination due to high blood pressure, in 2013. The ship had to deviate for 6 h to get to the port of Shanghai. The seafarer was found not-fit-for-duty and transported to his country of origin. The data from DMA provided no information on the sickness duration and it was assumed that the seafarer was ill for the full 18 week period that DMA reimburses. The average total costs were estimated at 47,597 euro. The main cost driver was the deviation cost, which accounted for 13,200 euro (27.7%) [25].

Case vignette no. 3

The appendicitis case vignette was comprised of the ships cook turning ill with severe abdominal pain in 2011. She was evacuated to the port of Malaga. The ship had to deviate for 12 h to get to the port of Malaga, where the seafarer was transported to the hospital for an appendectomy. As illustrated in Table 3 the majority of the average total costs were attributed to the direct costs. Of the total amount of 58,639 euro, about half (46.5%) was attributed to the ship deviation, with next higher the hospitalization cost at (17.7%).

Case vignette no. 4

The malaria case vignette comprised of a deck officer. The seafarer was evacuated to the port of Norfolk Virginia after a rapid malaria test shown a positive result and from the port to the hospital for further diagnosis and treatment. A boat service was utilized to get the seafarer from the vessel to shore. The patient was initiated

Table 2 Summary of cost estimates and assumptions

Category	Description	Estimates in EUR and source of estimations
Direct costs	Average cost per hour of ship diversion (100 ton/24*525 EUR)	2200 per hour of diversion [2]
Direct costs	Average costs per helicopter mission	25,000 [2]
Direct costs	Seafarer wage in the first month of absence	Depends on rank of the seafarer [25]
Indirect costs	Overtime for fellow seafarers 8 h per day spent working overtime	Based on salary [25]
Indirect costs	Replacement costs (1 flight ticket to the vessel)	1500 [22]
Indirect costs	Replacement costs (up front salary to new seafarer 2 months)	Same rank and monthly salary as the repatriated seafarer [25]
Indirect costs	Insurance premium increase [2]	10% of reimbursed costs [2]
Indirect costs	Captain of the vessel managing the case	100 Euro per contact with DMA and Radio Medical (assumption)

on malaria treatment and discharged from the hospital the following day. The seafarer was found not-fit-for-duty and had to be repatriated back to his home country. The total average cost amounted to 23,792 euro, with the main single cost driver the cost of a new recruitment, which accounted for 49.7% of the average total costs of this repatriation case equivalent to 11,825 euro.

Sensitivity analysis

A sensitivity analysis was carried out for all the four cases in order to investigate the robustness of the cost categories. The sensitivity analysis addressed the uncertainties regarding the cost estimates and assumptions [14]. The sensitivity analysis was carried out with an optimistic and a pessimistic case scenario. The inputs for the sensitivity analysis are provided in Table 4. The costing categories prone to sensitivity analysis were the cost of transportation, (helicopter or fuel consumption in case of ship deviations) compensation costs to the repatriated seafarer, the cost of managing the repatriation case, insurance premium increase and the cost of recruiting a new seafarer. The reimbursed costs by DMA were not prone to the sensitivity analysis, since no uncertainty surrounded these estimates.

The sensitivity analysis revealed that deviation and evacuation had major impact on the average total costs of repatriation. More specifically, in the appendicitis case the average total costs changed by as much as 23% by applying the pessimistic and optimistic costs for deviation. For the AMI case vignette the tornado diagram (Fig. 1) illustrates the changes in the estimates of the average total costs of repatriation in the optimistic and the pessimistic case scenario. In the optimistic case scenario the reduced costs of helicopter evacuation reduced

the estimated average total costs with 17%. The sensitivity analysis for the malignant hypertension case vignette the major cost categories were the costs of recruiting a new seafarer and deviating the vessel. In the optimistic case scenario reductions in the costs of recruiting a new seafarer led to an estimated reduction in the average total costs by 28% and in the pessimistic scenario increases in the costs of deviating the vessel led to an estimated increase in the average total costs by 14% (Fig. 2), similar results were seen in the appendicitis and malaria case vignette (Figs. 3 and 4 respectively). On the contrary, the costing categories compensation and insurance premium increase had an impact on the average total costs of repatriation of less than 10% in both sensitivity analysis scenarios for all the four case vignettes and the same applies to the management of the repatriation case with a no more than 3% impact in any of the scenarios.

Discussion

Limited published literature is available on the topic of repatriating seafarers [2], showing the relevance and meaningfulness of the estimates provided in this study. This survey applied a retrospectively micro-costing approach to estimate the financial burden of repatriation. Costs were measured by a local approach using company level data [13]. In some instances, such as the helicopter evacuation and deviation costs published data were used [2, 27]. Cost data were attributed to four cases vignettes. The case vignette approach assigns values to resources used in diagnoses – "vignette case" – and in this way comparisons among different countries can be made. In this study, the data yielded large variations in the average total costs of repatriation, where the costs ranged between 23,792 and 98,823 euros. This large gap in the

Table 3 Overview of the average direct, indirect and total costs of repatriation in 2013 Euro prices

Cost category	AMI	Malignant hypertension	Appendicitis	Malaria
Direct	77,255 (78%)	25,852 (54%)	43,114 (74%)	9560 (40%)
Indirect	21,567 (22%)	21,745 (46%)	15,523 (26%)	14,232 (60%)
Total	98,823 (100%)	47,597 (100%)	58,639 (100%)	23,792 (100%)

Table 4 Summary of cost estimates and assumptions

Category	Description	Optimistic assumption/estimate	Base case assumption/estimate	Pessimistic assumption/estimate
Direct costs	Average cost per ship diversion	1100 per hour of diversion (assumption)	2200 per hour of diversion [2]	3300 per hour of diversion (assumption)
Direct costs	Average costs per helicopter mission	9200 [34, 35]	25,000 [2]	37,500 (assumption)
Direct costs	Seafarer wage in the first month of absence	International Transport Workers Federation (ITF) minimal wage [37]	Marine Insight data [25]	PayScale Inc. data [38]
Indirect costs	Overtime	ITFminimal hourly wage [37]	Marine Insight data [25]	PayScale Inc. data [38]
Indirect costs	Replacement costs - 1 flight ticket (assumption)	500	1500	5000
Indirect costs	Replacement costs - salary	Two month salary up front, similar to repatriated seafarer (assumption)		
Indirect costs	Insurance premium increase (assumption)	None	10% of reimbursed costs	20% of reimbursed costs
Indirect costs	Master of the ship managing the case (assumption)	50 Euro per contact with DMA and Radio Medical	100 Euro per contact with DMA and Radio Medical	200 Euro per contact with DMA and Radio Medical

cost of repatriation indicates a great heterogeneity in repatriation cases. This variance was driven by large variations in the average direct costs. These differences were mainly due to large differences in; *I) the costs of evacuation (getting the seafarer from the vessel to shore) and II) differences in treatment costs.* The variations in indirect costs between the cases were mainly due to differences in the replacement costs. The average indirect costs varied between 14,000 euro in the malaria case and almost 22,000 euro in the malignant hypertension case vignette. The variation indicates that average indirect cost proportions ranges between 22 and 60% in the case vignettes. Indirect costs remain a substantial cost driver and outline the importance of estimating indirect costs, when estimating the total costs of repatriation.

In the AMI case vignette the data revealed, that the employer had costs which were not reimbursed by DMA and the estimate of 98,823 euro is, therefore, likely to be an underestimate of the financial burden held by the

employer in this repatriation case. This illustrates that using the data from DMA as a proxy for the direct costs held by the employer is not entirely accurate.

Previous data suggests that the annual number of repatriations amounts to nearly 10,000 with an annual cost of 760 million euro [2]. With the costs per repatriation case ranging between 24,000 and 99,000 euro the annual cost of 10,000 repatriations cases is somewhere between 240 million and 1 billion euros.

Results from similar studies using the case vignette approach to estimate the costs of AMI treatment in nine selected countries under DRG tariffs showed big differences among countries too. In France, The Netherlands and Italy, PCI was the standard of care intervention to treat AMI, with costs ranging between 3720 and 9374 euros [28]. In case vignette number one, the corresponding treatment for an AMI was PCI with a cost of nearly 43,000 euro, which makes the treatment of this case vignette much higher than the estimates

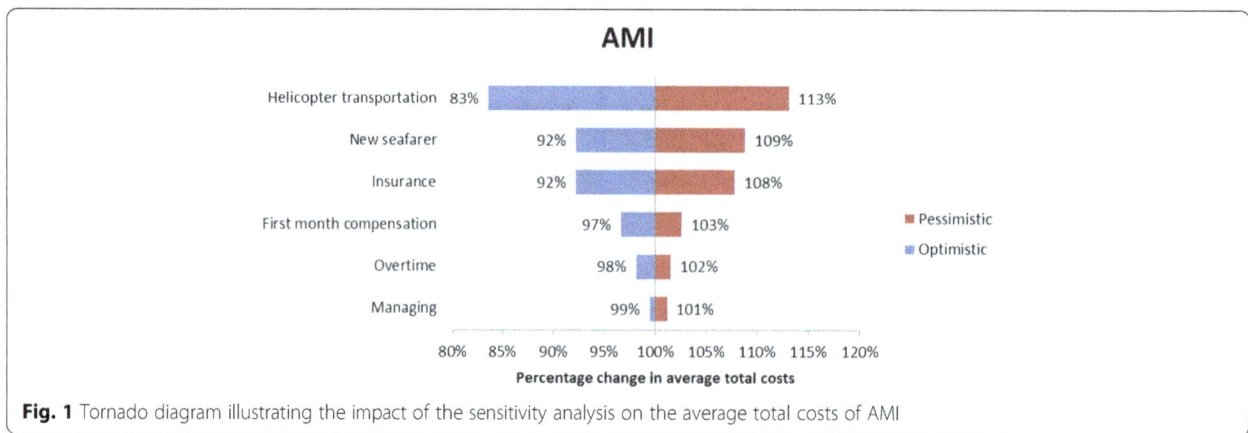

Fig. 1 Tornado diagram illustrating the impact of the sensitivity analysis on the average total costs of AMI

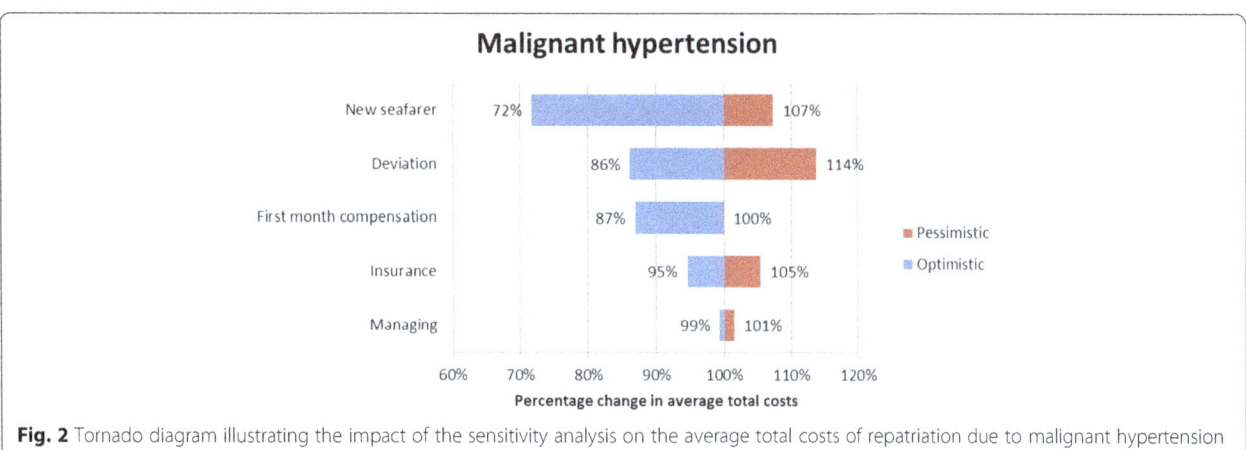

Fig. 2 Tornado diagram illustrating the impact of the sensitivity analysis on the average total costs of repatriation due to malignant hypertension

provided by the EU HealthBASKET project [28]. Similar studies found AMI treatment costs to range between 5434 and 7770 euros [29, 30].

Similar results were found with regards to the costs of treatment for appendicitis [18]. The mean total costs per case vignette across the selected countries were 1601 euro. Spain, was included in the selected countries of the EU HealthBASKET project, had a very low cost of treating appendicitis at a mean of 594 euro in DGR tariffs [31]. However, the findings of this survey showed the treatment costs for the case vignette number three were 10,076 euro, for the same country. Only in the United States, the most expensive health care system in the world treatment of appendectomy [32], was found to be similar to those found in this study [33].

This implies that in the case of seafarers – international employees not covered by any health system – market prices are used for the health services provided to them, contributing to a higher treatment cost.

The cost of helicopter evacuation at sea was estimated to be 25,000 euros per intervention [2]. Helicopter evacuation at sea has some similarities with remote area helicopter emergency services, which have average costs per mission varying between 6600 and 13,500 euros [34, 35].

A considerable amount of indirect cost represented the ship deviations depending on the distance from the nearest shore.

Any model is always a simplification of the reality [36], and since the available data did not cover all aspects of the model, several assumptions had to be made and assumptions come with uncertainty. In order to produce a robust cost analysis, special attention should be made in regards to properly estimate the major cost drivers [19]. The three major cost drivers for repatriation were transport from vessel to shore either by helicopter or ship deviation, treatment, and sickness benefits. Sickness benefits and treatment costs were reimbursed and are in the DMA records, which is why these estimates are fairly valid. The salary of the seafarers and transportation from sea to shore and insurance premium increase are all based on published literature and assumptions since no local level data were available and therefore they are surrounded by some degree of uncertainty. The companies should seek to routinely collect and make available these data.

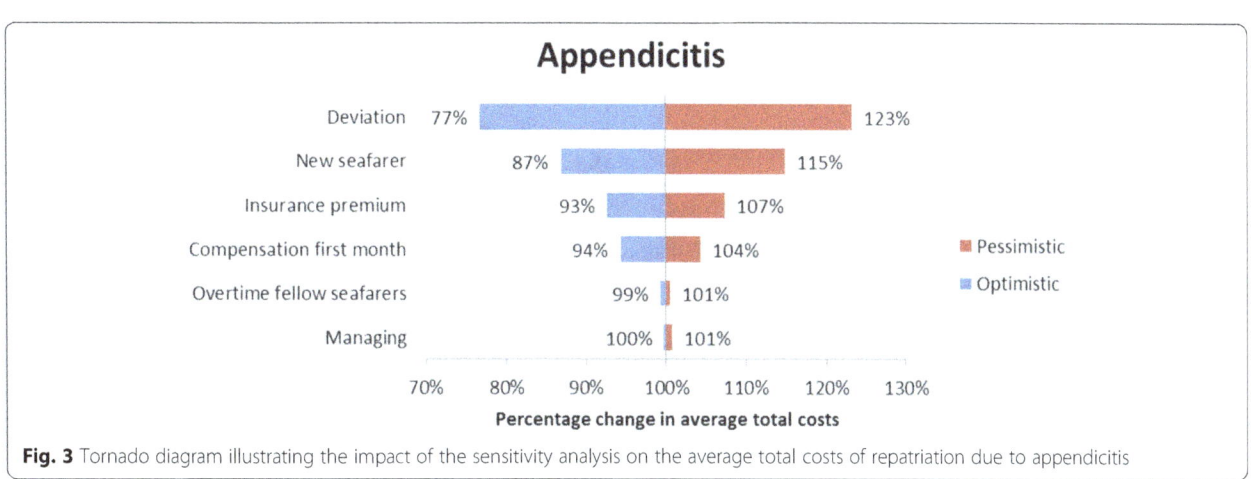

Fig. 3 Tornado diagram illustrating the impact of the sensitivity analysis on the average total costs of repatriation due to appendicitis

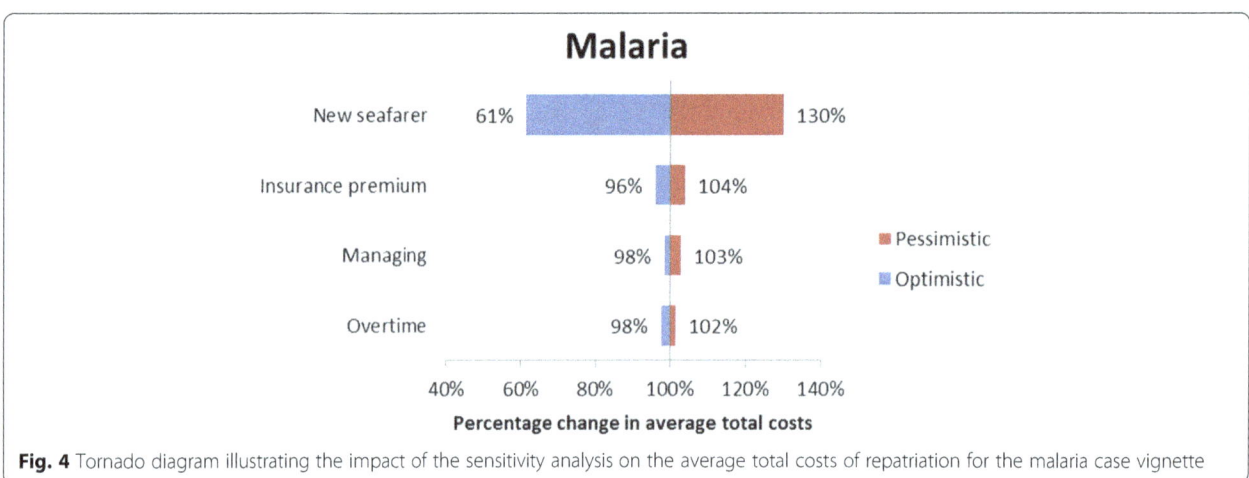

Fig. 4 Tornado diagram illustrating the impact of the sensitivity analysis on the average total costs of repatriation for the malaria case vignette

This study did not estimate any costs in terms of charterer loss penalties, which could imply that estimates of repatriation in the current study are conservative estimates of the true total costs.

By applying the case vignette approach, it was assumed that cases in each case vignette represents the typical repatriation case of this disease, however a more representative sample could provide more accurate cost data.

Conclusion

This study was a first attempt to map the relevant financial burden to the employer due to employee sickness on board merchant vessels. The objective was to estimate the costs of repatriation of ill seafarers based on four case vignettes; *I) acute myocardial infarction, II) malignant hypertension, III) acute appendicitis and IV) malaria*. The findings are a framework for investigating the average total costs of repatriation by applying a local level micro-costing approach. The cost formula included direct and indirect costs and the local approach proved to be a feasible approach to estimate the total costs of repatriation with an employer perspective.

Every case of repatriation poses a large financial burden on employers, and the results indicated a large variation in the average total costs of repatriation for the four case vignettes. These variations in the proportions of direct cost were mainly due to hospitalization and deviation expenses. It is worth noticing that fee-for-service contributed to higher prices for treating seafarers around the globe. This clearly shows how prices for treating the same diagnosis differentiate in different countries and give insight for introducing possible collective bargaining agreements.

With regards to the indirect costs the recruitment of a new employee was the main cost driver among the case vignettes. In our analysis, it was established that indirect costs are an important estimate from the employer's point of view, and a major cost driver for the total costs of repatriation. These indirect costs are not reimbursed,

and they all fall directly upon the employer. In order to estimate the total costs of repatriation, it would be beneficial if these cost data were collected regularly at the company level.

From the employers' point of view, it would be interesting to know these costs of repatriation, especially regarding helicopter evacuation, deviation and charterer loss. This could help the employers' insight and motivation for disease preventive and health promotion interventions on board.

Employers have a financial interest in promoting the health of seafarers by introducing or strengthening cost-effective prevention and health promotion programs, and hereby reducing the number of repatriations, as each repatriation of an ill seafarer is a heavy financial burden to the employer.

Endnotes

[1]Evacuation is a process of transporting the seafarer from the vessel to the nearest suitable port for medical treatment with repatriation be further transportation on to the home country, where additional treatment may be needed [9].

Abbreviations
AMI: Acute myocardial infarction; DKK: Danish Kroner; DMA: Danish Maritime Authority; EU: European Union; EUR: Euro; ITF: International Transport Workers Federation; MLC: Maritime Labour Convention; PCI: Percutaneous coronary intervention

Funding
This work was supported by the Danish Maritime Fund (grant number 2014-057).

Authors' contributions
MDF carried out the data gathering and data analyses as well as drafted the manuscript. DA and OCJ designed the study, applied for approval to the Danish Data Protection Agency, substantially contributed to the interpretation of the data and provided comments on all drafts. OCJ actively supported the

data gathering. DA developed the economic model. LH actively supported the data gathering and provided comments on all drafts. All authors confirm that this manuscript describes original work and has neither been published or submitted for publication elsewhere. All authors read and approved the final manuscript.

Competing interests
The authors declare that they have no competing interests.

References
1. United Nations Conference on Trade And Development. Review of maritime transport 2016. 2016.
2. Henny C, Hartington K, Scott S, et al. The business case for telemedicine. Int Marit Health. 2013;64:129–35.
3. Lefkowitz RY, Slade MD, Redlich CA. Risk factors for merchant seafarer repatriation due to injury or illness at sea. Int Marit Health. 2015;66:61–66.
4. Lefkowitz RY, Slade MD, Redlich CA. Injury, illness, and work restriction in merchant seafarers. Am J Ind Med. 2015;58:688–96.
5. Poulsen TR, Burr H, Hansen HL, et al. Health of Danish seafarers and fishermen 1970-2010: What have register-based studies found? Scand J Public Health. 2014;42:534–45.
6. Roberts SE, Nielsen D, Kotłowski A, et al. Fatal accidents and injuries among merchant seafarers worldwide. Occup Med Oxf Engl. 2014;64:259–66.
7. Baum F. The new public health. 3rd ed. Melbourne; New York: Oxford University Press; 2008.
8. International Transportation Workers' Federation. The maritime labour convention, 2006 - a seafarers' bill of rights. London: n.d. International Transportation of Worker' Federation; 2006.
9. Maritime Labour Convention. Repatriation. 2006.
10. Abaya ARM, Roldan S, Ongchangco JCE, et al. Repatriation rates in Filipino seafarers: a five-year study of 6,759 cases. Int Marit Health. 2015;66:189–95.
11. Tomaszunas S, Mroziński W. Diseases and injuries in Polish seafarers repatriated from ships. Bull Inst Marit Trop Med Gdynia. 1990;41:17–20.
12. The Danish Ministy of Health. Bekendtgørelse om rederiers bidrag til den særlige sygesikringsordning for søfarende. 2006.
13. Jallon R, Imbeau D, de Marcellis-Warin N. Development of an indirect-cost calculation model suitable for workplace use. J Saf Res. 2011;42:149–64.
14. Drummond MF, editor. Methods for the economic evaluation of health care programmes. 3rd ed. Oxford: Oxford Univ. Press; 2007.
15. Schreyögg J, Tiemann O, Stargardt T, et al. Cross-country comparisons of costs: the use of episode-specific transitive purchasing power parities with standardised cost categories. Health Econ. 2008;17:S95–103.
16. Rice DP. Cost of illness studies: What is good about them? Inj Prev. 2000;6:177–9.
17. Gavious A, Mizrahi S, Shani Y, et al. The costs of industrial accidents for the organization: developing methods and tools for evaluation and cost–benefit analysis of investment in safety. J Loss Prev Process Ind. 2009;22:434–8.
18. Busse R, Schreyögg J, Smith PC. Variability in healthcare treatment costs amongst nine EU countries – results from theHealthBASKET project. Health Econ. 2008;17:S1–8.
19. Mogyorosy Z, Smith P. The main methodological issues in costing health care services - a literature review. York: The University of York - Centre for Health Economics; 2005.
20. The Danish National Labour Market Authority. Bekendtgørelse om sygedagpenge til søfarende, vol. BE728K; 2012.
21. Retsinformation. Bekendtgørelse om den særlige sygesikringsordning for søfarende m.fl. 2006.
22. Andrioti D, Jensen O, Abaya A, et al. Designing a model to estimate the cost of repatriations, 14th International Symposium on Maritime Health, Manilla, Phillippines. 2017.
23. European Central Bank. Euro foreign exchange reference rates. 2017.
24. Statistics Denmark. Forbrugerprisindeks n.d; 2017.
25. Marine Insight. How much does an Indian seafarer officer earn? 2016.
26. Retsinformation. Bekendtgørelse om sygedagpenge til søfarende. 2012.
27. Hendriks ME, Kundu P, Boers AC, et al. Step-by-step guideline for disease-specific costing studies in low- and middle-income countries: a mixed methodology. Glob Health Action. 2014;7:23573.
28. Tiemann O. Variations in hospitalisation costs for acute myocardial infarction – a comparison across Europe. Health Econ. 2008;17:S33–45.
29. Häkkinen U, Rosenqvist G, Peltola M, et al. Quality, cost, and their trade-off in treating AMI and stroke patients in European hospitals. Health Policy Amst Neth. 2014;117:15–27.
30. Häkkinen U, Rosenqvist G, Iversen T, et al. Outcome, use of resources and their relationship in the treatment of AMI, stroke and hip fracture at European hospitals: treatment of AMI, stroke and hip fracture. Health Econ. 2015;24:116–39.
31. Schreyögg J. A micro-costing approach to estimating hospital costs for appendectomy in a cross-European context. Health Econ. 2008;17:S59–69.
32. Roehr B. Rise in US spending on healthcare in 2009 was twice that in UK. BMJ. 2012;344:e3274.
33. Wu JX, Dawes AJ, Sacks GD, et al. Cost effectiveness of nonoperative management versus laparoscopic appendectomy for acute uncomplicated appendicitis. Surgery. 2015;158:712–21.
34. Taylor CB, Stevenson M, Jan S, et al. A systematic review of the costs and benefits of helicopter emergency medical services. Injury. 2010;41:10–20.
35. Taylor CB, Stevenson M, Jan S, et al. An investigation into the cost, coverage and activities of helicopter emergency medical services in the state of New South Wales, Australia. Injury. 2011;42:1088–94.
36. Box GEP, Draper NR. Empirical model-building and response surfaces. New York: Wiley; 1987.
37. International Transportation Workers' Federation. What should my wages be? n.d; 2017.
38. PayScale Inc. Salary Data & Career Research Center (United States). Seattle: PayScale Inc; 2017.

6

Inequalities in child immunization coverage in Ghana: evidence from a decomposition analysis

Derek Asuman[1], Charles Godfred Ackah[1*] and Ulrika Enemark[2]

Abstract

Childhood vaccination has been promoted as a global intervention aimed at improving child survival and health, through the reduction of vaccine preventable deaths. However, there exist significant inequalities in achieving universal coverage of child vaccination among and within countries. In this paper, we examine rural-urban inequalities in child immunizations in Ghana. Using data from the recent two waves of the Ghana Demographic and Health Survey, we examine the probability that a child between 12 and 59 months receives the required vaccinations and proceed to decompose the sources of inequalities in the probability of full immunization between rural and urban areas. We find significant child-specific, maternal and household characteristics on a child's immunization status. The results show that children in rural areas are more likely to complete the required vaccinations. The direction and sources of inequalities in child immunizations have changed between the two survey waves. We find a pro-urban advantage in 2008 arising from differences in observed characteristics whilst a pro-rural advantage emerges in 2014 dominated by the differences in coefficients. Health system development and campaign efforts have focused on rural areas. There is a need to also specifically target vulnerable children in urban areas, to maintain focus on women empowerment and pay attention to children from high socio-economic households in less favourable economic times.

Keywords: Immunization coverage, Childhood, Vaccination, Health inequality, Decomposition, Rural-urban, Ghana

Background

Improving child health outcomes has been central to global development efforts over the last four decades. For example, the Millennium Development Goals (2000–2015) adopted by the United Nations in 2000 committed global agencies and national governments in Target 4 to reduce global child mortality rates. The succeeding Sustainable Development Goals (2016–2030) re-emphasizes the importance of improving child health and survival rates as an important global development objective. Such global commitments have led to increased public and private investments in promoting accessible and affordable child health intervention programs, particularly in nutrition and immunization services [18]. For example, GAVI has provided financial and technical support for the development of effective vaccines and low-cost immunization implementation programmes in developing countries [41].

The World Health Organisation (WHO) in 1974 launched the Expanded Programme on Immunization (EPI) as a public health initiative aimed at improving child health and survival through routine and universal immunization coverage. Generally, the EPI has been successful, increasing child immunization rates from 5% at the inception of the initiative to 83% in 2014 [14]. Despite these efforts, there exist substantial challenges to achieving universal coverage of child immunization in developing countries, especially within the Sub Saharan African (SSA) region [31]. The limited coverage of child immunisation programmes within the SSA region may attenuate the ability of countries in the region to improve child health outcomes [12]. For example, Liu et al. [31] estimates that SSA will account for 60% of global child deaths by 2030.

As such, there exist an urgent need to achieve universal coverage of full immunization as a mechanism to

* Correspondence: cakach@ug.edu.gh
[1]Institute of Statistical, Social and Economic Research, University of Ghana, E.N. Omaboe Building, P. O. Box LG 74, Legon, Ghana
Full list of author information is available at the end of the article

achieve the child mortality target of the SDGs. For policy purposes, it is imperative to examine and understand the factors that contribute to the utilization of immunization services in the sub-region for effective and targeted programme implementation. Achieving equity in immunization involves creating equal opportunities for all eligible children to have access to such services as well as identifying disadvantaged and vulnerable children who are at risk of being unvaccinated [29]. A number of socio-economic and demographic factors have been identified to influence child immunization coverage. Evidence from earlier studies have shown child-specific, parental and household-level characteristics as important predictors of child immunization coverage.

At the child-level, there exist conflicting evidence of gender gaps in immunization coverage which may reflect cultural specific differences in the status of women. Studies such as, Corsi et al. [16] and Pal [37] report significant gender disparities in India, with girls disadvantaged. Antai [5] on the other hand finds that girls are more likely to receive full immunization in Nigeria whilst Tsawe et al. [42] and Landoh et al. [28] do not find significant gender differentials in immunization coverage in Swaziland and Togo respectively. In addition to gender, other child-specific characteristics found to influence immunization status are birth order or parity [5, 19], age [38], and place of delivery [13, 36].

For parental-specific characteristics, studies on child immunization have focused extensively on maternal characteristics. Particularly, educational attainment and literacy [6, 7, 19, 36], employment status [13, 43], age and age at birth [5, 36], media exposure [13, 42], marital status [28] and religion [28, 36] have been found to have strong relationships with the immunization status of a child. The presence of such strong maternal effects on child immunization coverage is a reflection of the traditional childcare responsibility of mothers in most developing countries, which dovetails to the policy recommendation that empowering women in the household decision-making process, such as child health, may be crucial to achieving universal immunization coverage among underserved populations [5, 44].

Two household-level characteristics have been examined extensively in earlier studies on inequalities in child health outcomes – residence of the household and socioeconomic status measured by wealth or assets. The effects of these characteristics on child immunization coverage are however ambiguous, reflecting large cross-country differences. For example, Bugvi et al. [13], Olorunsaiye & Degge, [36] and Singh and Parasuraman [40] find inequalities in immunization coverage disfavoring children residing in households with lower socioeconomic status. On the other hand, Barata et al. [9] finds lower immunization rates among children from households with high socioeconomic status in Brazil. These findings may reflect differential opportunity of time costs that mothers or caregivers face in making regular visits to immunization centres [38, 40].

Equally, a number of studies have reported significant rural-urban disparities in child immunization coverage across developing countries. In developing countries where spatial inequalities in availability and access to health facilities and information are pervasive, rural communities remain underserved in a number of essential services. A group of studies such as Abadura et al. [1], Antai [5] and Bugvi et al. [13] report rural disadvantage in child immunization in Ethiopia, Nigeria and Pakistan. A second strand of studies has on the other hand reported lower immunization rates among children in urban areas, especially slum and informal settlements in Kampala [8] and Nairobi [19]. Such differences may arise from differences in development strategies as well as the definition of rural and urban areas.

There exist significant differences across countries and localities in the sources of inequalities in child immunizations due to significant variations in structural, cultural and institutional settings [26]. The presence of such differences require that further studies are undertaken to identify the country-specific extent and sources of inequalities in child immunization coverage. In this paper, we seek to contribute to the literature by examining rural-urban inequalities in child immunization coverage in Ghana. The objectives of the paper are twofold. First, we examine the determinants of full immunization coverage of children aged 12–59 months using a logistic regression technique. Specifically, the paper assesses the probability that a child receives the basic WHO required immunizations. The paper then proceeds to decompose the difference in the probability of full immunization coverage between rural and urban areas into a part attributable to differences in observed characteristics and an unexplained component, which may reflect structural and institutional differences in health systems between urban and rural areas.

We employ data from the fifth and sixth waves of the Ghana Demographic and Health Survey (GDHS) conducted in 2008 and 2014 respectively. The healthcare delivery systems in Ghana witnessed substantial transformation between 2008 and 2014, especially in the expansion of primary healthcare facilities in rural areas and access to health insurance. The period also saw stable economic growth, made significant gains towards poverty reduction and a rapid rate of urbanization. Using data from the two waves of the survey enables us to compare the changes in the nature and sources of inequalities in child immunization coverage within the structural and demographic transformations over the period.

The rest of the paper is organised as follows, Section 2 provides an overview of the child immunization programme in Ghana. Section 3 focuses on the estimation approaches including the decomposition analysis. Section 4 discusses the data source, description of variables and summary statistics of the sample. Section 5 consists of two parts. The first section discusses the results from the determinants of full immunization status whilst the second section focuses on the results of the inequality decomposition. The paper ends with a summary of the main findings and policy recommendations based on the findings.

Child immunization in Ghana

Ghana launched the Expanded Programme on Immunizations in 1978. The launch of the immunization programme was in response to a national strategy to reduce maternal and infant morbidity and mortality from vaccine preventable diseases. Six antigens were introduced at the inception of the immunization programme for expectant mothers and children. Child vaccinations included Bacillus Calmette-Guèrin (BCG) vaccination against tuberculosis; measles; Diphtheria-Pertusis-Tetanus (DPT) and oral polio for children under 12 months old and tetanus toxoid vaccination for pregnant women. In 1992, a yellow fever vaccination was added to the national immunization programme for children.

The National Immunization Programme has adopted the guidelines proposed by the WHO and UNICEF on child immunization. The guidelines recommend that a child receives one dose each of BCG and measles and three doses of DPT and polio. A dose of BCG vaccine is required at birth or at the first clinical contact. Equally, a dose of polio is recommended at birth or within 13 days of birth. The required doses of DPT and polio vaccines are recommended to be taken at 6, 10 and 14 weeks of age. The measles vaccines are required to be taken at 9 months of age. It is recommended that a child receives the basic required immunizations before 12 months of age.

The immunization programme in Ghana has been reviewed periodically since the inception of the programme. The DPT vaccine was replaced with a pentavalent vaccine (DPT-Hep B-Hib) in 2002 to include immunizations against Hepatitis B and *Haemophilus Influenza* type B. Two new vaccines – pneumococcal and rotavirus to protect children from pneumococcal diseases particularly pneumonia and diarrhoea respectively were introduced in 2012. A child is required to receive three doses of the pneumococcal vaccine at 6, 10 and 14 weeks of age and two doses of the rotavirus at 6 and 10 weeks old respectively. The measles only vaccine was replaced in 2013 with a measles-rubella vaccine also to be given at 9 months. A second dose of the measles-only vaccine was introduced in the same year to be given as a booster at 18 months.

Methods

Traditionally, studies examining socioeconomic inequalities in health outcomes have applied the concentration index and concentration graph approaches [27, 45]. These techniques though useful for measuring the health inequalities, do not explain the pathways through which socioeconomic factors influence observed inequalities in health outcomes between groups. Wagstaff et al. [46] proposes a methodology to decompose the concentration index into a part that shows the contribution of each characteristic to the concentration index and a component that is residual, which is the part of inequality that cannot be explained by the variations in contributing factors across socioeconomic groups. However, the approach proposed by Wagstaff et al. [46] is appropriate for decomposing ranked-based socioeconomic inequalities. The technique, however, may not be useful for examining subgroup inequalities in health such as rural-urban differences, not based on socioeconomic rankings (see [35] for a discussion).

This paper adopts an alternative approach. We estimate a logit model to examine the determinants of immunization status and proceeds to decompose the observed rural-urban differentials in immunization coverage based on a non-linear decomposition technique. This section consists of two parts and discusses the methodological approaches adopted for the empirical estimations. The first part is focused on the econometric technique employed to examine the determinants of full immunization status among children in the sample. The second part presents the decomposition technique applied to assess the source and extent of rural-urban inequalities in Ghana.

Determinants of child immunization status

The immunization status (I_{ijh}) of child i of mother j in household h is modelled as a non-linear function of child-specific characteristics(C_{ijh}), maternal characteristics (M_{jh}), household socioeconomic characteristics (Z_h) including region of residence, and an error term(ε_{ijh}).

$$I_{ijh} = F\left(C_{ijh}; M_{jh}; Z_h; \varepsilon_{ijh}\right)$$

A reduced form model is estimated, where the dependent variable is binary and takes the value of 1 if the child is fully immunized and 0 if otherwise. The reduced form model is specified as

$$I_{ijh} = \pi + \alpha_i C_{ijh} + \beta_i M_{jh} + \delta_i Z_h + \varepsilon_{ijh}$$

where π is a constant term and α, β, and δ are parameters to be estimated. The error term is random and assumed to be constant variance and mean of zero. For simplicity, we generalise the functional form of the reduced model to be estimated as

$$I = X'\beta$$

such that I is the immunization status of the child, X is a vector of explanatory variables and β is a vector of coefficient to be estimated. The probability of a child being fully immunized conditioned on the independent variables is obtained as

$$\Pr(I = 1|X) = \Lambda\left(X'\beta\right) = \frac{e^{X'\beta}}{1 + e^{X'\beta}}$$

where Λ is the cumulative density function of the logistic distribution.

The coefficient estimated by the logit regression technique, similar to other limited dependent variable estimation models, only show the direction of the relationship between the covariates and the probability of a full immunization. In such models, the marginal effects represent the effect of a change in a covariate on the predicted probability of full immunization. Thus, marginal effects of the logit model are presented for ease of interpretation and discussion. The marginal effect with respect to a change in a covariate (X_i) is computed as.

$$\frac{\partial \Pr(I = 1|X)}{\partial X_i} = \Lambda\left(X'\beta\right)\left[1 - \Lambda\left(X'\beta\right)\right]\beta_i$$

Separate logit regressions are estimated for each survey round.

Decomposition of inequalities in child immunization status

A common approach to examine differences in continuous outcomes between groups is the decomposition technique proposed by Oaxaca [34] and Blinder [10]. The Oaxaca-Blinder decomposition technique identifies two sources of outcome differentials between groups. The first component of the observed gap is the explained or endowment effect. The endowment effect captures differences in the outcome of interest that arises from observed differentials in the endowments or characteristics between the groups. The second components of sources of outcome differences is referred to as coefficient or return effect. The return effect is unexplained and is attributed to differences in the returns to endowments between groups. Thus, each group receives different returns for the same level of endowments. When applied to a labour market outcome such as wages, the returns effect has been attributed to discrimination against a disfavoured group. However, in the case of a health outcome, the returns effect may reflect the indirect effects of structural and institutional differences in health systems that affect the health seeking behaviours and attitudes differently between rural and urban areas [15].

The classical Oaxaca-Blinder decomposition technique has been extended to binary and other non-linear

outcomes. Fairlie [20] and Fitzenberger, Kohn and Wang [22] have applied the extended technique to decompose differentials between groups when outcomes are binary dependent variables. The non-linear decomposition model assumes that the conditional expectation of the probability of the immunization status of a child is a non-linear function of a vector of characteristics. Following the generalized structure of the reduced form of the model, separate models are estimated for rural and urban areas as.

$$I_r = \Lambda\left(X'_r\beta_r\right) \text{ for subsample of rural and}$$

$$I_u = \Lambda\left(X'_u\beta_u\right) \text{ for the subsample of urban areas.}$$

To decompose the rural-urban inequalities in immunization status (ΔI), is rewritten as:

$$\Delta I = I_r - I_u = \overline{\Lambda\left(X'_r\beta_r\right)} - \overline{\Lambda\left(X'_u\beta_u\right)}$$

Consider a counterfactual conditional probability of immunization status (I^*) which evaluates the conditional probability of immunization status if the coefficients for rural and urban areas are the same.

$$I^* = \overline{\Lambda(X'_r\beta_u)}$$

The decomposition of the gaps is obtained as

$$\Delta I = I_r - I^* + I^* - I_u = \overline{\Lambda\left(X'_r\beta_r\right)} - \overline{\Lambda\left(X'_r\beta_u\right)} \\ + \overline{\Lambda\left(X'_r\beta_u\right)} - \overline{\Lambda\left(X'_u\beta_u\right)}$$

The first term, $\overline{\Lambda(X'_r\beta_r)} - \overline{\Lambda(X'_r\beta_u)}$ measures the returns effect, whereas the second term $\overline{\Lambda(X'_r\beta_u)} - \overline{\Lambda(X'_u\beta_u)}$ represents endowment effect. The decomposition technique, in addition, assesses the contribution of each covariate to the rural-urban inequalities in immunization coverage in Ghana.

Data source, description of variables and summary statistics

Data source

The data used in this paper comes from the Ghana Demographic and Health Survey (GDHS), implemented by the Ghana Statistical Service (GSS), the Ghana Health Service (GHS) and the National Public Health Reference Laboratory of the GHS [24]. The primary objective of the GDHS is to generate reliable information on fertility, family planning, infant and child mortality, maternal and child health, and nutrition. In addition, the dataset contains information on the characteristics of the respondents and the household. To date, six rounds of the GDHS have been collected using similar procedures.

The surveys follow a two-stage sample design. The first stage involves selecting sample points or clusters, consisting of enumeration areas. The second stage involves a systematic listing of households in selected clusters. A pre-determined number of households are randomly selected from each cluster to constitute the total sample size of households. All women aged 15–49 years who are either permanent residents of the household or visitors who stayed in the household the night before the survey were eligible to be interviewed. The birth history of each woman was collected. For children under five years, the immunization status of each child was taken either from their vaccination or verbal recall from the mother. The working sample for this study is drawn from the children between 12 and 59 months old from the fifth and sixth waves of the survey collected in 2008 and 2014 respectively. The sample for the study includes 2147 children of 1781 mothers residing in 1700 households in 2008. The sample for 2014 on the other hand includes 4386 children of 3652 mothers in 3506 households.

Description of variables

The dependent variable is a binary indicator of immunization status of a child. The variable captures whether or not a child had received required basic immunizations. The WHO and UNICEF recommends that a child receives one dose each of BCG and measles and three doses each of polio vaccines and DPT. Full immunization is restricted to the basic immunizations to enable comparison between the two survey rounds as well as with studies from other countries and settings.

The explanatory variables, as stated earlier, include child-specific, maternal and household characteristics. The choice of these variables was influenced by the earlier studies. Child-specific characteristics include age in months, sex, birth order and place of delivery. Child age in months has been categorised into four groups, 12–23 months, 24–35 months, 36–47 months and 48–59 months. The youngest category (12–23 months) is adopted as the referenced category to compare age-differentials in immunization coverage. Similarly, the sex of the child is included to examine the presence of gender differentials. The birth order of the child captures the attitudes of mothers towards immunization as the number of children increases. Some of the immunizations are recommended at birth or first clinical contact. As such, the place of delivery of the child is important to determining whether a child will receive the required immunizations.

The maternal characteristics are crucial to immunization status as the mothers are the primary caregivers within the Ghanaian society. The maternal characteristics included are the age at birth, years of completed schooling and marital status. Religious affiliation of the mother is included as an explanatory variable to examine religious differences in immunization status. Health authorities embark on media campaigns to educate mothers on the importance of child immunization as well as the schedule of immunization programmes. Thus, a mother's exposure to media may be important to immunization coverage. A dummy of variable of media exposure is therefore included. A mother is defined to be exposed to the media if she has access to information through newspapers and magazines, radio and television. To capture other informal access to information on immunization, the number of women of reproductive age resident in the household is included as an additional variable.

Other maternal characteristics include ownership of a valid health insurance policy, which is adopted as a proxy to capture the health seeking behaviour of the mother. Membership of a health insurance has been found to increase demand for outpatient services through the provision of protection against the financial risk [2]. Mothers who make the effort to obtain a health insurance card, demonstrate, ceteris paribus, a stronger underlying preference for health and health care than others. This further materializes in higher use of health services among those insured. The nature of the economic activity of the mother is categorised into unemployed, self-employed and working for family or others and included as an explanatory variable. This variable is important as it may be adopted to capture time use and opportunity cost of waiting at immunization centres for mothers as well as the capacity to pay for other services such as transportation. Though child immunization services in Ghana are free, mothers may face significant costs to access health and immunization centres. Therefore, the ease of access to health facilities, captured by whether distance poses a challenge to women, is included as a dummy variable.

One of the objectives of this paper is to examine rural-urban inequalities in child immunization coverage. The main variable of interest is therefore the location of the household. A dummy variable that indicates whether a household is located in a rural or urban area is included to capture the rural-urban differentials. Household socioeconomic status is measured by a composite wealth index based on household ownership of selected assets, housing conditions and access to water and sanitation facilities. Three categories of household socioeconomic status are created – low, middle and high. The low category is adopted as the reference category to compare socioeconomic differences in immunization coverage. Lastly, regional dummies are included to capture variations in health attitudes and behaviours, social and cultural norms and belief and health systems across the ten administrative regions.

Descriptive statistics

Summary statistics of the variables utilized for the empirical analysis is presented in Table 1. In both rounds of

Table 1 Summary statistics of child-specific, maternal and household characteristics[a]

Characteristics	2008	2014
	Percentage	
Immunization coverage	71.7	71.4
Female child	48.4	48.3
Child delivered at health facility	56.7	73.0
Marital or consensual union	88.1	84.1
Distance to health facility is a problem	28.8	26.8
Has valid health insurance	39.1	65.2
Exposed to media	84.4	90.1
Rural	59.8	53.8
Age category of child		
12–23 months	26.1	26.1
24–35 months	23.5	25.6
36–47 months	24.0	24.8
48–59 months	26.5	23.5
Religious affiliation of mother		
No/Other religion	10.9	7.1
Christian	70.9	76.2
Moslem	18.2	16.7
Labour market status of mother		
Unemployed	9.5	15.7
Family/Other employee	18.6	20.6
Self-employed	71.9	63.7
Household wealth index		
Low	45.1	40.5
Middle	19.1	20.5
High	35.8	39.0
	Mean	
Mother's age at birth	28.2	28.7
Mother's years of completed schooling	5.8	6.0
Number of co-resident women	0.4	0.3
Number of observations	2147	4386

[a]Estimates adjusted for survey settings

the survey, over two-thirds of the children aged 12–59 months had received the required basic immunizations. Females constitute about 48% of the sample in 2008 and 2014. The proportion of children delivered at health facilities increased from 57% in 2008 and 73%. Equally, the proportion of mothers with valid health insurance policies increased from 39% to 65% between 2008 and 2014. A free health insurance membership policy for pregnant women was initiated in 2008 as a mechanism to achieve the maternal and child health target of the MDG. The policy was aimed to improve access to prenatal, delivery and postnatal healthcare. This resulted in increased health insurance coverage for women and increased facility based delivery.

The summary statistics shows significant changes in the nature of employment of mothers between 2008 and 2014. The proportion of mothers unemployed increased to nearly 16% in 2014 from 10% in 2008, whilst mothers in self-employment declined from 72% in 2008 to 64% in 2014. The shifts in employment status of mothers reflect the macroeconomic challenges such as a debilitating energy crisis that resulted in a decline in economic activity especially in the non-agricultural informal sector. The years of completed schooling for mothers remain low, at 6 years – corresponding to primary school completion in both 2008 and 2014.

The proportion of households in rural areas decreased from 60% in 2008 to 54% in 2014, a reflection of the rapid urbanisation witnessed in Ghana, a reflection of a demographic shift witnessed in Ghana as well as other countries within the SSA region. The summary statistics shows that the differences in household socioeconomic status in 2008 and 2014 rounds of the survey. 45% of households in 2008 had low socioeconomic status, whilst 36% fell within the high socioeconomic status category. In 2014, the proportion of households within the low socioeconomic category was 41% whilst 39% of households were high socioeconomic status. The shifts in the socioeconomic status of households between 2008 and 2014 is reflective of the relatively stable economic growth witnessed over the period and the resulting decrease in poverty in the country.

Results and discussions
Determinants of child immunization status
Table 2 presents the marginal effects of the logit regressions. The findings show the presence of significant rural-urban differences in the probability of a child being fully immunized in both survey rounds. Specifically, the results show that compared to children in urban areas, children residing in rural households are about 8% and 4% more likely to have received the basic required immunizations in 2008 and 2014 respectively. The finding departs from earlier studies in developing countries that report statistically significant rural disadvantage in child immunization coverage [1, 5, 13]. On the other hand, studies such as Awasthi et al. [7], Babirye et al. [8], and Egondi et al. [19] report that in spite of the physical access to health facilities and immunization centres in urban areas, there exist substantial barriers to immunization coverage in urban settings, with large underserved populations in slum and informal settings.

Demographic and health systems development may have contributed to the urban immunization disadvantage in Ghana. Over the last two decades, Ghana has witnessed a rapid pace of urbanisation, with substantial growth in slum

Table 2 Determinants of Full Childhood Immunizations, 2008–2014

VARIABLES	2008			2014		
	Full	Urban	Rural	Full	Urban	Rural
Rural	0.0770**			0.0448**		
	(0.0306)			(0.0191)		
23–35 months	−0.0137	0.0418	−0.0388	− 0.0207	− 0.0469	0.0039
	(0.0249)	(0.0414)	(0.0312)	(0.0177)	(0.0286)	(0.0224)
36–47 months	−0.1208***	− 0.0644	− 0.1489***	−0.0667***	− 0.0848***	−0.0516**
	(0.0261)	(0.0454)	(0.0323)	(0.0186)	(0.0303)	(0.0236)
48–59 months	− 0.1392***	− 0.1195***	− 0.1513***	− 0.1170***	− 0.1306***	− 0.1065***
	(0.0257)	(0.0457)	(0.0311)	(0.0191)	(0.0309)	(0.0244)
Female	−0.0081	−0.0060	− 0.0076	0.0049	0.0093	0.0037
	(0.0187)	(0.0315)	(0.0232)	(0.0132)	(0.0214)	(0.0168)
Birth order	−0.0056	− 0.0060	− 0.0028	− 0.0095*	−0.0067	− 0.0101
	(0.0072)	(0.0159)	(0.0082)	(0.0054)	(0.0094)	(0.0067)
Delivered at health facility	−0.0024	0.0423	−0.0136	0.0356**	0.0765**	0.0241
	(0.0225)	(0.0448)	(0.0263)	(0.0169)	(0.0379)	(0.0187)
Mother's age at birth	0.0048**	0.0073*	0.0029	0.0056***	0.0070***	0.0045**
	(0.0022)	(0.0042)	(0.0027)	(0.0016)	(0.0026)	(0.0020)
Years of schooling	0.0038***	0.0041	0.0033**	0.0054***	0.0042	0.0056**
	(0.0015)	(0.0029)	(0.0016)	(0.0020)	(0.0030)	(0.0027)
Number of co-resident women	−0.0181	−0.0136	−0.0179	−0.0179*	−0.0344*	−0.0063
	(0.0131)	(0.0203)	(0.0169)	(0.0101)	(0.0179)	(0.0122)
Married/Consensual union	0.0254	0.0318	0.0181	0.0716***	0.0809**	0.0568**
	(0.0328)	(0.0534)	(0.0429)	(0.0215)	(0.0333)	(0.0282)
Christian	0.0741**	0.0833	0.0790**	0.0320	0.0266	0.0284
	(0.0315)	(0.0952)	(0.0351)	(0.0262)	(0.0567)	(0.0293)
Moslem	0.0806**	0.0610	0.0962**	0.0807***	0.0198	0.1044***
	(0.0349)	(0.1010)	(0.0402)	(0.0284)	(0.0605)	(0.0328)
Media exposure	0.0162	0.0265	0.0152	0.0303	0.0327	0.0274
	(0.0268)	(0.0663)	(0.0302)	(0.0214)	(0.0506)	(0.0232)
Employed – family/others	0.1169***	0.0449	0.1439***	−0.0097	−0.0338	0.0116
	(0.0386)	(0.0623)	(0.0502)	(0.0230)	(0.0356)	(0.0306)
Employed - self	0.1068***	0.0587	0.1228***	0.0306	0.0122	0.0493*
	(0.0349)	(0.0513)	(0.0469)	(0.0197)	(0.0299)	(0.0264)
Has valid health insurance	0.0585***	0.0955***	0.0449*	0.0458***	0.0617**	0.0343*
	(0.0210)	(0.0359)	(0.0265)	(0.0148)	(0.0249)	(0.0185)
Distance to facility is a problem	−0.0174	−0.0801*	−0.0037	−0.0213	−0.0289	− 0.0160
	(0.0212)	(0.0474)	(0.0242)	(0.0156)	(0.0290)	(0.0183)
Middle	0.0612**	0.0549	0.0600*	−0.0337	0.0003	−0.0410
	(0.0301)	(0.0662)	(0.0354)	(0.0208)	(0.0362)	(0.0267)
High	0.0926***	0.0638	0.1055**	−0.0878***	−0.0433	− 0.1313***
	(0.0328)	(0.0668)	(0.0424)	(0.0263)	(0.0377)	(0.0444)
Regional dummies	Yes	Yes	Yes	Yes	Yes	Yes
Observations	2147	709	1438	4386	1743	2643

Standard errors in parentheses ***$p < 0.01$, **$p < 0.05$, *$p < 0.1$

and informal settlements. Thus, the growing number of underserved children in slum and informal settlements in urban areas in Ghana have contributed to the observed urban disadvantage in the coverage of child immunizations. Given the existence of large spatial disparities in access and utilization of health services and facilities, the child immunization strategy in Ghana appears to have place emphasis on rural areas, much to the neglect of underserved populations in urban areas. In line with this, there has been much emphasis on expanding basic health services in rural areas through the Community-based Health Planning and Services (CHPS) program. The urban-based CHPS has turned out to be much more challenging to implement as the population is more volatile and less well demarcated [4].

In terms of child-specific characteristics, there are no gender disparities in the immunization status of children in Ghana. Indeed, evidence of gender differences in child immunization status have largely been reported by studies from southern Asian countries where son preference are endemic [16, 37]. However, there exist statistically significant age differentials in the immunization status of children. Compared to children 12–23 months old, children between 36 and 47 months and 48–59 months olds are less likely to receive fully the basic immunizations. Age differentials in childhood immunization coverage have been reported in earlier studies. Such age disparities reflect the increasing trend in coverage with recent cohorts of children being fully immunized.

The results indicate a negative effect of the birth order of a child on the probability of a child receiving immunization in 2014. Adedokun et al. [1] and Antai [5] report that children of higher birth order are less likely to complete the required immunizations in Nigeria, and Corsi et al. [16] report same for India. The results suggest *"immunization fatigue"* of mothers as their interest to immunize their children as the number of children increases wanes [3]. Antai [5] on the other hand posits that the reduced likelihood of full immunization coverage of children of higher birth order reflects inter-sibling competition for parental care and limited household resources, leading to neglect.

There may be alternative explanations to the negative effect of child's birth order on the probability of complete basic immunizations. First, the result may reflect the increased opportunity cost of time. The *indirect wage* of mothers in home production increases as the number of children increases. As such, as the high opportunity cost of time spent at a health centre to vaccinate a child of higher birth order reduces the probability of the child being fully immunized. Secondly, younger mothers may be better educated and informed on family planning and child health. The improved education thus reflects in fewer number of children and increased probability of

complete immunization. Lastly, the results may be a reflection of a cohort effect – children with siblings have older mothers and the probability of taking children to vaccination decreases over time. The effect may be higher among old mothers than new mothers.

The place of delivery of a child shows a significant positive relationship with the probability of full immunization in 2014. The likelihood of full immunization is about 4% higher for children delivered in health facilities compared to children delivered at home. The importance of place of delivery to child immunization status is consistent to earlier studies such as Adedokun et al. [3] and Bugvi et al. [13]. Delivery at a health facility enables a child to receive the immunizations required at birth and provides an opportunity for the mother to be informed of the immediate schedules. The emergence of a significant relationship between the place of delivery of the child and probability of full immunization reflects the effects of improved access and utilisation of health services on child health. The reduction of the financial barriers to the demand for maternal and child health through the fee exemption policy under the National Health Insurance Scheme has contributed to achieving equity in child vaccinations in Ghana. Disaggregated by the place of residence, we find that the effect of the place of delivery is significant for urban areas only. This finding suggests the relative success of outreach programmes in rural areas where home vaccinations have been promoted through CHPS.

Religion is an important determinant of health seeking behaviours as well as health outcomes [28, 36]. The results indicate the presence of significant religious effects on the probability of full immunization status in 2008. Compared to mother with no or other religious backgrounds, children with Christian or Moslem mothers are more likely to be fully immunized. The effects of religion, however, appear to have been attenuated in 2014. The significant difference between the immunization of children born to Christian mothers and mothers with no and other religious affiliations disappears, whilst, Moslem mothers are more likely to complete the required immunization routine for their children.

The significant relationships between maternal characteristics and the probability of full childhood immunization indicate the importance of maternal characteristics to child immunization status. Similar to Adedokun et al. [3] and Antai [5], the results indicate a positive relationship between the age at birth of the mother and the probability of the child being fully immunized in 2008 and 2014. Given pervasive cultural disapproval of early childbirth, the results may reflect the attitude of health workers and community members towards teenage mothers leading such mothers to drop-out of the routine child immunization [5]. The effects of mother's age at childbirth, thus, sheds light on the possible barriers that cultural values and belief systems impose on child immunization attitudes in Ghana. In addition, younger mothers have been found to have limited bargaining power in intra-household decision making, as young mothers may be required to seek the permission of other household members regarding decision concerning the health of the child [30, 39]. Thus, delays in household decision making may have negative consequences for child health outcomes.

Improving female and maternal education has been promoted globally as a mechanism to enhance child health outcomes, especially in developing countries. Indeed, there is a growing body of empirical literature that show significant effects of increased maternal education on improved child health outcomes [25, 32]. The results from the logit estimations are consistent with the findings of these previous studies such as Abadura et al. [1], Adedokun et al. [3] and Ataguba, Ojo and Ichoku [6]. An additional year of completed schooling of a mother exerts a positive effect of the probability of a child receiving the basic immunizations. Educational attainment of the mother enhances the access and reception of information as well as facilitates communication between the mother and health workers, leading to better understanding of immunization schedules and practices [28].

The labour market status of the mother is included as a proxy for the mothers' time use as well as the opportunity cost of waiting at health and immunization centres. The variable may also capture the effect of the socioeconomic status of a woman on the immunization status of the child. Uthman et al. [43] finds that the probability that a child receives the full basic required immunizations is lower for children with unemployed mothers. Bugvi et al. [13] suggest that unemployed mothers and those in low paying occupations do not find the time and resources to travel to health centres for the immunization of their children, leading to incomplete immunization routines. On the other hand, employed mothers may face high opportunity cost of time foregone, thus causing them to forego routine visits to complete the basic immunization requirements. Our results in this paper are consistent with Uthman et al. [43]. The probability of full immunization coverage is higher for children with employed mothers in 2008. However, there exist no significant effect of maternal employment on immunization status of children in 2014 except for children in rural areas with self-employed mothers. The changes observed in the labour market status of mothers between 2008 and 2014 appear to have shifted the effects on the probability of full vaccination of children. An increase in unemployment increases the opportunity cost of foregone wages. As such, employed mothers faced higher opportunity cost for waiting time at vaccination centres in 2014. Other things equal, this would reduce the propensity of employed mothers to

spend time at vaccination centres, thereby eroding the higher likelilhood of having their children fully immunized observed in 2008.

Enrolment in a health insurance scheme has been found to increase the utilisation of outpatient services and reduction of out-of-pocket expenditures [21]. Brugiavini and Pace [11] finds a positive effect of health insurance membership on maternal health in Ghana. Our results show that mothers with valid health insurance policy are more likely to complete the basic immunizations for their children. Thus, there exists a spill-over effect of mother's attitude to their own health to the health outcomes of their children. Mothers with health insurance may generally seek care more often when ill or when their child is ill. Health workers may use this opportunity to catch up on missing immunizations, thus resulting in the higher coverage in this group. Equally, the positive relationship between health insurance policy and completed basic child immunization may reflect possible financial barriers to child immunization. Child immunizations are offered for free in Ghana. However, mothers without valid health insurance coverage may be deterred by the fear of financial payments for immunization services.

Previous studies have reported significant socioeconomic inequalities in the coverage of child immunization across developing countries. The socioeconomic status of the household is an indicator of standard of living and has been adopted as a proxy for opportunity cost of women's time as well as financial access to healthcare. Ataguba, Ojo and Ichoku [6], Olorunsaiye and Degge, [36] and Singh and Parasuraman [40] report a disadvantage against children residing in households with low socioeconomic status. The present results from logit regressions reveal changes in the socioeconomic inequalities in child immunization coverage in Ghana between 2008 and 2014. Whilst children in high socioeconomic households are more likely to receive the full basic required immunizations compared to children from low socioeconomic households.

The results reveal a reversal of the disadvantage faced by households with low socioeconomic status in 2014 as there exist a significant negative effect of high household socioeconomic status and the probability of full childhood immunization. The presence of inequalities in child immunization against high socioeconomic households departs from a majority of studies on socioeconomic inequalities in child health outcomes. The results, however, reflect changing economic conditions witnessed between 2008 and 2014. A slowdown of economic activity exerted pressure on the time of women as such women may be required to engage in market activities to smoothen household standards of living. The increased demand for mother's time in market activities may have led to an increase in the opportunity cost of time for mothers potentially leading mothers to pursue income-generating activities instead of completing the immunization routines for their children. Equally, the expansion of services and coverage through the CHPS initiative have also contributed to better access for least wealthy populations especially in rural areas.

Decomposition of rural-urban inequalities in child immunization, 2008/2014

A summary of sources of rural-urban inequalities in child immunization coverage in Ghana in 2008 and 2014 obtained from the decomposition analysis are presented in Table 3. The rural subsample is the reference category for the decomposition of the gaps in immunization coverage. The findings reveal the existence of rural-urban disparities in the probability of a child receiving the basic immunizations. Unlike logit estimates, the decomposition analysis reveals that the direction of disparities in child immunization coverage changes between 2008 and 2014.

In 2008, the average probability of a child in a rural household to receive the full basic immunization is 0.6940 compared to an average probability of 0.735 for a child in an urban area. The rural-urban differential in the average probability of a children being fully immunized in 2008 is statistically significant at 5%. In terms of the source of the disparities in the probability of full immunization, the results further indicates that the endowment or explained effect contributes about 59% of the gap. Indeed, differences in the endowments or characteristics favours urban resident children. This suggests that on average, children residing in urban areas possess higher levels of endowments compared to their counterparts in rural areas. The coefficient or unexplained effect, however, favours children in rural areas. This result

therefore, implies that the health system in Ghana, in terms of child immunization services reward rural households higher for the same level of characteristics compared to urban households. Given the disparities in access to health care services and facilities, the child immunization program in Ghana has adopted strategies that aim at reaching the most vulnerable households, especially in rural areas. This strategy, however, appear to neglect vulnerable children in fast growing slums and informal settlements in urban areas.

Table 4 shows the contribution of each group of characteristics to the rural-urban gap in child immunization coverage. The decomposition reveals that maternal and household characteristics are the significant contributors to the endowment effect. The locational differences in both group of characteristics contribute to widening the gap in the probability of a child being fully immunized between rural and urban areas.

In 2014 however, the average probability of a child in a rural area to be immunized was 0.728 compared to 0.701 for a child in an urban area. The difference in the average probability of fully immunization between rural and urban areas is statistically significant at 10%. However, the coefficient or unexplained component of the gap dominates in 2014, accounting for 70.2% of the estimated rural-urban differentials in the probability of a full immunization of a child. The dominance of the coefficient effect may be attributed to the expansion of primary healthcare in rural Ghana between the periods though the CHPS programme The CHPS programme aims at improving access to primary healthcare and family planning services through community participation and mobilization. The number of functional CHPS facilities increased from 409 in 2008 to 2948 in 2014 [23]. The programme has

Table 3 Summary of Oaxaca-Blinder Decomposition Results

Sources	Overall 2008	Overall 2014
Rural	0.6940***	0.7276***
	(0.0121)	(0.0086)
Urban	0.7348***	0.7011***
	(0.0165)	(0.0109)
Difference	−0.0408**	0.0265*
	(0.0205)	(0.0139)
Endowment / Explained	−0.1335***	−0.0196***
	(0.0286)	(0.0154)
Coefficient / Unexplained	0.0926**	0.0461**
	(0.0362)	(0.0204)
Coefficient / Unexplained (%)	41.0	70.2
Observations	2147	4386

Robust standard errors in parentheses ***p < 0.01, **p < 0.05, *p < 0.1

Table 4 Sources of contributions to rural-urban inequalities in child immunization coverage

Characteristics	2008		2014	
	Endowment	Return	Endowment	Return
Child	−0.0075	−0.1042	−0.0260***	−0.0254
	(0.0139)	(0.1060)	(0.0089)	(0.0564)
Maternal	−0.0379***	−0.1687	−0.0398***	−0.0276
	(0.0117)	(0.2629)	(0.0101)	(0.1133)
Household	−0.0701***	0.0274	0.0602***	−0.0295
	(0.0262)	(0.0687)	(0.0231)	(0.0268)
Region dummies	−0.0180	−0.0454	−0.0140**	−0.1415**
	(0.0141)	(0.1416)	(0.0070)	(0.0701)
Constant		0.3835		0.2701**
		(0.2928)		(0.1339)
Observations	2147		4386	

Robust standard errors in parentheses ***p < 0.01, **p < 0.05, *p < 0.1

achieved considerable success in rural areas whilst the implementation in urban areas has been challenging.

The endowment effects in 2014 arises from significant differences in child, maternal, household and regional characteristics. Child, maternal and regional differences favor children in urban households, thus, contributing to widening the gap in immunization coverage between rural and urban areas. Household characteristics, which includes the number of resident women of reproductive age and household socioeconomic status, contribute to the endowment effect in favour of rural-resident children. On the other hand, returns to region of residence – contribution to the unexplained or coefficient component – is positive in favour of children in urban areas. This implies that in each region, the health system rewards children in urban areas higher in terms of probability of full immunization than children in rural areas.

Conclusion and policy recommendations

The objective of this paper was to investigate rural-urban inequalities in child immunization coverage in Ghana between 2008 and 2014. Improving child health outcomes constitute a primary development objective in developing countries, especially in SSA. Global development efforts over the last two decades – MDGs (2000–2015) and SDGs (2016–2030) - have emphasized the centrality of child health improvements to economic growth and development. Investments in early childhood health have been found to be essential to later-life outcomes such as cognitive ability, education, income and productivity [15]. Thus, socioeconomic disparities in health investments in early childhood may perpetuate intergenerational poverty and inequalities as well as deride the objective of equitable and inclusive growth.

The paper focuses on a sample of children between 12 and 59 months old, drawn from the two recent rounds of the Ghana Demographic and Health Survey conducted in 2008 and 2014. First, the paper examines the determinants of the probability of a child receiving the basic required immunizations of one dose each of BCG and measles and three doses each of polio vaccines and DPT using a logit regression technique. The second part of the paper decomposes the rural-urban inequalities in coverage of full child immunizations into a component attributed to differences in observed characteristics and a component arising from differences in returns to these characteristics using the Oaxaca-Blinder technique extended to non-linear outcomes.

The findings of the paper reveal significant rural-urban differentials in the probability of a child receiving the required immunization. Specifically, children in rural households are more likely to have completed the required immunizations compared to children in urban areas in both 2008 and 2014. In addition, child-specific,

maternal and household characteristics exert significant effects on the probability of a child's immunization status. The effects of maternal education and employment suggest the importance of women empowerment to child health outcomes in developing countries. The effect of household socioeconomic status on the probability of a child receiving the required immunizations changed between 2008 and 2014. The probability of full immunization was positive for children residing in households with high socioeconomic status in 2008. However, the effect of household socioeconomic status in 2014 shows that the probability of a child receiving the required immunizations is lower for children in households with high socioeconomic status.

The decomposition analysis of the rural-urban inequalities in child immunization coverage reveals the existence of significant disparities in the probability of a child receiving the full immunization. The direction of the disparities, however, differs in 2008 and 2014. In 2008, there exist a rural disadvantage in child immunization coverage. The gap in immunization coverage is dominated by endowment or explained effect. In 2014, there exist an urban disadvantage in child immunization. The emerging urban disadvantage may reflect the neglect of primary healthcare delivery in fast growing slums and informal settlements in urban areas. The coefficient or unexplained effect is the dominant source of the coverage gap in 2014, reflecting the concentration on immunization campaigns and improvement in access to primary healthcare in rural areas.

The findings of the paper provide insights for achieving universal child immunization coverage in Ghana. A number of policy recommendations may be drawn from the findings of this paper. First, and most importantly, policies aimed at reducing socioeconomic inequalities in child health in Ghana need to adjust focus and increasingly target vulnerable children in urban areas, particularly in slum and informal settlements. The rapid pace of urbanization in Ghana requires that public health policies incorporate strategies that address the demands of a growing urban population. Recent systematic reviews of the literature up to 2016 assessing interventions to improve routine immunization coverage in urban areas [33] and in low income urban or slum areas [17] identified only few studies in low and middle income countries, of which only 7 in total from SSA and only 4 of them less than ten years old. Both reviews point towards the need across low and middle income countries for further development and testing of interventions in view of the local context and with communities. National immunization campaigns should be targeted at mothers and children in slums and informal settlements in urban areas through community participation and mobilization as a means to increase coverage of immunization services in such areas. For example, the school vaccination program must be intensified and expanded to improve immunization coverage in urban areas. Similarly, our findings underscores the urgency of developing and upscaling user-friendly close-to-client health care options (parallel, but not similar, to CHPS) that can work in the more complex urban environment.

In addition, immunization campaigns should focus attention on women and children in higher socioeconomic households to address the emerging gaps in immunization coverage. Lastly, the findings highlight the importance of women empowerment, for example, through education and employment to child health outcomes. As such, child health interventions should be situated within broader strategies of women empowerment and decision making within the household through improving female education and employment. This paper amplifies recommendations that have also been identified in previous studies. Implementation, however, has been slow and may call for application of more diverse research methods for achieving an in-depth understanding of the factors promoting or hindering uptake of routine childhood immunization.

Abbreviations
BCG: Bacillus Calmette-Guèrin; CHPS: Community-based Health Planning and Services; DPT: Diphtheria-Pertusis-Tetanus; EPI: Expanded Programme on Immunizations; GAVI: Global Alliance for Vaccines and Immunizations; GDHS: Ghana Demographic and Health Survey; GHS: Ghana Health Services; GSS: Ghana Statistical Service; MDGs: Millennium Development Goals; SDGs: Sustainable Development Goals; SSA: Sub-Saharan Africa; UNICEF: United Nations Children's Emergency Fund; WHO: World Health Organisation

Funding
This study was not funded.

Authors' contributions
The authors contributed equally to the development of the study. All authors read and approved the final manuscript.

Competing interests
The authors declare that they have no competing interests.

Author details
[1]Institute of Statistical, Social and Economic Research, University of Ghana, E.N. Omaboe Building, P. O. Box LG 74, Legon, Ghana. [2]Section for Health Promotion and Health Services Research, Department of Public Health, Aarhus University, Bartholins Alle 2, 8000 Aarhus C, Denmark.

References
1. Abadura SA, Lerebo WT, Kulkarni U, Mekonnen ZA. Individual and community level determinants of childhood full immunization in Ethiopia: a multilevel analysis. BMC Public Health. 2015;15(1):972.
2. Acharya A, Vellakkal S, Taylor F, Masset E, Satija A, Burke M, Ebrahim S. The impact of health insurance schemes for the informal sector in low-and middle-income countries: a systematic review. The World Bank Research Observer. 2012;28(2):236–66.
3. Adedokun ST, Uthman OA, Adekanmbi VT, Wiysonge CS. Incomplete childhood immunization in Nigeria: a multilevel analysis of individual and contextual factors. BMC Public Health. 2017;17(1):236.
4. Adongo PB, Phillips JF, Aikins M, Arhin DA, Schmitt M, Nwameme AU, Tabong PT, Binka FN. Does the design and implementation of proven innovations for delivering basic primary health care services in rural communities fit the urban setting: the case of Ghana's community-based health planning and services (CHPS). Health research policy and systems. 2014;12(1):16.
5. Antai D. Gender inequities, relationship power, and childhood immunization uptake in Nigeria: a population-based cross-sectional study. Int J Infect Dis. 2012;16(2):e136–45.
6. Ataguba JE, Ojo KO, Ichoku HE. Explaining socio-economic inequalities in immunization coverage in Nigeria. Health Policy Plan. 2016;31(9):1212–24.
7. Awasthi A, Pandey CM, Singh U, Kumar S, Singh TB. Maternal determinants of immunization status of children aged 12–23 months in urban slums of Varanasi, India. Clinical Epidemiology and Global Health. 2015;3(3):110–6.
8. Babirye JN, Engebretsen IM, Rutebemberwa E, Kiguli J, Nuwaha F. Urban settings do not ensure access to services: findings from the immunisation programme in Kampala Uganda. BMC Health Serv Res. 2014;14(1):111.
9. Barata RB, de Almeida Ribeiro MC, de Moraes JC, Flannery B. Socioeconomic inequalities and vaccination coverage: results of an immunisation coverage survey in 27 Brazilian capitals, 2007–2008. J Epidemiol Community Health. 2012;66(10):934–41.
10. Blinder AS. Wage discrimination: reduced form and structural estimates. J Hum Resour. 1973;8(4):436–55.
11. Brugiavini A, Pace N. Extending health insurance in Ghana: effects of the National Health Insurance Scheme on maternity care. Heal Econ Rev. 2016;6(1):7.
12. Bryce J, Terreri N, Victora CG, Mason E, Daelmans B, Bhutta ZA, Bustreo F, Songane F, Salama P, Wardlaw T. Countdown to 2015: tracking intervention coverage for child survival. Lancet. 2006;368(9541):1067–76.
13. Bugvi AS, Rahat R, Zakar R, Zakar MZ, Fischer F, Nasrullah M, Manawar R. Factors associated with non-utilization of child immunization in Pakistan: evidence from the demographic and health survey 2006-07. BMC Public Health. 2014;14(1):232.
14. Chan M. Beyond expectations: 40 years of EPI [Margaret Chan]. Lancet. 2014;383(9930):1697–8.
15. Charasse-Pouélé C, Fournier M. Health disparities between racial groups in South Africa: a decomposition analysis. Soc Sci Med. 2006;62(11):2897–914.
16. Corsi DJ, Bassani DG, Kumar R, Awasthi S, Jotkar R, Kaur N, Jha P. Gender inequity and age-appropriate immunization coverage in India from 1992 to 2006. BMC International Health and Human Rights. 2009;9(1):S3.
17. Crocker-Buque T, Mindra G, Duncan R, Mounier-Jack S. Immunization, urbanization and slums–a systematic review of factors and interventions. BMC Public Health. 2017;17(1):556.
18. Currie J, Almond D. Human capital development before age five. Handbook of Labor Economics. 2011;4:1315–486.
19. Egondi T, Oyolola M, Mutua MK, Elung'ata P. Determinants of immunization inequality among urban poor children: evidence from Nairobi's informal settlements. Int J Equity Health. 2015;14(1):24.
20. Fairlie RW. An extension of the blinder-Oaxaca decomposition technique to logit and probit models. J Econ Soc Meas. 2005;30(4):305–16.
21. Fink G, Robyn PJ, Sié A, Sauerborn R. Does health insurance improve health?: evidence from a randomized community-based insurance rollout in rural Burkina Faso. J Health Econ. 2013;32(6):1043–56.
22. Fitzenberger B, Kohn K, Wang Q. The erosion of union membership in Germany: determinants, densities, decompositions. J Popul Econ. 2011;24(1):
23. Ghana Health Service. Annual Report. Accra: Ghana Health Service, 2016: 2017.
24. Ghana Statistical Service, Ghana Health Service, and ICF Macro. Accra: Ghana Demographic and Health Survey, 2014: 2014.
25. Grépin KA, Bharadwaj P. Maternal education and child mortality in Zimbabwe. J Health Econ. 2015;44:97–117.
26. Holte JH, Mæstad O, Jani JV. The decision to vaccinate a child: an economic perspective from southern Malawi. Soc Sci Med. 2012;75(2):384–91.
27. Kakwani N, Wagstaff A, Van Doorslaer E. Socioeconomic inequalities in health: measurement, computation, and statistical inference. J Econ. 1997;77(1):87–103.

28. Landoh DE, Ouro-Kavalah F, Yaya I, Kahn AL, Wasswa P, Lacle A, Nassoury DI, Gitta SN, Soura AB. Predictors of incomplete immunization coverage among one to five years old children in Togo. BMC Public Health. 2016;16(1):968.

29. Lauridsen J, Pradhan J. Socio-economic inequality of immunization coverage in India. Heal Econ Rev. 2011;1(1):11.

30. Lépine A, Strobl E. The effect of women's bargaining power on child nutrition in rural Senegal. World Dev. 2013;45:17–30.

31. Liu L, Oza S, Hogan D, Chu Y, Perin J, Zhu J, Lawn JE, Cousens S, Mathers C, Black RE. Global, regional, and national causes of under-5 mortality in 2000–15: an updated systematic analysis with implications for the sustainable development goals. Lancet. 2017;388(10063):3027–35.

32. Makate M, Makate C. The causal effect of increased primary schooling on child mortality in Malawi: universal primary education as a natural experiment. Soc Sci Med. 2016;168:72–83.

33. Nelson KN, Wallace AS, Sodha SV, Daniels D, Dietz V. Assessing strategies for increasing urban routine immunization coverage of childhood vaccines in low and middle-income countries: a systematic review of peer-reviewed literature. Vaccine. 2016;34(46):5495–503.

34. Oaxaca R. Male-female wage differentials in urban labor markets. Int Econ Rev. 1973;14(3):693–709.

35. O'Donnell O, Van Doorslaer E, Wagstaff A, Lindelow M. Analyzing health equity using household survey data. Washington, DC: World Bank; 2008.

36. Olorunsaiye CZ, Degge H. Variations in the uptake of routine immunization in Nigeria: examining determinants of inequitable access. Global Health Communication. 2016;2(1):19–29.

37. Pal R. Decomposing inequality of opportunity in immunization by circumstances: evidence from India. The European Journal of Development Research. 2016;28(3):431–46.

38. Pande RP. Selective gender differences in childhood nutrition and immunization in rural India: the role of siblings. Demography. 2003;40(3):395–418.

39. Richards E, Theobald S, George A, Kim JC, Rudert C, Jehan K, Tolhurst R. Going beyond the surface: gendered intra-household bargaining as a social determinant of child health and nutrition in low and middle income countries. Soc Sci Med. 2013;95:24–33.

40. Singh PK, Parasuraman S. 'Looking beyond the male–female dichotomy'–sibling composition and child immunization in India, 1992–2006. Soc Sci Med. 2014;107:145–53.

41. Storeng KT. The GAVI Alliance and the 'gates approach' to health system strengthening. Global Public Health. 2014;9(8):865–79.

42. Tsawe M, Moto A, Netshivhera T, Ralesego L, Nyathi C, Susuman AS. Factors influencing the use of maternal healthcare services and childhood immunization in Swaziland. Int J Equity Health. 2015;14(1):32.

43. Uthman OA, Adedokun ST, Olukade T, Watson S, Adetokunboh O, Adeniran A, Oyetoyan SA, Gidado S, Lawoko S, Wiysonge CS. Children who have received no routine polio vaccines in Nigeria: who are they and where do they live? Human Vaccines & Immunotherapeutics. 2017;13(9):2111–22.

44. Wado YD, Afework MF, Hindin MJ. Childhood vaccination in rural southwestern Ethiopia: the nexus with demographic factors and women's autonomy. The Pan African Medical Journal. 2014;17(Suppl 1):9.

45. Wagstaff A, Paci P, Van Doorslaer E. On the measurement of inequalities in health. Soc Sci Med. 1991;33(5):545–57.

46. Wagstaff A, Van Doorslaer E, Watanabe N. On decomposing the causes of health sector inequalities with an application to malnutrition inequalities in Vietnam. Journal of Econometrics. 2003;112(1):207–23.

7

Potential gains in life expectancy by eliminating deaths from cardiovascular diseases and diabetes mellitus in the working life ages among Slovak population

Beata Gavurova*⃝ and Tatiana Vagasova

Abstract

Background: In recent years, high mortality from cardiovascular diseases (chronic ischemic heart disease, acute coronary syndrome, cerebrovascular diseases, atherosclerosis, hypertensive diseases) and diabetes mellitus have burdened economic and health system of the Slovak Republic considerably. By eliminating these deaths, the life expectancy could be prolonged. Since the mortality of population during working period has higher importance in terms of economic consequences of diseases, this article aims to assess the potential gains in life expectancy (PGLEs) of the Slovak population comparing the entire life span and working life-time.

Methods: Data are obtained from the National Health Information Center mortality reports by sex during 1996–2014, and the method of constructing abridged life tables is used to compute the corresponding PGLEs. The added years, which would be gained by eliminating causes of deaths, are decomposed by the two sets of working age groups population (25–44 and 45–64 years).

Results: The highest impact on life expectancy was recorded in chronic ischemic heart disease for both sexes aged 45–64 years (0.078 for males, 0.019 added years for females) over 1996–2014. However, they showed a small declining trend (− 16%) for males and even an increasing trend (2%) for females. At present, the labour force potential of working group (25–44 years) is most threatened by deaths from cerebrovascular diseases, while population of working age (45–64 years) by deaths from chronic ischemic heart disease. Relative importance of acute coronary syndrome for males (45–64 years) increased, when comparing the entire with working time life.

Conclusions: The findings pose new and immediate challenges to policy makers and provoke discussion about prevention program strategies leading to increasing the life expectancy.

Keywords: Life expectancy, Potential gains in life expectancy at birth, Working age groups, Mortality, Cardiovascular diseases, Diabetes mellitus

Background

Cardiovascular diseases (CVD), as the main causes of death in developed countries, represent the most frequent causes of death in Slovakia. In particular, chronic ischemic heart disease, acute coronary syndrome, cerebrovascular diseases, atherosclerosis, hypertensive diseases. The number of deaths caused by CVD is estimated to 3.9 million per year in Europe, what accounts for 45% of all deaths in

Europe [1]. The CVD mortality rates have been falling since 1970 in Western Europe [2], but in Eastern Europe remain comparatively high [3]. Specifically, CVD mortality rates decreased by 17–18% in Slovakia between 2001 and 2010, however, they decreased by 32–33% in France and by 31–34% in Germany during approximately the same time period [4].

Diabetes mellitus represents a very strong risk factor for CVD. The prevalence of diabetes mellitus for all age-groups worldwide was around 2.8% in 2000 and is estimated to be around 4.4% in 2030. The total number

* Correspondence: beata.gavurova@tuke.sk
Faculty of Economics, Technical University of Kosice, Nemcovej 32, 040 01 Kosice, Slovakia

of people with diabetes is projected to rise from 171 million in 2000 to 366 million in 2030. The prevalence of diabetes is higher in men than women, however, in absolute terms there are more women with diabetes than men. The most important demographic change to diabetes prevalence across the world appears to be an increase in the proportion of people 65 years of age [5]. In 2012, there were 1.5 million of deaths due to diabetes mellitus and more than 2.2 million of deaths related to cardiovascular complications of diabetes mellitus. WHO predicts diabetes mellitus as 7th most common death by year 2030 [6]. In Slovakia we have around 400,000 patients with diabetes mellitus (7% of total population) and probably another 20–30% in pre-diabetes or with latent form of diabetes mellitus, and our predictions are around 15% by year 2030 [7]. The annual mortality rates from diabetes mellitus have been decreasing by 19.2% since 1990, an average of 0.8% a year [8].

In recent two decades, an overall decrease in mortality has contributed to the extension of life expectancy by 4 years in Slovakia, from 72.9 in 1996 to 76.9 years in 2014. It raises a question if it is a suitable growth of life expectancy, and how many additional years of life expectancy would be gained, if the main causes of deaths were eliminated. This issue can be measured by the potential gain in life expectancy (PGLE). The fall in mortality has changed according to a particular cause of death, sex, or age group of population. Therefore, an examination of the impact of the major causes of death on the life expectancy provides valuable information about the burden of these diseases on health system and economy of a particular country. Although, the high occurrence of morbidity and mortality in the group of retired people burdens the health system financing in a large extent, the mortality of population during working period has higher importance in terms of economic consequences of diseases. The high mortality among people of working age (the most 15–64 years) leads to the lower labour productivity as well as decelerating economic growth. Hence, the investigation of mortality in the working age groups may be a more relevant mortality indicator for a country compared with the group of retired people over age 65. In addition, the determination of underlying cause of deaths for older people can be difficult due to the high occurrence of comorbidities.

Costs of interventions related to CVD annually reach almost 200 billion EUR in the European Union. Diagnostics and treatment of cardiovascular diseases represent large economic burden on the health system in Slovakia. The European Union has set objectives with which the Slovak Republic identified and those contributed to better understanding of mechanisms supporting health, occurrence and development of diseases, improvements of possibilities of diagnostics, treatment and management

of diseases leading to the healthy ageing [9]. Despite the advances in preventive cardiology, the cardiovascular mortality remains high. Metabolic syndrome is defined as simultaneous presence of lipid and non-lipid related cardiovascular and cardio-metabolic risk factors that significantly increase the risk of cardiovascular disorders, as well as diabetes type 2 and hypertension as compounds of metabolic syndrome [10].

There are several ways how to measure the burden of diseases on population [11, 12]. Previous studies [13–18] have explored the life tables containing the potential gains in life expectancy as a research method to determine the impact of diseases with the highest prevalence causing death on the life expectancy of population. However, most of these studies have focused on the overall groups of causes of death with relation to the demography but no with the specific implications on health interventions. For instance, Lai and Hardy [14] compared the PGLEs with the years of potential life lost by race and gender group from HIV, heart diseases, and cancer for US population. They found that better indicator for the measuring impact of disease deaths on a population is the PGLE because it is not influenced by the age and size population structure. In China, Liu et al. [15] proved that deaths from accidental injuries together with chronic diseases play a major role in influencing life expectancy. Conti et al. [13] found that AIDS and accidents have higher impact on life expectancy when considering working group (15–64 years), rather than 50% reduction in cardiovascular diseases deaths. Generally, it is necessary to observe a potential of the main causes of death and to encourage steps in the increase of life expectancy.

The aim of this paper is to analyse the influence of the deaths from CVD and diabetes mellitus on the life expectancy of the Slovak population comparing the entire life span and working life-time by sex from 1996 to 2014. These findings have a great potential for the creation of targeted prevention programs in Slovakia.

Methods

Under the conditions of the contract, data on the number of deaths by five-year age groups for the period 1996–2014 were obtained from National Health Information Centre of Slovakia. Data on the mid-year population at the age groups in every year were downloaded from the Statistical Office of the Slovak Republic.

The PGLE reflects how many years on average a person would still live, if a given cause of death was eliminated. In other words, PGLE expresses years of life lost resulting from a certain disease in an age group. So, life expectancy could be extended for these years. The higher PGLE, the higher impact of the disease on life expectancy is.

For calculation of PGLEs it was needed to construct the life tables and the specific life tables regarding causes of deaths in the Slovak Republic in every year and an age group separately according to the methodical tutorials of Demographic Research Centre by Mészáros [19] and the National Vital Statistics Reports by Arias et al. [20]. We examined the life expectancy (e_x) expressing the all causes of deaths and cause-eliminated life expectancy ($e_x^{(-i)}$) by elimination of the certain causes of deaths. The Tenth Revision of the International Classification of Disease (ICD-10) was used to specify causes of death included in this analysis: diabetes mellitus (E10-E14), hypertensive diseases (I10-I13), acute coronary syndrome (I20-I22), chronic ischemic heart disease (I25), cerebrovascular diseases (I60-69), atherosclerosis, aortic aneurysm and dissection (I70-I72).

Cause-eliminated life expectancy ($e_x^{(-i)}$) was the result from analysis of deaths caused by a certain disease and was calculated from the abridged life table minus causes of death.

According to the Mészáros [19], the first step is the calculation of the probabilities of survival ($_np_x$) from the all-caused abridged life tables with the formula:

$$_np_x = 1 - {_nq_x} \tag{1}$$

where x – the exact age; n – the number of years in the age interval; $_nq_x$ - the probability of dying between the beginning of an age interval and before reaching the end of that age interval.

Then, the probabilities of death eliminating the i_{th} cause ($_nq_x^{(-i)}$) were estimated by:

$$_nq_x^{(-i)} = 1 - {_np_x}^{\left(\frac{_nD_x - {_nD_x^i}}{_nD_x}\right)} \tag{2}$$

where $_nD_x$ - the number of deaths in the age interval x to $x+n$ for all causes; $_nD_x^i$ - the number of deaths in the age interval x to x + n attributable to the i_{th} cause of death.

Arias et al. [20] report the number of person-years lived ($_nL_x^{(-i)}$) in the age interval x to $x+n$ was estimated for ages 0, 1, 5, 10,......, 95 by the formula:

$$_nL_x^{(-i)} = \left(n - {_nf_x}\right) \cdot l_x^{(-i)} + {_nl_x} \cdot l_{x+n}^{(-i)} \tag{3}$$

where $n = 1$ for x = 0, $n = 4$ for x = 1, and $n = 5$ for x = 5, 10, ..., 95; $_nl_x$ – the number of persons from the original life table who survive to the beginning of each age interval; $l_x^{(-i)}$ - the number of survivals from life table due to the i_{th} causes; L_x – the number of person-years from the original life table within an age interval x to $x + n$, and the quantities $_nf_x$ were estimated from the all-cause life table by:

$$_nf_x = \frac{n \cdot {_nl_x} - {_nL_x}}{l_x - l_{x+n}} \tag{4}$$

The last step is to calculate the number of person-years lived after exact age x ($T_x^{(-i)}$) by:

$$T_x^{(-i)} = L_x^{(-i)} + L_{x+1}^{(-i)} + ... + L_{95+}^{(-i)} \tag{5}$$

Finally, the cause-eliminated life expectancy ($e_x^{(-i)}$) is calculated as:

$$e_x^{(-i)} = \frac{T_x^{(-i)}}{l_x^{(-i)}} \tag{6}$$

Subsequently, the PGLE of a disease in a certain year is calculated as the difference between cause-eliminated life expectancy ($e_x^{(-i)}$) and life expectancy (e_x) in the same year.

$$PGLE = e_x^{(-i)} - e_x \tag{7}$$

The PGLEs for the working age group (the most 15–64 years) are those added years that would be gained, in the case of a particular cause of death elimination, before reaching the end of the working life span at age 65. In our analysis, we divided this general working group on two more particular age groups: young adults (25–44 years) and adults (45–64 years). It was carried out in compliance with the age classifications used for the topics of labour force participation and usage of health services recommended by United Nations [21].

To find out the PGLE in the working age groups of young adults (25–44 years) as well as adults (45–64 years), the partial life expectancies ($e_{25,44}$ and $e_{45,64}$) in the ages between 25 and 44 years as well as 45 and 64 years are calculated as:

$$e_{25,44\ (45,64)} = \frac{T_{25\ (45)} - T_{44\ (64)}}{l_{25(45)}} \tag{8}$$

where $T_{25(45)}$ – $T_{44(64)}$ are the number of person-years lived in the age intervals 25–44 or 45–64, and $l_{25(45)}$ are the number of survivors at 25 or 45 years of age in the life table. Similarly, the partial life expectancies in both age intervals after elimination of a particular cause of death are estimated. Finally, the PGLEs for the working life ages are expressed as the differences between cause-eliminated partial life expectancy and partial life expectancy for the working population aged 25–44 and 45–64 years separately.

Results

Trends of potential gains in life expectancy in the working age groups from 1996 to 2014

The PGLEs for the Slovak males and females in the working age groups 25–44 and 45–64 are plotted in Fig. 1. During the time span 1996–2014, the highest impacts of deaths from each of the examined diseases on life expectancy were recorded for males in the older age group (M_45–64), followed by females (F_45–64), young adult males (M_25–44), and young adult females (F_25–44). The PGLEs for young adults are approaching zero, that seems to be a negligible impact of deaths elimination on added years in life expectancy, even lower than 1 day added.

Considering men aged 45–64 years, the highest average PGLEs were recorded for chronic ischemic heart disease (0.078 years added), followed by acute coronary syndrome (0.075 years), cerebrovascular diseases (0.042 years), atherosclerosis (0.024 years), hypertensive diseases (0.022 years), and diabetes mellitus (0.009 years) from 1996 to 2014. For instance, after elimination of

chronic ischemic heart disease deaths, a person at age 45 could be expected to live an average of 0.078 years longer before reaching the end of the working range at age 65. After the conversion potential gained years into days, 29 days of life could be added for men of older working age. We can see that the burdens of chronic ischemic heart disease and acute coronary syndrome are almost the same, while the burden of cerebrovascular diseases is lower by 45% on average. Considering women aged 45–64 years, the highest average PGLEs were also recorded for chronic ischemic heart disease (0.019 years, in other words 7 days added), cerebrovascular diseases (0.017 years), acute coronary syndrome (0.016 years), hypertensive diseases (0.009 years), atherosclerosis (0.006 years), and diabetes mellitus (0.004 years). For females, the PGLEs differences between the examined causes of death are not so remarkable than those for males.

Between 1996 and 2014, the PGLEs for males aged 45–64 years decreased for each of causes of deaths, similarly for females, except the small increase of chronic

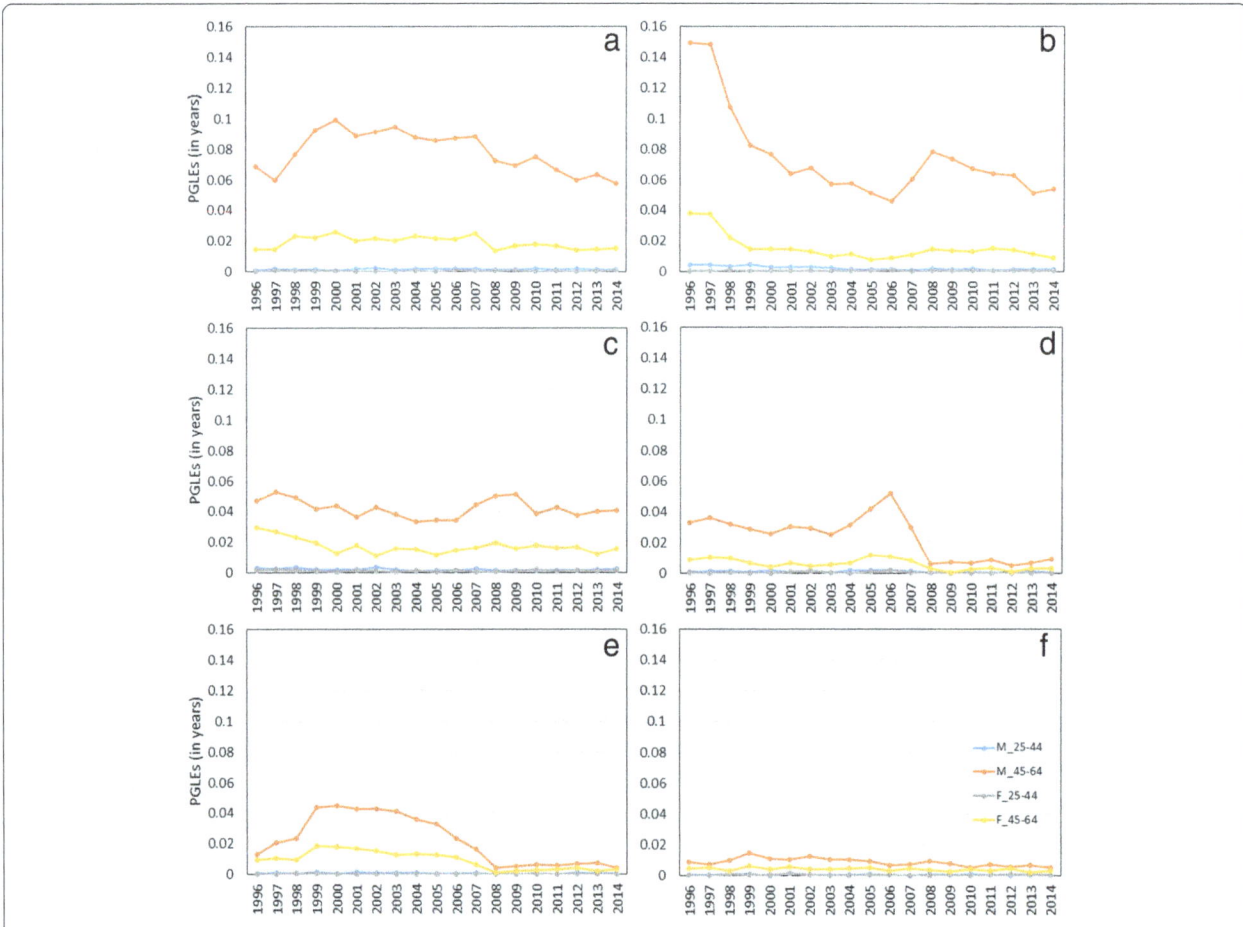

Fig. 1 Trends of potential gains in life expectancy (PGLEs) by elimination of deaths from chronic ischemic heart disease (**a**), acute coronary syndrome (**b**), cerebrovascular diseases (**c**), atherosclerosis (**d**), hypertensive diseases (**e**), diabetes mellitus (**f**) for males (**M**) or females (**F**) Slovak population in the working age groups 25–44 or 45–64, 1996–2014

ischemic heart disease for females. Despite the fact that deaths from chronic ischemic heart disease had the highest impact on life expectancy, showed a small declining trend (– 16%) for males and even an increasing trend (2%) for females. The highest falls of PGLEs was recorded for atherosclerosis from 0.033 in 1996 to 0.01 in 2014 (– 71%), hypertensive diseases from 0.013 to 0.004 (– 68%), and acute coronary syndrome from 0.15 to 0.054 (– 64%) for males. The disease rank order is opposite for females aged 45–64 years, for acute coronary syndrome from 0.038 to 0.009 (– 77%), hypertensive diseases from 0.01 to 0.003 (– 69%), atherosclerosis from 0.009 to 0.003 (– 63%). As one could notice, the beginning of the economic crisis dated approximately from 2006 to 2008 might contribute to the rapid increase of deaths from acute coronary syndrome. On the contrary, the fast drop for atherosclerosis was showed in the same time span. As the above results show, the differences in PGLEs between the sexes still existed and men were more burdened of each disease than women. The highest

gaps were found in acute coronary syndrome (4.8 times more for men) and chronic ischemic heart disease (4.1 times more for men), on the other hand, the lowest gap was resulted from diabetes mellitus (2.1 times more for men). The differences between the sex groups have been most reduced for atherosclerosis and hypertensive diseases since 2008.

Potential gains in life expectancy in total expectation of life and in the working life ages

Table 1 shows the potential added years of life at birth, as well as of working life ages 25–44 and 45–64, through the elimination in mortality from six examined causes of death according to the sex. The PGLE is presented as an average value for the past 3 years 2012–2014. Moreover, when comparing the working age groups and entire life span, a relative importance of the disease is reported in Table 1. The relative weight is expressed as a share between the PGLE expected for the working group and the PGLE during entire life span.

Table 1 Added years of life at birth and for working ages after eliminating causes of death by sex, 2012–2014

Cause of death	Potential gains in life expectancy (in years)				
	Age group			(%)	
Sex	at birth	25–44	45–64	25–44/at birth	45–64/at birth
Chronic Ischemic Heart Disease (I25)					
Total population	3.55	0.0013	0.0377	0.04	1.06
Males	2.93	0.0019	0.0602	0.07	2.05
Females	3.97	0.0005	0.0148	0.01	0.37
Cerebrovascular Diseases (I60-I69)					
Total population	1.11	0.0018	0.0273	0.16	2.47
Males	1.03	0.0021	0.0394	0.21	3.81
Females	1.12	0.0015	0.0150	0.13	1.34
Acute Coronary Syndrome (I20-I22)					
Total population	0.70	0.0011	0.0340	0.16	4.89
Males	0.85	0.0017	0.0561	0.20	6.61
Females	0.49	0.0005	0.0116	0.11	2.36
Hypertensive Diseases, exc. Secondary (I10-I13)					
Total population	0.18	0.0004	0.0048	0.24	2.65
Males	0.16	0.0008	0.0063	0.50	3.93
Females	0.19	0.0001	0.0033	0.03	1.71
Atherosclerosis, Aortic Aneurysm and Dissection (I70-I72)					
Total population	0.16	0.0005	0.0050	0.30	3.14
Males	0.15	0.0009	0.0073	0.59	4.76
Females	0.15	0.0000	0.0026	0.01	1.69
Diabetes Mellitus (E10-E14)					
Total population	0.14	0.0006	0.0047	0.45	3.48
Males	0.12	0.0004	0.0060	0.35	5.04
Females	0.15	0.0008	0.0034	0.55	2.32

The highest values of PGLE at birth among all Slovak population are stated from the elimination of chronic ischemic heart disease (3.55 years), followed by cerebrovascular diseases (1.11 years), acute coronary syndrome (0.7 years), hypertensive diseases (0.18 years), atherosclerosis (0.16 years), and diabetes mellitus (0.14 years). The impacts of deaths from chronic ischemic heart disease, cerebrovascular diseases, hypertensive diseases and diabetes mellitus on the length of life are higher for females than those for males. On the other hand, males would live longer than females, if mortality of acute coronary syndrome was eliminated. In the case of atherosclerosis elimination, the PGLEs at birth of both sexes are the same. It is worth noting that women are more burdened of chronic heart disease than men, while the burden of acute heart disease is higher for men compared with women. Thus, after elimination of chronic ischemic heart disease deaths, a woman at birth could be expected to live 3.97 years longer than the actual life expectancy at birth for females. While a man at birth could be expected to live 2.93 years longer than the actual life expectancy at birth for males.

When working ages are compared, the impacts of deaths from the each of diseases are higher for males than females, except the impact of diabetes mellitus in the age group 25–44. Consideration population of young adults (25–44 years), its labour force potential is most threatened by mortality of cerebrovascular diseases. By eliminating the deaths from cerebrovascular diseases, the duration of remaining working life of young adults would be prolonged by 0.0018 years of life. As for population of adults (45–64 years), its labour force potential is most threatened by chronic ischemic heart disease as well as acute coronary syndrome.

As one would notice, in spite of the PGLE of chronic ischemic heart disease (0.0602 years) for males of adults is higher than the PGLE of acute coronary syndrome (0.0561 years), the PGLE for working age 45–64 by elimination of chronic ischemic heart disease represents only 2.05% of the PGLE at birth, as compared with 6.61% for acute coronary syndrome. The same finding is seen when the PGLE at birth of chronic ischemic heart disease (2.93 years) is higher than the PGLE at birth of acute coronary syndrome (0.85 years) for males, however, the PGLE for working age 45–64 by elimination of chronic ischemic heart disease represents less contribution than acute coronary syndrome. Similar results are observed for people aged 25–44 years by eliminating two mentioned causes of death, although, a highest relative weight accounting for 0.59% is found for males by eliminating atherosclerosis.

Discussion

The aim of this analysis was to quantify the impact of deaths from cardiovascular diseases and diabetes mellitus on life expectancy of the Slovak population in the working age groups by sex from 1996 to 2014 and to reveal the relative importance of causes of deaths when comparing the entire life span and working life-time.

According to results, the main problem, that should be primarily solved by health policy planners, relates to the deaths from chronic ischemic heart disease in the working age (45–64 years) for males as well as females. The finding results from the long-term observation during the last two decades. It is one of the ways by which the life expectancy could be faster prolonged and also the economic production could be higher. When consideration past three examined years in terms of the PGLE at birth, life expectancy could be most extended by elimination of deaths from chronic ischemic heart disease for females, and acute coronary syndrome for males. In this case, we have to take into account that the PGLE at birth considers the entire life span, hence, additionally the people aged 65 over. In terms of the PGLE for both sexes of working group (25–44 years), the labour force potential is most threatened by deaths from cerebrovascular diseases, while deaths from chronic ischemic heart disease for population of working age (45–64 years).

In addition, we revealed that a relative importance of some diseases can change when comparing the entire with working time life. The relative importance of acute coronary syndrome for males aged 45–64 years increased when the share of PGLE (45–64 years) on PGLE at birth was calculated. Our findings suggest that it is very important to determinate whether the PGLEs at birth or working life time are considered, and then decide about the most burdens of diseases. Obviously, the years gained during the two sets of working life do not have the same weight in terms of economic costs of diseases.

One of the reasons for the high differences in the CVD between males and females, supported by previous studies [22–24], may be the fact that women in reproductive age are protected by hormones, thus have a lower prevalence of CVD. On the other hand, women in menopause are at a higher risk than men.

Nevertheless, there are any specific CVD prevention or treatment procedures that would take into account gender differences in Slovakia. Henceforth, the health policy makers should focus on eliminating risk factors (e.g. LDL cholesterol, dietary habits, physical activity, smoking) and compensation of already existing diseases (hypertension, diabetes mellitus – type 2, dyslipidemia atherogenic, metabolic syndrome).

Unfortunately, a national program of CVD prevention as well as treatment guidelines do not exist in Slovakia.

Concurrently, the general practitioners are ageing and they do not have a motivation for education, that leads to the incorrect treating patients. This interpretation is consistent with the DYSIS study by Pella et al. (not published yet), who found that only a fifth patients had met the target for LDL-C and achieved optimal levels of other screened lipids.

Our surprising findings, that the labour force potential of working group (25–44 years) is most threatened by deaths from cerebrovascular diseases and working group (45–64 years) by the deaths from chronic ischemic heart disease, can be explained by gradually shifting morbidity into the younger age groups of the Slovak population [25].

Our result also suggests that women aged 25–44 are more threatened by deaths from diabetes mellitus than men aged 25–44. This finding appears to reflect the fact that women in younger age suffer from gestational diabetes or subsequent development of postpartum diabetes, obesity, higher weight after a childbirth, metabolic syndrome, insulin resistance. Our statements are in agreement with the studies by Martinka et al. [7], Šulcová et al. [26], Wild et al. [5].

To reduce the prevalence of diabetes mellitus can help these possible strategies: reducing preventable risk factors, such as obesity; screening; improve the diagnosis and monitoring of blood glucose diabetics; improve the treatment of vascular complications, including diseases of the kidney, retinopathy, diabetic legs and other neuropathies; and improved monitoring of cardiovascular risk.

Additionally, the potential gain expected for males working age 25–44 by elimination deaths from atherosclerosis represents 0,59% of the expected gain for the entire life span, while the lower shares are observed in other diseases. As for men in working age 45–64, the highest share was found in acute coronary syndrome. These results confirm that atherosclerosis is the main risk factor associated with an increased risk of acute coronary syndrome, and it is a warning signal indicating the expected increase in deaths from acute coronary syndrome.

Limitations

While the potential gains in life expectancy seems to be a beneficial indicator for measuring the burden of diseases, it has some limitations. According to this indicator, life expectancy is extended by elimination of deaths. However, life expectancy is also affected by many other factors, e.g. quality of health care, life style, crime rates, economy, state military status, environment, and others. Moreover, total elimination of a certain cause of death is not likely, on the other hand, it provides the real strength to the other competing risks of causes of death.

It may seem that the extension of life expectancy through eliminating deaths from a disease in the working age groups by several days is negligible and unimportant. However, we have mentioned in introduction section that life expectancy prolonged by 4 years from 1996 to 2014, that is quite a long duration, therefore an extension of life expectancy only by a few days means a substantial progress.

Conclusions

Based on the observed law values of the potential gains in life expectancy for the working population, we can assume that the substantial part of the burden of examined diseases refers to the people aged 65 over. However, from the term of sustainability of health system financing and economic growth, it is desirable to highlight the relative importance of causes of death during the working life of Slovak population.

In spite of limitations, the PGLE is an innovative indicator for measurement the competing risks of causes of death expressing the value to which the lifetime could be extended. Comprehensive analysis is a basis for creating the strategic solutions in prevention, diagnostics and treatment guidelines in the Slovak Republic.

Abbreviations
CVD: Cardiovascular diseases; ICD-10: The Tenth Revision of the International Classification of Disease; PGLEs: Potential gains in life expectancy

Acknowledgements
Our acknowledgments belong to the Ministry of Health of the Slovak Republic and the Health Policy Institute for their cooperation and support in creating new conceptions and methodologies, and for their support of our research activities.
Our thanks also goes out to the National Health Information Center (NHIC) of Slovakia for providing access to the central mortality database for the studied period as well as other studied data along with the Statistical Office of the Slovak Republic.

Funding
This study was funded by the VEGA Project No. 1/0846/18: *"Evaluation of the efficiency of public procurement of selected commodities in healthcare facilities in the Slovak Republic"* from The Ministry of Education, Science, Research and Sport of the Slovak Republic.

Authors' contributions
BG and TV participated in the conceptualisation of the study, data analysis, statistical methods and interpretation. BG participated in the discussion and explanation of the results. TV participated in the drafting the manuscript. BG and TV participated in the acquisition of funding. All authors read and approved the final manuscript.

Competing interests
The authors declare that they have no competing interests.

References

1. Wilkins E, Wilson L, Wickramasinghe K, Bhatnagar P, Leal J, Luengo-Fernandez R, et al. European Cardiovascular Disease Statistics 2017. European Heart Network 2017. http://www.ehnheart.org/cvd-statistics.html. Accessed 16 April 2017.

2. Kesteloot H, Sans S, Kromhout D. Dynamics of cardiovascular and all-cause mortality in western and Eastern Europe between 1970 and 2000. Eur Heart J. 2006; https://doi.org/10.1093/eurheartj/ehi511.

3. Graham I, Atar D, Borch-Johnsen K, Boysen G, Burell G, Cifkova R, et al. European guidelines on cardiovascular disease prevention in clinical practice: full text. Fourth Joint Task Force of the European Society of Cardiology and other societies on cardiovascular disease prevention in clinical practice (constituted by representatives of nine societies and by invited experts). Eur J Cardiovasc Prev Rehabil. 2007; https://doi.org/10.1097/01.hjr.0000277984.31558.c4.

4. Nichols M, Townsend N, Scarborough P, Rayner M. Cardiovascular disease in Europe 2014: epidemiological update. Eur Heart J. 2014; https://doi.org/10.1093/eurheartj/ehu299.

5. Wild S, Roglic G, Green A, Sicree R, King H. Global prevalence of diabetes: estimates for the year 2000 and projections for 2030. Diabetes Care. 2004;27:1047–53.

6. Mathers CD, Loncar D. Projections of global mortality and burden of disease from 2002 to 2030. PLoS Med. 2006; https://doi.org/10.1371/journal.pmed.0030442.

7. Martinka E, et al. National Diabetes Program. Slovakian Diabetes Society. 2012. http://www.diaslovakia.sk/contentData/0225/Národný_diabetologický_program_predložený_MZSR.pdf. Accessed 16 March 2017 (In Slovak.).

8. Murray CJL, et al. Global, regional, and national age–sex specific all-cause and cause-specific mortality for 240 causes of death, 1990–2013: a systematic analysis for the global burden of disease study 2013. Lancet. 2015; https://doi.org/10.1016/S0140-6736(14)61682-2.

9. Nichols M, Townsend N, Luengo-Fernandez R, Leal J, Gray A, Scarborough P, Rayner M. European Cardiovascular Disease Statistics 2012. European Heart Network and European Society of Cardiology 2012. http://www.escardio.org/static_file/Escardio/Press-media/press-releases/2013/EU-cardiovascular-disease-statistics-2012.pdf. Accessed 15 March 2017.

10. Merkovska L, Jedlickova L, Jackova L, Pella D. Effects of hypolipidemc therapy on the endothelial dysfunction in patients with metabolic syndrome. Atherosclerosis. 2015; https://doi.org/10.1016/j.atherosclerosis.2015.04.826.

11. CJL M, Lopez AD, editors. The global burden of disease: a comprehensive assessment of mortality and disability from diseases, injuries, and risk factors in 1990 and projected to 2020, Global burden of disease and injury series. Cambridge: Harvard University Press; 1996.

12. WHO. The global burden of disease: 2004 update. WHO Press. 2008. http://www.who.int/healthinfo/global_burden_disease/2004_report_update/en/. Accessed 03 January 2017.

13. Conti S, Farchi G, Masocco M, Toccaceli V, Vichi M. The impact of the major causes of death on life expectancy in Italy. Int J Epidemiol. 1999; https://doi.org/10.1093/ije/28.5.905.

14. Lai D, Hardy RJ. Potential gains in life expectancy or years of potential life lost: impact of competing risks of death. Int J Epidemiol. 1999;28:894–8.

15. Liu P, Li C, Wang Y, Zeng W, Wang H, Wu H, et al. The impact of the major causes of death on life expectancy in China: a 60-year longitudinal study. BMC Public Health. 2014; https://doi.org/10.1186/1471-2458-14-1193.

16. Mackenbach JP, Kunst AE, Lautenbach H, Oei YB, Bijlsma F. Gains in life expectancy after elimination of major causes of death: revised estimates taking into account the effect of competing causes. J Epidemiol Community Health. 1999;53:32–7.

17. Tsai SP, Lee ES, Hardy RJ. The effect of a reduction in leading causes of death: potential gains in life expectancy. Am J Public Health. 1978;68:966–71.

18. Wang GD, Lai DJ, Burau KD, Du XL. Potential gains in life expectancy from reducing heart disease, cancer, Alzheimer's disease, kidney disease or HIV/AIDS as major causes of death in the USA. Public Health. 2013; https://doi.org/10.1016/j.puhe.2013.01.005.

19. Mészáros J. Methodological guide. The calculation of life tables. The calculation of Potential Years of Life Lost. INFOSTAT Demographic Research Centre. 2000. http://www.infostat.sk/vdc/pdf/metodika_ut.pdf. Accessed 04 January 2017 (In Slovak.).

20. Arias E, Heron M, Tejada-Vera B. United States life tables eliminating certain causes of death, 1999–2001. In: National vital statistics reports. National Center for Health Statistics. 2013. https://www.cdc.gov/nchs/data/nvsr/nvsr61/nvsr61_09.pdf. Accessed 03 January 2017.

21. United Nations. Provisional guidelines on standard international age classifications. Department of International Economic and Social Affairs 1982. https://unstats.un.org/unsd/publication/SeriesM/SeriesM_74e.pdf. Accessed 03 January 2017.

22. Fedacko J, Pella D, Jarcuska P, Sabol F, Kmec J, Lopuchovsky T, et al. Slovak trial on cardiovascular risk reduction following national guidelines with CaDUET® (the STRONG DUET study). Adv Ther. 2013; https://doi.org/10.1007/s12325-012-0075-z.

23. Gavurová B, Vagašová T. Regional differences of standardised mortality rates for ischemic heart diseases in the Slovak Republic for the period 1996–2013 in the context of income inequality. Health Econ Rev. 2016; https://doi.org/10.1186/s13561-016-0099-1.

24. Maas AHEM, Appelman YEA. Gender differences in coronary heart disease. Neth Heart J. 2010;18:598–602.

25. Gavurová B, Kováč V, Vagašová T. Standardised mortality rate for cerebrovascular diseases in the Slovak Republic from 1996 to 2013 in the context of income inequalities and its international comparison. Health Econ Rev. 2017; https://doi.org/10.1186/s13561-016-0140-4.

26. Šulcová M, Čižnár I, Fabianová E, et al. Public Health. Bratislava: VEDA; 2012. (In Slovak.)

8

Association of Child Maltreatment with South African Adults' Wages: Evidence from the Cape Area Panel Study

Xiaodong Zheng[1], Xiangming Fang[1,2*], Deborah A. Fry[3], Gary Ganz[4], Tabitha Casey[3], Celia Hsiao[5] and Catherine L. Ward[4]

Abstract

Child maltreatment is a prevalent public health problem in both developed and developing countries. While many studies have investigated the relationship between violence against children and health of the victims, little is known about the long term economic consequences of child maltreatment, especially in developing countries. Using data from the Cape Area Panel Study, this paper applies Heckman selection models to investigate the relationship between childhood maltreatment and young adults' wages in South Africa. The results show that, on average, any experience of physical or emotional abuse during childhood is associated with a later 12% loss of young adults' wages. In addition, the correlation between physical abuse and economic consequence (14%) is more significant than the relationship between emotional abuse and wages (8%) of young adults; and the higher the frequency of maltreatment, the greater the associations with wages. With respect to gender differences, wage loss due to the experience of childhood maltreatment is larger for females than males. Specifically, males' wages are more sensitive to childhood emotional abuse, while females' wages are more likely to be affected by childhood physical abuse. These results emphasize the importance of prioritizing investments in prevention and intervention programs to reduce the prevalence of child maltreatment and to help victims better overcome the long-term negative effect.

Keywords: Child maltreatment, Physical abuse, Emotional abuse, Wages, Heckman selection model, South Africa

JEL classification: I18, J30, J31

Background

Child maltreatment remains a prevalent public health problem in both developed and developing countries. In South Africa, violence against children, abuse, and neglect are widespread. According to the household survey of the Optimus Study South Africa, a nationally representative study of 15–17-year olds, 18% had experienced physical abuse and 26.1% emotional abuse, in their lifetimes [1]. Across Africa, more than half of children have experienced maltreatment in their lifetime, and more than one fourth report lifetime multiple abuse victimization [2, 3].

There is increasing evidence that child maltreatment is associated with serious consequences for child development, including mental health [4–7], physical health [8–10], and academic, social, and behavioral functioning [11–14]. Little is known, however, about the association between childhood maltreatment and wages of adults, especially in developing countries. The purpose of this paper is therefore to explore the long-term consequences of child maltreatment on adulthood wages in South Africa.

Evidence of the link between child maltreatment and economic consequences is important for several reasons. First, the long-term consequences of child maltreatment on adult wages should improve the understanding of the economic burden of child maltreatment to society [15–17]. Second, the lifelong economic consequences of child maltreatment provide another key element for the comprehension of the formation of inequality and its persistence. Evidence shows

* Correspondence: xmfang@cau.edu.cn
[1]College of Economics and Management, China Agricultural University, Beijing, China
[2]School of Public Health, Georgia State University, 140 Decatur Street, Atlanta, GA 30303, USA
Full list of author information is available at the end of the article

that socioeconomic status is an important risk factor for child maltreatment [18–20]. If child maltreatment is associated with later adverse socioeconomic attainment, then it would be crucially linked to income and class inequality [21]. Third, estimating the variation in adult wages caused by childhood maltreatment will help policymakers and government officials prioritize funding and develop services to reduce or prevent child maltreatment.

Child maltreatment can cause gross physical trauma to the brain, including hypothalamic-pituitary-adrenal axis dysregulation, as well as parasympathetic and catecholamine responses [22, 23]. Therefore, it is not surprising that child maltreatment leads to consequences such as adverse mental health, physical health, and educational outcomes [24, 25]. These consequences may in turn have an effect on later economic productivity and socioeconomic attainment of the victims [26, 27].

Several studies used data from developed countries such as the USA and New Zealand to investigate this issue. Among them, Macmillan examined the relationship between adolescent victimization, which can broadly be understood as a form of child maltreatment, and later income in adulthood [28]. The results indicated that adolescent violent victimization reduced hourly income by an average of 14%. Mullen and colleagues and Hyman studied the socioeconomic consequences of childhood sexual abuse [29, 30]. They found that childhood sexual abuse had a significant adverse effect on the earnings of women. Zielinski found that adults who had experienced maltreatment in childhood had significantly higher rates of unemployment, poverty, and Medicaid usage in the USA [27]. Currie and Widom applied a prospective cohort design to examine the adult economic status and productivity consequences of early victimization of child maltreatment, and found that individuals with histories of maltreatment had lower levels of education, employment, and earnings, and fewer assets in middle age [26].

Several studies from South Africa have shown associations between child maltreatment with psychosocial and educational outcomes as well as quality of life [1, 31–33]. However, to date very few studies have focused on the relationship between childhood maltreatment and economic well-being of adults in developing countries like South Africa.

Using the Heckman Selection Model to overcome problems of self-selection bias, this study empirically examined the association of maltreatment during childhood with adult wages in South Africa. Because previous studies indicated that child maltreatment was more detrimental to the health and educational outcomes of girls [34–37] and frequency of abuse was an important marker of severity [38, 39], which may affect subsequent economic consequences, we also investigated the the impact of gender and frequency of maltreatment on the relationship between child maltreatment and young adults' wages.

Methods
Data

The data used in this study is from the Cape Area Panel Study (CAPS). CAPS is a longitudinal study that follows the lives of a representative sample of youth and young adults as they undergo the multiple transitions from adolescence to adulthood in Cape Town, South Africa. The study commenced in 2002 as a collaborative project of the Universities of Cape Town and Michigan. The CAPS household sample was drawn through a two-stage process. First, a sample of primary sampling units (PSUs) was selected within each population group stratum with probability proportional to size. Second, a sample of 25 screener households was drawn within each PSU, and the adolescents aged 14–22 in each selected family were the respondents in Wave 1 [40]. Currently, CAPS includes five waves from 2002 to 2009 [41] and the dataset has been increasingly used in recent years to examine issues related to education, employment, and health of youth and young adults in South Africa [42–46].

We used two sets of indicators, from Waves 1 and 5. Child maltreatment indicators are included in Wave 1, in which young adults aged 14–22 were asked to recall their childhood abuse; and socioeconomic outcomes in Wave 5 when the age of young adults was 21–29. Wave 1 of CAPS successfully interviewed 4752 youth or young adults in face-to-face interviews, and Wave 5 successfully followed 2915 respondents [41]. Because of missing data in Wave 5, the final sample size in our study was 2644. Bivariate analyses across gender, age, race, education levels and marital status were conducted to examine the differences between excluded missing cases in Wave 5 and non-missing cases, and no significant differences were found. In addition to unweighted data, we also used weighted CAPS data to provide results that were based on a more reasonably representative sample. The weighted distribution of participants was generated in line with population group distribution in Cape Town, which was within one percentage point bias from the 1996 census [40].

Measures
Child maltreatment

The key dependent variables of physical and emotional abuse used in this study are retrospective questions about child maltreatment from the first wave of CAPS in 2002. Respondents were asked to reflect on their family life up until they were 14 years of age. The questions with regard to child maltreatment, which were adapted from the Conflict Tactics Scale (CTS) [47], included how often a perpetrator had sworn at or insulted them, or put them down ("put down"); made them afraid that they might be physically hurt ("afraid of hurt"); pushed, grabbed, slapped, or thrown something at them ("push");

and hit them so hard that they had marks or were injured ("hit hard"). The respondents were also asked whether a parent, stepparent, or an adult living in their home was the perpetrator. Following Chapman et al. and Dube et al. [48, 49], "put down" and "afraid of hurt" are considered as emotional abuse, while "push" and "hit hard" are regarded as physical abuse. The respondents were asked to report the frequency of maltreatment on a five-point Likert scale: never, once or twice, sometimes, often, very often.

From each answer to the questions relevant with child maltreatment, we generated two types of child maltreatment variables. The first type was a dummy variable which was scored 0 if the respondent answered "never," otherwise scored 1. The second type was composed of two dummy variables: whether the respondent answered "once or twice" or "sometimes" (low frequency maltreatment), and whether the respondent answered "often" or "very often" (high frequency maltreatment). Type 1 indicates whether the respondent has been maltreated or not, whereas Type 2 divides the respondents into three categories (non-maltreated, low frequency maltreatment, and high frequency maltreatment). In order to differentiate the association of physical abuse and emotional abuse with young adults' wages, we generated dummy variables for "emotional abuse": scored 1 if the young adult had once suffered from "put down" or "afraid of hurt," otherwise scored 0; "physical abuse": scored 1 if the young adult had once suffered from "push" or "hit hard", otherwise scored 0; and "any child maltreatment": scored 1 if the respondent had suffered from any kind of maltreatment in childhood, scored 0 if the respondent had never been maltreated.

Although the retrospective measures of child maltreatment can almost rule out the possibility of reverse causation [50], several biases are possible. First, recall bias exists if young adults forget childhood maltreatment or do not recognize what they experienced as a child as maltreatment. Second, reporting bias may exist if young adults choose not to disclose such private information; this may particularly be true of males [1]. Third, selection bias may occur if young adults refuse to answer the question. Pieterse used the same data to test the possible biases and found that recall bias and selection bias were not a serious problem [25]. Although females are more likely to report experiences of childhood maltreatment, there was no evidence to determine whether that was reporting bias or a genuine gender difference. Other studies have shown that the childhood maltreatment CAPS data is properly collected and thus provides a valid and reliable measure of maltreatment in childhood [48, 49, 51].

Economic outcome
The respondent's monthly wages (measured in South African Rands, ZAR) in the fifth wave of CAPS in 2009,

were used as the economic outcome variable. Young adults were asked to report take-home pay after taxes and other deductions in a typical month.

Control variables
Various factors are associated with the wages of young adults, including personal and household characteristics. Omitting variables which are both correlated with child maltreatment and adulthood wages would bias estimates in the regression models. Since family environment in childhood may both be correlated with adulthood wages and an important determinant of child maltreatment, we used childhood household characteristics in Wave 1 rather than that in Wave 5 to reduce the possibility of endogeneity problems as far as possible. Therefore, in the empirical analyses, we controlled for individual characteristics from Wave 5 and household characteristics from Wave 1. The controls included gender, race, age, age squared, education levels, marital status, home language, household size, the gender of household head, mother's education (and also whether an observation of mother's education was missing) and the family income per capita. Compared to existing relevant studies [25–27], this study controlled more relevant variables, especially childhood household characteristics.

The measures of variables used in this study were summarized in Appendices A1 (available at https://drive.google.com/open?id=1TW54hbQ7dt4PKQ86bwfd2p8hC5ZJRlWP).

Descriptive analyses
The descriptive statistics for childhood maltreatment of young respondents in the CAPS are reported in Table 1, with t-tests for different groups by gender and race. The overall prevalence of child maltreatment in the sample was 59%: 34% of young adults reported having been physically abused, and 54% having been emotionally abused. From t-test results, a significantly higher proportion of females have been "put down" and "afraid of hurt" by adults compared to males. The prevalence of child maltreatment of Colored youth is significantly higher than that of Black adolescents.

Table 2 presents the monthly wages of the young adults who worked in 2009, and shows t-tests for groups by gender and race. The average monthly wages of young adults in the Cape Town area was ZAR 3058.55 (nearly $413 USD) in 2009. Results of t-tests show that males earned more than females, and Colored people had higher wages than Black people. Descriptive statistics for respondents' individual and household characteristics are reported in Table 3. The weighted means show that the adolescents were predominately female (51%), Colored (56%), single (82%) and not well educated (only 14% percent of the sample had graduated from college). 24% of household heads were female and 38% of families' home language was English. The mean

Table 1 Childhood maltreatment by gender and race (unweighted)

Variable	Total (N = 2644)	Gender			Race		
		Female (N = 1447)	Male (N = 1197)	t-test	Black African (N = 1219)	Colored (N = 1310)	t-test
Put down	0.49	0.51	0.47	1.80*	0.42	0.57	−7.77***
Afraid of hurt	0.29	0.30	0.27	1.96**	0.32	0.27	3.18***
Push	0.31	0.31	0.32	−0.20	0.24	0.39	−8.09***
Hit hard	0.12	0.12	0.13	−0.07	0.09	0.16	−5.48***
Put down (high)	0.08	0.09	0.07	2.47**	0.04	0.12	−7.73***
Afraid of hurt (high)	0.04	0.04	0.03	1.42	0.02	0.06	−3.97***
Push (high)	0.05	0.05	0.04	0.92	0.02	0.07	−5.60***
Hit hard (high)	0.02	0.02	0.02	−0.97	0.01	0.03	−2.15**
Physical abuse	0.34	0.34	0.34	0.16	0.26	0.42	−8.56***
Emotional abuse	0.54	0.55	0.52	1.54	0.47	0.61	−6.92***
Any child maltreatment	0.59	0.60	0.57	1.25	0.51	0.66	−7.70***

Note: Statistics in t-test column are t values. The terms "Black African" and "Colored" date from the Apartheid era in South Africa. Our use of them does not imply support for these racialised categories; rather, we report them because of their continuing association with health and other inequalities [52]. The term Black African means Black people; the terms Colored means mixed-race South Africans. Since there were too few observations of White and Indian peoples, the table does not report statistics for these groups in the "Race" column. "High" refers to high frequency
*** $p < 0.01$, ** $p < 0.05$, * $p < 0.1$

household size and household income per capita were 5.55 and 831.44 ZAR, respectively.

Empirical analyses

Our econometric analysis took place in three steps. First, we used a probit model to estimate the probability of adulthood employment as a function of child maltreatment and control variables. Second, we use an ordinary least square (OLS) model to estimate the association of child maltreatment with adulthood wages, as follows:

$$
\begin{aligned}
lnwage_i = \; & \beta_0 + \beta_1 maltreated_i + \beta_2 male_i + \beta_3 african_i \\
& + \beta_4 colored_i + \beta_5 age_i + \beta_6 agesqr_i + \beta_7 coll_i \\
& + \beta_8 collab_i + \beta_9 marr_i + \beta_{10} sepa_i + \beta_{11} hlang_i \\
& + \beta_{12} hsize_i + \beta_{13} hheadfe_i + \beta_{14} moedu_i \\
& + \beta_{15} moedumiss_i + \beta_{16} lnfaminc_i + \varepsilon_{1i}
\end{aligned}
$$

$$(1)$$

where $lnwage_i$ represents natural logarithm of the ith respondent's monthly wages; and $maltreated$ is an indicator for the ith respondent who had a substantiated

case of a type of maltreatment in childhood; ε represents the random error term; and β_i, the coefficient of $maltreated$, is the elasticity of wage to child maltreatment.

However, the OLS model does not take into account possible sample selection bias because our study has access to wage observations for only those who work, who are not randomly selected from the population. For example, adult respondents who did not work were more likely to have lower education, to be students, or to have a child, especially for women [53, 54]. Estimating the association of child maltreatment with adulthood wages from subpopulation who work by using OLS regressions may introduce bias. Therefore, in our third phase of econometric analyses we applied Heckman selection models [55–57] to correct for such sample selection bias. The Heckman selection model takes place in two stages: the selection equation, and then and the outcome equation. In the first stage, we formulated a selection equation using probit regression to estimate the probability of working. The extended form of the selection equation is as follows:

Table 2 Young adults' monthly wage by gender and race (unweighted)

Variable	Total (N = 1786)	Gender			Race		
		Female (N = 934)	Male (N = 852)	t-test	African (N = 732)	Colored (N = 1006)	t-test
Monthly wages (ZAR)	3058.55	2929.04	3200.52	−2.55**	2326.62	3440.99	−11.69***
	(3515)	(2125.06)	(2365.67)		(1567.09)	(2192.43)	

Note: Standard deviation in parentheses
*** $p < 0.01$, ** $p < 0.05$, * $p < 0.1$

Table 3 Individual and household characteristics ($N = 2644$)

Variable	Symbol	Mean (sample)	Mean (weighted)	Standard deviation	Wave
Individual Characteristics					
Male	male	0.45	0.49	0.50	Wave 5
African	african	0.46	0.29	0.50	Wave 5
Colored	colored	0.50	0.56	0.50	Wave 5
Age	age	24.47	24.67	2.58	Wave 5
Age square	age_sqr	605.42	615.11	127.54	Wave 5
College degree	coll	0.07	0.12	0.25	Wave 5
College degree above	coll_ab	0.02	0.02	0.13	Wave 5
Married	marr	0.14	0.16	0.35	Wave 5
Separated	sepa	0.02	0.02	0.13	Wave 5
In school	school	0.09	0.11	0.28	Wave 5
Have a child	child	0.33	0.29	0.47	Wave 5
Household Characteristics					
Home language English	hlang	0.16	0.24	0.36	Wave 1
Household size	hsize	5.77	5.55	2.50	Wave 1
Female-headed household	hhead_fe	0.40	0.38	0.12	Wave 1
Mother's education	mo_edu	0.12	0.10	0.33	Wave 1
Mother's education missing	mo_edu_miss	0.82	0.85	0.38	Wave 1
Household income per capita (log)	lnfaminc	6.11	6.47	0.02	Wave 1

$$\text{Prob}(\text{wage}_i > 0) = \beta_0 + \beta_1 maltreated_i + \beta_2 male_i$$
$$+ \beta_3 african_i + \beta_4 colored_i$$
$$+ \beta_5 age_i + \beta_6 agesqr_i + \beta_7 coll_i$$
$$+ \beta_8 collab_i + \beta_9 marr_i + \beta_{10} sepa_i$$
$$+ \beta_{11} hlang_i + \beta_{12} hsize_i + \beta_{13} hheadfe_i$$
$$+ \beta_{14} moedu_i + \beta_{15} moedumiss_i$$
$$+ \beta_{16} lnfaminc_{i+} \beta_{17} school_i$$
$$+ \beta_{18} child_i + \varepsilon_{2i}$$

$$(2)$$

where *school* and *child* are the unique regressors in the selection equation, and.

$$\varepsilon_1 \sim N(0, \sigma) \tag{3}$$

$$\varepsilon_2 \sim N(0, 1) \tag{4}$$

$$corr\left(\varepsilon_1, \varepsilon_2\right) = \rho \tag{5}$$

where ρ represents the correlation of error term ε_1 and ε_2. The simple OLS regression technique yields biased results when $\rho \neq 0$, which demonstrates the observed young adults are not randomly selected. In such circumstance, the Heckman selection model estimates are consistent and asymptotically efficient.

In the second stage, we corrected for self-selection in the outcome equation, which is the same as eq. (1), by incorporating a transformation of the predicted probabilities in the first stage as an additional explanatory variable. We firstly used two types of Heckman selection model: Heckman Two-Step (H2S) procedure, and maximum likelihood estimation (MLE). The non-selection hazard or Inverse Mill's Ratio (λ) is computed and used as an additional explanatory variable in outcome equation in H2S estimation, while σ and ρ are indirectly estimated by $\ln\sigma$ and $atahn\rho$ in the MLE to correct sample selection bias in the outcome equation.

In addition to H2S and MLE, we also used weighted Heckman maximum likelihood estimation (weighted MLE) to check the robustness of the model results.

Results and discussion
Different subtypes and frequency of child maltreatment and adulthood wages

Table 4 shows the probit and OLS regression estimates of the relationship between different subtypes (with different frequency levels) of childhood maltreatment and adulthood employment and wages in South Africa. Estimates from the probit models show that any experience of different subtypes of childhood maltreatment is not significantly correlated with the employment status (employment vs. unemployment) of the young adults. However, higher

Table 4 Estimates of probit and OLS regressions

Variables	probit: whether at work				OLS: wages			
	Coefficient	Standard error	Coefficient	Standard error	Coefficient	Standard error	Coefficient	Standard error
Put down	0.00	(0.05)			−0.06**	(0.03)		
Put down (low)			0.01	(0.05)			−0.04	(0.03)
Put down (high)			− 0.06	(0.10)			−0.14***	(0.05)
R^2 / Pseudo-R^2	0.059		0.058		0.21		0.21	
Observations	2644		2644		1786		1786	
Afraid of hurt	−0.03	(0.06)			− 0.08***	(0.03)		
Afraid of hurt (low)			−0.03	(0.06)			−0.08**	(0.03)
Afraid of hurt (high)			−0.07	(0.13)			−0.14*	(0.07)
R^2 / Pseudo-R^2	0.059		0.058		0.21		0.21	
Observations	2644		2644		1786		1786	
Push	−0.06	(0.05)			− 0.12***	(0.03)		
Push (low)			−0.02	(0.06)			−0.11***	(0.03)
Push (high)			−0.26**	(0.13)			−0.24***	(0.07)
R^2 / Pseudo-R^2	0.059		0.060		0.21		0.21	
Observations	2644		2644		1786		1786	
Hit hard	−0.05	(0.08)			− 0.06	(0.04)		
Hit hard (low)			−0.02	(0.08)			−0.05	(0.04)
Hit hard (high)			−0.22	(0.19)			−0.16*	(0.10)
R^2 / Pseudo-R^2	0.059		0.059		0.21		0.21	
Observations	2644		2644		1786		1786	

Note: Coefficients for each subtype of child maltreatment come from separated regressions. In both models, the following controls were included: gender, race, age, age squared, education level, marital status, home language, household size, female-headed household, mother's education, and household per capita income. Standard error in parentheses

*** $p < 0.01$, ** $p < 0.05$, * $p < 0.1$

frequency of physical abuse such as "push" is associated with lower probability of working, showing that child maltreatment may also correlate with lower levels of labor supply, which coincides with Zielinski's study [27]. The OLS regressions were applied only to the subsample of respondents who worked and earned income. All subtypes of child maltreatment except "hit hard" were significantly correlated with lower wages. The estimates show that any experience of "put down", "afraid of hurt" and "push" were associated with 6%, 8% and 12% loss of young adults' wages respectively, indicating that the relationship between "push" and economic consequence is stronger. Compared to low frequency of childhood maltreatment, high frequency of childhood violence resulted in more adverse economic situations for young adults.

Table 5 presents the results of Heckman selection models with different subtypes and frequency of child maltreatment. To economise on space, we only report the estimates of the coefficients of the child maltreatment variables. The full information estimation results of Heckman selection models are presented in Appendices A2 to A10 (available at https://drive.google.com/open?id=1TW54hbQ7dt4PKQ86bwfd2p8hC5ZJRlWP).

In all cases, the selective terms (atahnρ, lnσ) are statistically significant, which shows that the estimates in OLS regressions are biased and the application of the Heckman selection model is the more reasonable and reliable approach. The results in the left side of Table 5 show that all measures of child maltreatment are significant except "hit hard" in the MLE column. The estimates of child maltreatment in the three types of Heckman selection model are relatively close. The results of weighted MLE estimation indicate that any experience of physical abuse ("push" or "hit hard") in childhood is associated with more adverse economic consequences than emotional abuse ("put down" or "afraid of hurt"). Overall, "put down", "afraid of hurt", "push" and "hit hard" are associated with 8%, 10%, 14% and 7% wages loss, implying that the estimates in OLS regressions are underestimated. In addition, low frequency and high frequency child maltreatment are associated with 7% to 13%, and 15% to 25%, more loss of wages than that of young adults who have never been abused in childhood, which also demonstrates that the higher frequency of being maltreated in childhood is associated with more negative economic earning ability in adulthood.

Table 5 Estimates of association between each subtype of child maltreatment and adulthood wages (N = 2644)

Variables	H2S		MLE		Weighted MLE	
	Coefficient	Standard error	Coefficient	Standard error	Coefficient	Standard error
Child maltreatment: never vs. at least once						
Put down	−0.08**	(0.03)	−0.06**	(0.03)	−0.08**	(0.03)
Afraid of hurt	−0.10***	(0.03)	−0.08***	(0.03)	−0.09**	(0.04)
Push	−0.14***	(0.03)	−0.13***	(0.03)	−0.15***	(0.03)
Hit hard	−0.07*	(0.04)	−0.06	(0.04)	−0.12***	(0.05)
Child maltreatment: never vs. low frequency; never vs. high frequency						
Put down (low)	−0.07*	(0.03)	−0.05	(0.03)	−0.06	(0.04)
Put down (high)	−0.16***	(0.06)	−0.14***	(0.05)	−0.16**	(0.06)
Afraid of hurt (low)	−0.09***	(0.03)	−0.08**	(0.03)	−0.08**	(0.04)
Afraid of hurt (high)	−0.15**	(0.08)	−0.14*	(0.07)	−0.20**	(0.08)
Push (low)	−0.13***	(0.04)	−0.12***	(0.03)	−0.14***	(0.04)
Push (high)	−0.25***	(0.08)	−0.24***	(0.07)	−0.27***	(0.06)
Hit hard (low)	−0.06	(0.05)	−0.05	(0.04)	−0.10*	(0.05)
Hit hard (high)	−0.17*	(0.10)	−0.16*	(0.10)	−0.22**	(0.10)

Note: Coefficients for each subtype of child maltreatment come from separated regressions. Regressions in Heckman outocme equation with controls including gender, race, age, age squared, education level, marital status, home language, household size, female-headed household, mother's education and household per capita income. Controls in Heckman selection equation are the same elements plus "have a child" and "in school". "low" and "high" refer to low frequency and high frequency respectively. Standard error in parentheses
*** $p < 0.01$, ** $p < 0.05$, * $p < 0.1$

Table 6 reports the Heckman selection model estimates of the associations of overall physical abuse, emotional abuse, and any maltreatment in childhood with wages of young adults. The selectivity terms in all cases, and each coefficient of child maltreatment in the Heckman selection model, are also significant, and the results in three types of Heckman selection model are almost the same. The estimates show that, compared to those respondents who did not report the corresponding type of child maltreatment, having experience of physical abuse, emotional abuse, and any child maltreatment are associated with 12%–14%, 7%–9%, and 11%–13% loss of wages respectively, which also shows that the long-term negative economic consequences of physical abuse are more severe than the effect resulting from emotional abuse. This result is consistent with related studies [26, 27]. Previous studies suggest that

physical abuse is particularly associated with behavior problems, marital breakdown, and low educational levels, while emotional abuse is correlated with low self-esteem and psychological distress [25, 29, 58, 59]. The more adverse social, educational and health consequences of physical abuse may explain why physical abuse in childhood is more detrimental to the later economic consequences than emotional abuse.

Child maltreatment and adulthood wages: Gender differences

Table 7 reports the estimates of Heckman selection models by gender, which indicates the relationship between different subtypes of childhood maltreatment and young adults' wages. Overall, the negative correlations between all subtypes of childhood maltreatment and females' wages are higher. The associations between

Table 6 Estimates of association between child maltreatment and adulthood wages (N = 2644)

Variables	H2S		MLE		Weighted MLE	
	Coefficient	Standard error	Coefficient	Standard error	Coefficient	Standard error
Physical abuse	−0.13***	(0.03)	−0.12***	(0.03)	−0.14***	(0.03)
Emotional abuse	−0.09***	(0.03)	−0.07**	(0.03)	−0.08**	(0.04)
Any child maltreatment	−0.13***	(0.04)	−0.11***	(0.03)	−0.12***	(0.04)

Note: Coefficients for each subtype of child maltreatment come from separated regressions. Regressions in Heckman outocme equation with controls including gender, race, age, age squared, education level, marital status, home language, household size, female-headed household, mother's education and household per capita income. Controls in Heckman selection equation are the same elements plus "have a child" and "in school". "low" and "high" refer to low frequency and high frequency respectively. Standard error in parentheses
*** $p < 0.01$, ** $p < 0.05$, * $p < 0.1$

Table 7 Estimates of association between each subtype of child maltreatment and adulthood wages: gender difference

Variables	H2S		MLE		Weighted MLE	
	Coefficient	Standard error	Coefficient	Standard error	Coefficient	Standard error
Male (N = 1197)						
Put down	−0.06	(0.04)	−0.06	(0.04)	−0.05	(0.05)
Afraid of hurt	−0.06	(0.04)	−0.06	(0.04)	−0.07	(0.05)
Push	−0.08[*]	(0.04)	−0.07[*]	(0.04)	−0.09[**]	(0.04)
Hit hard	−0.06	(0.06)	−0.05	(0.06)	−0.09	(0.07)
Physical abuse	−0.07[*]	(0.04)	−0.07[*]	(0.04)	−0.08[*]	(0.05)
Emotional abuse	−0.05	(0.04)	−0.05	(0.04)	−0.03	(0.05)
Any child maltreatment	−0.07	(0.04)	−0.06	(0.04)	−0.06	(0.05)
Female (N = 1447)						
Put down	−0.10[*]	(0.05)	−0.06	(0.04)	−0.11[**]	(0.05)
Afraid of hurt	−0.13[***]	(0.05)	−0.10[**]	(0.04)	−0.11	(0.07)
Push	−0.20[***]	(0.05)	−0.18[***]	(0.04)	−0.21[***]	(0.05)
Hit hard	−0.08	(0.06)	−0.07	(0.06)	−0.13[*]	(0.07)
Physical abuse	−0.19[***]	(0.05)	−0.17[***]	(0.04)	−0.20[***]	(0.05)
Emotional abuse	−0.14[**]	(0.06)	−0.09[**]	(0.04)	−0.14[**]	(0.06)
Any child maltreatment	−0.21[**]	(0.09)	−0.15[***]	(0.04)	−0.19[***]	(0.06)

Note: Coefficients for each subtype of child maltreatment come from separated regressions. Regressions in Heckman outocme equation with controls including gender, race, age, age squared, education level, marital status, home language, household size, female-headed household, mother's education and household per capita income. Controls in Heckman selection equation are the same elements plus "have a child" and "in school". "low" and "high" refer to low frequency and high frequency respectively. Standard error in parentheses
*** $p < 0.01$, ** $p < 0.05$, * $p < 0.1$

"put down" and "afraid of hurt" and the wages of male adults are not significant, while they are significant for females. Both "push" and "hit hard" in childhood are significantly negative for both male and female young adults. On average, as shown in the estimates of the weighted MLE models, the proportion of wage loss for young female adults is, respectively, 6%, 4%, 12%, and 4% higher than males, for any experience of being put down, afraid of being hurt, pushed and hit hard.

Table 7 also presents the estimates of the associations of overall physical abuse, emotional abuse and child maltreatment with young adults' wages. For males, estimates show that physical abuse is more significantly associated with lower wages in adulthood, while emotional abuse and overall maltreatment are less strongly correlated with wages. For females, all the coefficients of physical abuse, emotional abuse, and overall child maltreatment are significantly negative. Specifically, experiencing physical abuse, emotional abuse and overall child maltreatment are associated with 8%, 3% and 6% loss of young male adults' monthly wages respectively, and 20%, 14%, 19% loss of wages respectively for females. In other words, the proportion of wages lost from any experience of the three types of child maltreatment is more than twice as great for females as for males. While many studies exploring the consequences of sexual abuse control for gender rather than exploring outcomes by

gender, some studies do find risks that may explain this. For instance, compared to males, females who have been maltreated in childhood are at increased risk of alcohol abuse and health problems [26, 60]. A global systematic review and meta-analysis has also found that child maltreatment impacts differentially on boys and girls in terms of educational absenteeism, which may have subsequent impact on employment and wage earnings [34]. However, other studies find that, while genders may differ in the kind of outcome they experience (for instance, females are more likely to experience internalizing disorders and males externalizing disorders), both kinds of outcome are likely to affect earning capacity [24]. Future studies should explore the variables that mediate and moderate the relationship between child maltreatment and adult wages.

Table 8 presents the three types of Heckman selection model estimates of the associations of different frequency of child maltreatment with young adults' wages. Estimation results indicate that high frequency of "afraid of hurt," on the one hand, is more significantly correlated with lower wages of young male adults, compared to young female adults. On the other hand, the proportion of wage loss for females is higher than that of young male adults for the high frequency of "push" and "hit hard." We also find the coefficients of low frequency and high frequency "afraid of hurt" for males and "hit hard"

Table 8 Estimates of association between different frequency of each subtype of child maltreatment and adulthood wages: gender difference

Variables	H2S		MLE		Weighted MLE	
	Coefficient	Standard error	Coefficient	Standard error	Coefficient	Standard error
Male (N = 1197)						
Put down (low)	−0.04	(0.04)	−0.04	(0.04)	−0.03	(0.05)
Put down (high)	−0.17**	(0.08)	−0.16**	(0.08)	−0.14*	(0.08)
Afraid of hurt (low)	−0.04	(0.05)	−0.03	(0.05)	−0.03	(0.05)
Afraid of hurt (high)	−0.23**	(0.11)	−0.23**	(0.11)	−0.30***	(0.11)
Push (low)	−0.07	(0.04)	−0.06	(0.04)	−0.09*	(0.05)
Push (high)	−0.18*	(0.10)	−0.17*	(0.10)	−0.19	(0.12)
Hit hard (low)	−0.06	(0.06)	−0.05	(0.06)	−0.09	(0.08)
Hit hard (high)	−0.02	(0.13)	−0.01	(0.13)	−0.10	(0.16)
Female (N = 1447)						
Put down (low)	−0.09	(0.06)	−0.04	(0.04)	−0.09*	(0.05)
Put down (high)	−0.16*	(0.09)	−0.11	(0.07)	−0.17*	(0.09)
Afraid of hurt (low)	−0.13**	(0.06)	−0.10**	(0.05)	−0.12**	(0.06)
Afraid of hurt (high)	−0.12	(0.11)	−0.10	(0.10)	−0.14	(0.11)
Push (low)	−0.20***	(0.06)	−0.17***	(0.04)	−0.19***	(0.05)
Push (high)	−0.30**	(0.13)	−0.31***	(0.09)	−0.35***	(0.06)
Hit hard (low)	−0.05	(0.07)	−0.04	(0.06)	−0.10	(0.07)
Hit hard (high)	−0.27*	(0.14)	−0.28**	(0.14)	−0.29***	(0.09)

Note: Coefficients for each subtype of child maltreatment come from separated regressions. Regressions in Heckman outocme equation with controls including gender, race, age, age squared, education level, marital status, home language, household size, female-headed household, mother's education and household per capita income. Controls in Heckman selection equation are the same elements plus "have a child" and "in school". "low" and "high" refer to low frequency and high frequency respectively. Standard error in parentheses
*** $p < 0.01$, ** $p < 0.05$, * $p < 0.1$

for females are greatly different, which implies that there may be a big variation of the effect between different frequencies of child maltreatment. Future studies should explore differences in effect between long-term and frequent child maltreatment, and short-term, less frequent maltreatment.

Conclusion and policy implications

Using data from the Cape Area Panel Study (CAPS), this study applied three types of Heckman selection model, including Heckman Two-Step estimation, and weighted and unweighted Heckman maximum likelihood estimation, to study the association of child maltreatment with young adults' monthly wages in South Africa. The results are consistent across the three types of model: on average, compared to an individual who has no history of childhood maltreatment, any experience of child maltreatment is associated with a 12% loss of young adults' wages. At the same time, physical abuse is more strongly correlated with adverse economic consequence than emotional abuse, which coincides with Zielinski's findings [27]. In addition, young adults appear to be more

strongly affected by high frequency childhood maltreatment than low frequency childhood maltreatment.

Consistent with some studies (e.g., [26]), but not with others (e.g., [24]), we identified gender differences in the association of child maltreatment with wages. Females were more strongly affected by the experience of childhood maltreatment than males. Also, compared to young female adults, high-frequency emotional abuse had a more severe adverse impact on the wages of young male adults, while the proportion of wages lost for females was higher than that of males for high frequency physical abuse. Future research should explore whether our findings are replicated in other samples and contexts, given that some studies find otherwise. The mechanisms by which this relationship comes about should also be explored in future research, so as to inform the development and implementation of prevention and intervention programs that are gender-sensitive. In addition, we also encourage future studies to investigate the possible relationship between child maltreatment and economic inequality, which would help to expand our knowledge of the effect of violence against children.

Our findings also bear significant policy implications. First, implementing support programs for parents, teachers, and other caregivers that provide alternatives to violent punishment and prevent child maltreatment, is an urgent need. In the area of child maltreatment, parent training programs including parent-infant home-visiting programs and group parent-training programs for parents of older children, have demonstrated effectiveness for reducing child maltreatment in other contexts [61, 62]. Importantly, several parent training programs have demonstrated cost-effectiveness for reducing child maltreatment in high-income countries such as the USA and are showing promise in South Africa [63, 64]. Such programs should urgently be introduced into low- and middle-income contexts, such as South Africa, and their cost-effectiveness investigated in the new contexts, as a tool for advocating with governments for their use. Recommendations feeding into such plans must be based on sound evidence, and will only be implementable if adequately resourced. Evidence from this study can contribute to building a strong case for state funding of violence prevention programs to be prioritized.

Second, a national policy, which aims at providing sufficient, subsidised healthcare services to children at risk and special education and rehabilitation services for victims of maltreatment, is urgently required, in order to assist victims of maltreatment to overcome the mental and physical health consequences of such abuse.

There are several limitations in this study. First, there may be measurement error in the data on maltreatment and, since the prevalence of maltreatment was reported in retrospect, it could be underreported. This underreporting could results from unwillingness to disclose such private information in an interview, but it is also possible that respondents have repressed traumatic memories or do not recognize that what they experienced as a child was actually maltreatment. The difference between actual maltreatment and disclosed maltreatment may cause underestimation of the association between childhood maltreatment and adults' wages in South Africa. Second, because the CAPS does not provide information on sexual abuse and neglect, which also constitute forms of child maltreatment, this study was unable to investigate these forms of child maltreatment. These forms of child maltreatment also have serious consequences, similar to emotional and physical abuse, and future studies should also address them. Third, the respondents in the Wave 5 of CAPS were aged 21–29 and wages in the twenties probably are not the most informative of how these people will fare later in life, which is more interesting and instructive to the relationship of child maltreatment and economic consequences of adults. Longer-term studies should therefore also be conducted. Despite these limitations, this study contributes to the understanding of the economic loss and inequality caused by child maltreatment in a middle-income country, and may advance awareness of policy makers of the relationship between the national fiscus, and investments in intervention programs to reduce the prevalence of child maltreatment and help the victims better overcome the long-term negative effect of childhood violence.

Overall, our findings suggest a long-term economic consequence of child maltreatment – lower wages – that plays a key role in the economic burden and socioeconomic inequality of child maltreatment on developing countries. Developing countries cannot afford any loss to the economy, let alone one that results from a human rights violation, and it is clear that prevention and intervention programs in low- and middle-income countries like South Africa are urgently needed.

Abbreviations
CAPS: Cape Area Panel Study; CTS: Conflict Tactics Scale; H2S: Heckman Two-Step Estimation; MLE: Maximum Likelihood Estimation; OLS: Ordinary Least Square; PoA: Programme of Action; USA: United States of America; USD: United States Dollar

Author details
[1]College of Economics and Management, China Agricultural University, Beijing, China. [2]School of Public Health, Georgia State University, 140 Decatur Street, Atlanta, GA 30303, USA. [3]Moray House School of Education, University of Edinburgh, Edinburgh, Scotland. [4]Department of Psychology, University of Cape Town, Cape Town, South Africa. [5]Save the Children South Africa, Johannesburg, South Africa.

References
1. Ward CL, Artz L, Leoschut L, Kassanjee R, Burton P. Sexual violence against children in South Africa: a nationally representative cross-sectional study of prevalence and correlates. Lancet Glob Health. 2018;6:e460–8. https://doi.org/10.1016/S2214-109X(18)30060-3.
2. Lemanski C. Residential responses to fear (of crime plus) in two Cape Town suburbs: implications for the post-apartheid city. J Int Dev. 2006;18(6):787–802.
3. Meinck F, Cluver LD, Boyes ME, Loening-Voysey H. Physical, emotional and sexual adolescent abuse victimisation in South Africa: prevalence, incidence, perpetrators and locations. J Epidemiol Community Health. 2016;70(9):910–6.
4. Edwards VJ, Holden GW, Felitti VJ, Anda RF. Relationship between multiple forms of childhood maltreatment and adult mental health in community respondents: results from the adverse childhood experiences study. Am J Psychiatr. 2003;160(8):1453–60.
5. Fang X, Fry DA, Brown DS, Mercy JA, Dunne MP, Butchart AR, et al. The burden of child maltreatment in the East Asia and Pacific region. Child Abuse Negl. 2015;42:146–62.
6. Kaplow JB, Widom CS. Age of onset of child maltreatment predicts long-term mental health outcomes. J Abnorm Psychol. 2007;116(1):176–87.
7. Kimcohen J, Caspi A, Taylor A, Williams B, Newcombe R, Craig IW, et al. MAOA, maltreatment, and gene-environment interaction predicting children's mental health: new evidence and a meta-analysis. Mol Psychiatry. 2006;11(10):903–13.

8. Springer KW, Sheridan J, Kuo D, Carnes M. Long-term physical and mental health consequences of childhood physical abuse. In: National Institutes of Health; 2007.

9. Norman RE, Byambaa M, De R, Butchart A, Scott J, Vos T. The long-term health consequences of child physical abuse, emotional abuse, and neglect: a systematic review and meta-analysis. PLoS Med. 2012;9(11):e1001349.

10. Frias-Armenta M. Long-term effects of child punishment on Mexican women: a structural model. Child Abuse Negl. 2002;26(4):371–86.

11. Gameros TA, Gameros TA. Social functioning of survivors of child sexual abuse: an analysis of childhood experiences and long-term effects. Texas Tech University. 2000;

12. Harter S, Alexander PC, Neimeyer RA. Long-term effects of incestuous child abuse in college women: social adjustment, social cognition, and family characteristics. J Consult Clin Psychol. 1988;56(1):5–8.

13. Lansford JE, Dodge KA, Pettit GS, Bates JE, Crozier J, Kaplow J. A 12-year prospective study of the long-term effects of early child physical maltreatment on psychological, behavioral, and Academic Problems in Adolescence. Arch Pediatr Adolesc Med. 2002;156(8):824–30.

14. Shen CT. Long-term effects of interparental violence and child physical maltreatment experiences on PTSD and behavior problems: a national survey of Taiwanese college students. Child Abuse Negl. 2009;33(3):148–60.

15. Fang X, Brown DS, Florence CS, Mercy JA. The economic burden of child maltreatment in the United States and implications for prevention. Child Abuse Negl. 2012;36(36):156–65.

16. Fang X, Fry DA, Ji K, Finkelhor D, Chen J, Lannen P, et al. The burden of child maltreatment in China: a systematic review. Bulletin of the World Health Organization. 2015;93(3):176–185.

17. Fang X, Zheng X, Fry DA, Ganz G, Casey T, Hsiao C, et al. The economic burden of violence against children in South Africa. Int J Environ Res Public Health. 2017;14(11):1431.

18. Herrenkohl TI, Klika JB, Herrenkohl RC, Russo MJ, Dee T. A prospective investigation of the relationship between child maltreatment and indicators of adult psychological well-being. Violence & Victims. 2012; 27(5):764.

19. Kaslow NJ, Thompson MP. Associations of child maltreatment and intimate partner violence with psychological adjustment among low SES, African American children. Child Abuse & Negl. 2008;32(9):888–96.

20. Laskey AL, Stump TE, Perkins SM, Zimet GD, Sherman SJ, Downs SM. Influence of race and socioeconomic status on the diagnosis of child abuse: a randomized study. J Pediatr. 2012;160(160):1003–8.

21. Macmillan R. The life course consequences of abuse, neglect, and victimization: challenges for theory, data collection, and methodology. Child Abuse Negl. 2009;33(10):661–5.

22. Glaser D. Child abuse and neglect and the brain—a review. J Child Psychol Psychiatry. 2000;41(1):97–116.

23. Lewis DO. From abuse to violence: psychophysiological consequences of maltreatment. J Am Acad Child Adolesc Psychiatry. 1992;31(3):383–91.

24. Chandy JM, Blum RW, Resnick MD. Gender-specific outcomes for sexually abused adolescents. Child Abuse Negl. 1996;20(12):1219–31.

25. Pieterse D. Childhood Maltreatment and Educational outcomes: evidence from South Africa. Health Econ. 2015;24(7):876–94.

26. Currie J, Widom CS. Long-term consequences of child abuse and neglect on adult economic well-being. Child Maltreatment. 2010;15(2):111–20.

27. Zielinski DS. Child maltreatment and adult socioeconomic well-being. Child Abuse Negl. 2009;33(10):666–78.

28. Macmillan R. Adolescent victimization and income deficits in adulthood: rethinking the costs of criminal violence from a life-course perspective. Criminology. 2000;38(2):553–88.

29. Mullen PE, Martin JL, Anderson JC, Romans SE, Herbison GP. The long-term impact of the physical, emotional, and sexual abuse of children: a community study. Child Abuse Negl. 1996;20(1):7–21.

30. Hyman B. The economic consequences of child sexual abuse for adult lesbian women. J Marriage Fam. 2000;62(1):199–211.

31. Barbarin OA, Richter L, Dewet T. Exposure to violence, coping resources, and psychological adjustment of south African children. Am J Orthopsychiatry. 2001;71(1):16–25.

32. Ward CL, Flisher AJ, Zissis C, Muller M, Lombard C. Exposure to violence and its relationship to psychopathology in adolescents. Injury Prevention. 2001; 7(4):297–301.

33. West BO. Quality of life among south African informal, non-familial caregivers of childhood sexual abuse survivors. 2016.

34. Fry D, Fang X, Elliott S, Casey T, Zheng X, Li J, et al. The relationships between violence in childhood and educational outcomes: a global systematic review and meta-analysis. Child Abuse Negl. 2018;75:6–28.

35. Moeller TP, Bachmann GA, Moeller JR. The combined effects of physical, sexual, and emotional abuse during childhood: long-term health consequences for women. Child Abuse Negl. 1993;17(5):623–40.

36. Thompson MP, Kingree JB, Desai S. Gender differences in long-term health consequences of physical abuse of children: data from a nationally representative survey. Am J Public Health. 2004;94(4):599–604.

37. Ullman SE, Filipas HH. Gender differences in social reactions to abuse disclosures, post-abuse coping, and PTSD of child sexual abuse survivors. Child Abuse Negl. 2005;29(7):767–82.

38. Manly JT, Cicchetti D, Barnett D. The impact of subtype, frequency, chronicity, and severity of child maltreatment on social competence and behavior problems. Dev Psychopathol. 1994;6(1):121–43.

39. Sugaya L, Hasin DS, Olfson M, Lin KH, Grant BF, Blanco C. Child physical abuse and adult mental health: a national study. J Trauma Stress. 2012;25(4):384–92.

40. Lam D, Seekings J. The cape area panel study (CAPS): technical documentation for wave 1. 2008.

41. Lam D, Ardington C, Branson N, Case A, Leibbrandt M, Maughan-Brown B, et al. The cape area panel study: overview and technical documentation waves 1–2–3-4-5 (2002–2009). Cape Town: University of Cape Town; 2012.

42. Ardington C, Case A, Islam M, Lam D, Leibbrandt M, Menendez A, et al. The impact of AIDS on intergenerational support in South Africa: evidence from the cape area panel study. Research on Aging. 2009;32(3):405–12.

43. Lam D, Leibbrandt M, Mlatsheni C. Dynamics of labor market entry and youth unemployment in South Africa: evidence from the cape area panel study. 2007.

44. Lekena M. Youth employment in the Cape Town area: insights from the cape area panel study. 2006.

45. Oyedokun AO. Young People's smoking behaviour; determinants and health consequences: evidence from cape area panel study (CAPS). Asian Journal of Humanities & Social Studies. 2014;

46. Ward JL, Viner RM. Secondary Education and Health outcomes in young people from the cape area panel study (CAPS). PLoS One. 2016;11(6)

47. Straus MA. Measuring intrafamily conflict and violence: the conflict tactics (CT) scales. J Marriage Fam. 1979:75–88.

48. Chapman DP, Whitfield CL, Felitti VJ, Dube SR, Edwards VJ, Anda RF. Adverse childhood experiences and the risk of depressive disorders in adulthood. J AFFECT DISORDERS. 2004;82(2):217–25.

49. Dube SR, Felitti VJ, Dong M, Chapman DP, Giles WH, Anda RF. Childhood abuse, neglect, and household dysfunction and the risk of illicit drug use: the adverse childhood experiences study. Pediatrics. 2003;111(3):564–72.

50. Tenkorang EY, Obeng Gyimah S. Physical abuse in early childhood and transition to first sexual intercourse among youth in Cape Town, South Africa. J sex res. 2012;49(5):508–17.

51. Allen JP, Leadbeater BJ, Aber JL. The development of problem behavior syndromes in at-risk adolescents. Dev Psychopathol. 1994;6(2):323–42.

52. Coovadia H, Jewkes R, Barron P, Sanders D, McIntyre D. The health and health system of South Africa: historical roots of current public health challenges. Lancet. 2009;374(9692):817–34.

53. Mulligan CB, Rubinstein Y. Selection, investment, and women's relative wages over time. Q J Econ. 2005;123(3):1061–110.

54. Schultz TP. Investments in the schooling and health of women and men: quantities and returns. J Hum Resour. 1993:694–734.

55. Gronau R. Wage Comparisons-A Selectivity Bias. J Polit Econ. 1974;82(6): 1119–43.

56. Heckman JJ, Robb JR. Alternative methods for evaluating the impact of interventions: an overview. J Econ. 1985;30(1–2):239–67.

57. Lewis HG. Comments on selectivity biases in wage comparisons. J Polit Econ. 1974;82(6):1145–55.

58. Bourassa C. Co-occurrence of Interparental violence and child physical abuse and its effect on the Adolescents' behavior. J Fam Violence. 2007; 22(8):691–701.

59. Weiss JA, Waechter R, Wekerle C. The impact of emotional abuse on psychological distress among child protective services-involved adolescents with borderline-to-mild intellectual disability. Journal of Child & Adolescent Trauma. 2011;4(2):142–59.

60. Currie A, Shields MA, Price SW. The child health/family income gradient: evidence from England. J Health Econ. 2007;26(2):213–32.

61. Hsiao C, Fry D, Ward C, Ganz G, Casey T, Zheng X, Fang X. Violence against children in South Africa: the cost of inaction to society and the economy. BMJ Global Health. 2018;3(1):e000573.

62. Ward C, Sanders MR, Gardner F, Mikton C, Dawes A. Preventing child maltreatment in low-and middle-income countries: parent support programs have the potential to buffer the effects of poverty. Child Abuse Negl. 2015;54:97–107.

63. Lee S, Aos S, Drake E, Pennucci A, Miller M, Anderson L. Return on investment: evidence-based options to improve statewide outcomes. Olympia: Washington state institute for. Public Policy. 2012;

64. Lachman J, Cluver L, Ward CL, Hutchings J, Mlotshwa S, Wessels IM, Gardner F. Randomized controlled trial of a parenting program to reduce the risk of child maltreatment in South Africa. Child Abuse Negl. 2017;72:338–51. https://doi.org/10.1016/j.chiabu.2017.08.014.

9

Extension of mandatory health insurance to informal sector workers in Togo

Dosse Mawussi Djahini-Afawoubo[*] (iD) and Esso-Hanam Atake

Abstract

Background: About 90.4% of Togolese workers operate in the informal sector and account for between 20 and 30% of Togo's Gross Domestic Product. Despite their importance in the Togolese economy, informal sector workers (ISW) do not have a health insurance scheme. This paper aims to estimate the willingness-to-pay (WTP) of ISW in order to have access to Mandatory Health Insurance (MHI), and to analyze the main determinants of WTP.

Methods: This study used data from the Community-Based Monitoring System (CBMS) project implemented in 2015 by the Partnership for Economic Policy (PEP). It focusses on 4,296 ISW (2,374 in urban areas and 1,922 in rural areas, respectively). The contingent valuation method was used to determine the WTP for the MHI while the Tobit model is used to analyze its determinants.

Results and discussion: Findings indicate that about 92% of ISW agreed to have access to MHI, like for formal sector workers. Overall, ISW are willing to pay 2,569 FCFA (USD 4.7) per month. ISW in the poorest quintiles are willing to allocate a higher proportion of their income (15%) to the premium than the richest quintiles (2.5%). Generally, women are more interested in MHI than men, although men are willing to pay higher premiums (3,168.9 FCFA or USD 5.8) than women (2,077 FCFA or USD 3.8). Women's lower WTP can be explained by their low levels of education and income, and a lack of employment opportunities compared to men. The gender of the head of the household, the size of the household and the education and income levels are the main determinants of WTP.

Conclusion: We conclude that it is possible to extend MHI to ISW as long as their premiums are subsidized. The annual subsidy is estimated at 4.1% of the state current general budget or 96% of the health sector budget. In setting the premium, policy makers should take into account the MHI benefits package, subsidies from the government, and information about the WTP. It is important to emphasize that resource mobilization and management, as well as health services delivery, would be effective only in a context of improved governance.

Keywords: Informal sector worker, Health insurance, Contingent valuation, Willingness-to-pay, Togo

Background

Access to health care can be extremely expensive and few people can afford to pay their own medical expenses [1, 2]. Governments should put in place policies that enable people to access health care services without incurring catastrophic health expenditures. Universal health insurance may therefore be a fundamental tool for improving people's welfare [1]. Access to universal health insurance could impact households in a number of ways. Firstly, it would lead to better health by protecting households from health shocks that reduce their capacity to generate income [3].

Secondly, access to health insurance is supposed to reduce out-of-pocket payments [4, 5]. In other words, households that are not insured have to allocate a large part of their budget to solving health problems which reduces the resources available for other goods [6, 7]. Finally, health insurance is essential in supporting the high costs of childbirth [8]. Access to health insurance should, therefore, contribute greatly to the individual and collective well-being.

Unfortunately, in developing countries, experiences have shown that it is difficult to group risks by including vulnerable populations such as Informal Sector Workers (ISW) into existing health insurance schemes [9]. The informal sector is characterised by low and irregular

* Correspondence: dossedjahini@gmail.com; samidosse@yahoo.fr
Department of Economic Sciences, University of Lomé (Togo), Lome, West africa, Togo

incomes which make it difficult to pay for health care in advance [10]. The existing prepayment systems, including government financing in least developed countries, exclude informal sector workers either because of inadequate resources or because they are too weak to afford the insurance premiums [10, 11]. This problem is particularly crucial in Togo, a Sub-Saharan African country ranked among the least developed countries.

The analysis of the determinants of the ISW's willingness to pay for Mandatory Health Insurance (MHI) is a major concern in the case of Togo for at least two reasons. First, a significant proportion of the Togolese workforce (90.4%) works in the informal sector [12]. Secondly, the utilization of health care services is very limited in Togo because of the high out-of-pocket payments [13]. Despite their importance in the Togolese economy, ISW do not have health insurance. In order for a greater number of workers to benefit from health insurance, a MHI scheme was instituted by Law n° 2011–003 of 18 February 2011. The scheme's main objective is to provide better financial access to quality healthcare for its beneficiaries. Currently, ISW are excluded from this health insurance scheme. As a result, it covers only 4% of the Togolese population [14]. In order to extend the MHI to ISW, it is necessary to determine their WTP for a health insurance premium and to identify the determinants of their WTP. Indeed, if the premium amount is higher than what ISW are willing to pay, they would be disadvantaged and a real problem of social justice would arise. The identification of the determinants of informal sector workers' willingness-to-pay for health insurance could help policymakers in setting the premium. The objective of this paper is to examine the determinants of ISWs' willingness to pay for MHI as is the case for formal sector workers in Togo. The paper aims specifically to estimate the ISWs' willingness to pay for MHI, and to analyze the main determinants of the WTP.

Several studies have analyzed the determinants of WTP for health insurance [12, 15–18]. Donfouet et al. [16] investigated the determinants of WTP for a community-based prepayment healthcare scheme in rural Cameroon using a contingent valuation method. They found that age, religion, knowledge of community-based health insurance, awareness of usual practice in rural areas, involvement in association and disposable income are key determinants of WTP. Dong et al. [17] and Onwujekwe et al. [18] found that WTP is influenced by household characteristics, such as location, household size and age composition. However, very few studies have focused on the specific case of ISW [18, 19]. Bärnighausen et al. [15] analyzed ISWs' willingness to pay for a health insurance scheme in China. They found that income and past expenditures on healthcare had a positive effect on WTP. They also found that being male, a migrant, with or without permanent employment significantly decreased WTP. As for Atake and Agbodji [12], they analyzed the ISW's willingness to pay for social protection in Togo. Their results reveal that 90.9% of Togolese ISW are willing to join social protection services. They also found that income and education were the main determinants of WTP for social protection.

The present paper differs from Atake and Agbodji [12] for at least two reasons. First, Atake and Agbodji [12] analyzed the WTP for a social protection scheme. Unfortunately, the Togolese social protection scheme includes only benefits available to households with children, pensions, workplace accidents and occupational diseases. Consequently, health insurance has been neglected. The second difference is methodological. Atake and Agbodji [12] used a logit model to analyze the determinants of ISWs' willingness to pay for social protection in Togo. However, in their analysis, it was important to consider the censored nature of the dependent variable since some individuals may not be willing to pay. Under these circumstances, a Tobit model would be more appropriate.

Overview of the social protection system and the health insurance scheme in Togo

The social protection scheme in Togo is offered by the National Social Security Fund (CNSS) and the National Pensions Fund (CRT). Private sector workers depend on the CNSS while civil servants depend on the CRT. The benefits cover only three domains namely: households with children, pensions (invalidity, old age, death and the survivors), workplace accidents and occupational diseases. The law on the social security code in Togo was adopted by the National Assembly in 2011 (Law n° 2011–006 enacted on 21 February 2011). This law theoretically extends social protection to ISW. However, it is yet to be applied by the CNSS. As a result, ISW are still deprived of social security protection. The implementation of the MHI offered by the National Health Insurance Institute (INAM) in 2012 has not been favorable to ISW. In 2012, INAM covered approximately 300,000 people for a population of more than 6,000,000 individuals. Its mission is to provide coverage of risks related to illness, non-professional accidents and motherhood to its main beneficiaries who are workers of public administrations, and their legal beneficiaries: civil servants, magistrates, military and paramilitary forces, contract staff working with parastatals and local government officials. It also includes members of the institutions of the Republic during their term in office. In order to meet the requirements of universal health insurance, INAM plans to extend its services in the coming years to ISW and vulnerable population. In this regard, it is important to set up a healthcare financing mechanism that will allow ISW to be involved in the health insurance program.

Methods
Data
Study setting

This study uses data from the Community-Based Monitoring System (CBMS) project implemented in 2015 by the Partnership for Economic Policy (PEP), in partnership with the Department for International Development (DFID) of the United Kingdom (UK Aid) and the International Development Research Center (IDRC) of Canada. The main objective of the project was to set up a system to locally monitor the various dimensions of poverty in the informal sector, in an attempt to explore feasibility of a social protection mechanism that would provide sufficient financial protection for workers in the informal sector. Data were collected in a district (Tokoin-Wuiti) of Lomé, the capital of Togo, and in two rural cantons, namely Gblainvié and Dalavé not far from Tokoin-Wuiti. These two rural communities are characterised by poor housing conditions, poor access to safe drinking water, poor hygiene and sanitation conditions, high unemployment and informal employment rates, low levels of education, and high prevalence of disease. Tokoin-Wuiti is an urban area located near industrial and commercial areas and comprises high and middle-income households with acceptable conditions of hygiene, sanitation and housing. This area is also characterised by better access to public infrastructure (health, education, market, etc.) and a high rate of informal employment.

Data collection

The CBMS data is all the more important for policy development as it left no one behind. In other words, data were collected from all households in the target localities. This data collection strategy makes it possible to generalize the results at the community and national levels. The three areas concerned included a total of 7846 households. In total, the data were collected from 7436 households, including 4296 ISW (2374 in urban areas and 1922 in rural areas, respectively). Uninhabited houses and refusals to answer questionnaires accounted for about 5.22% of the target households. The data were collected by interviewers who were originally from these areas, in order to facilitate questionnaire administration in the local language or mother tongue in case the respondent was illiterate. The final questionnaires were first prepared in French and then translated into the local languages during the training of enumerators. Trained enumerators conducted in-person, face-to-face interviews. They went into every household and interviewed only the heads of household or their spouses.

Three survey questionnaires were submitted to the respondents: the household profile questionnaire (HPQ), the rider questionnaire (individual questionnaire) and the community profile questionnaire (CPQ). The HPQ included information on household/member characteristics, education, health and nutrition, housing and tenure, water sources and sanitation, etc. The RQ was designed to collect additional information on social protection, and included an assessment of the ISWs' willingness to pay for access to social protection services such as health insurance, old-age social security, workmen's compensation, maternity benefits, etc. As soon as the respondents were identified as informal sector workers, they were asked to answer the RQ. Finally, the CPQ was responded by chiefs/representatives of districts/areas and by resource persons in health, education and other sectors. The CPQ contains information at the community level that was used to complement the information from the HPQ, such as physical and demographic characteristics of the village/community, demographic reference, service institutions and infrastructure, programs, projects and activities, etc.

Main variables

The RQ was used to collect data on the income of household members during the last four weeks preceding the survey. For workers with a daily or weekly income, we adjusted the income to its monthly value using an appropriate multiplier (26 or 04 respectively). Income data was collected in WAEMU francs (CFA francs). The average exchange rate during the survey period, July 2015 and September 2015, was 550 CFA francs per US dollar. With regard to data on social protection and willingness to pay, this study used the parametric approach of the referendum format. According to Arrow et al. [20], the referendum "refers to a choice mechanism that asks each respondent how he would vote if faced with a particular program and the prospect of paying for the program through some means such as higher taxes". First, the interviewers explained at length the advantages of each type of social protection service, using the national language and/or mother tongue. Information was then collected on the value they attributed to each social protection service, their availability to access it and the value of their willingness to pay. If the respondent was interested in the social protection services offered and answered "yes" to the first price proposed, the interviewer increased the offer slightly until the respondent answered "no". If the initial answer was "no" to the first price proposed, the interviewer gradually reduced the amount until the respondent answered "yes".

Empirical strategy

In order to extend the mandatory health insurance scheme to ISW, in a context characterized by an insufficient budget and where barely 4% of the population is covered, it is important to hear from the household heads working in the informal sector about their willingness or unwillingness to participate in the mandatory health insurance scheme and the maximum amount they are willing to pay (WTP).

Generally, the WTP of a household head depends on his own characteristics, the characteristics of his/her household and the availability of health services. In the light of previous studies [9, 15, 21], WTP is expected to increase with age [22], income, and education [23]. Other variables such as household composition (measured by the number of adults aged over 60 and the number of children aged under five), marital status of the household head, sex of the household head, as well as distance to the nearest health facility are also included. This last variable is introduced to take into account the availability of health facilities. Thus, WTP is expected to decrease proportionally to the increase in distance to the closest health facility. The general model is as follows:

$$WTP = f(AGE, GENDER, EDU, MAT, COMP, INCOME, RESIDENCE, DIST) \tag{1}$$

with WTP, the willingness to pay; AGE, the age of the household head; $GENDER$, the sex of the household head; EDU, the educational level of the household head; $COMP$, the household composition; MAT, the marital status of the household head; $INCOME$, the income level; $DIST$, the distance to the nearest health facility, $RESIDENCE$, the location of residence.

Because some individuals may not be willing to pay for pre-financing healthcare, our dependent variable (WTP for MHI) is a censored variable. Under these circumstances, the use of the ordinary least squares method is inappropriate because it leads to biased and inconsistent estimates [24]. A limited dependent variable model is therefore more appropriate. For this reason, the Tobit model [25] is chosen. The econometric model of willingness-to-pay for the MHI is then:

$$L_h = X'_h \beta + \xi_h \tag{2}$$

where L_h is a latent variable close to the maximum premium that a household head h is willing to pay. We assume that L_h linearly depends on X_h -the household head's characteristics and the characteristics of his/her household as well as the availability of health facilities (distance to the nearest health facility as described above) - via a parameters vector β; ξ_h is a normally distributed error term (with average equal to zero and a constant variance σ^2) to capture random influences on this relationship.

Let us suppose that Y_h is the total premium that an individual h is willing to pay. Y_h (the observed variable) is

defined to be equal to the latent variable whenever the latent variable is above zero and zero otherwise.

$$Y_h = \begin{cases} X'_h \beta + \xi_h & if \quad L_h > 0 \\ 0 & if \quad L_h \leq 0 \end{cases} \tag{3}$$

The Tobit model makes it possible to value the parameters β and σ^2 from the observations of Y_h and X_h. Since the total amount of WTP Y_h can be either positive or zero, the likelihood function can be expressed as follows:

$$L(\beta, \sigma^2/Y, X) = \prod_{Y_h=0} \left[1 - \Phi\left(\frac{X'_h \beta}{\sigma}\right) \right] \prod_{Y_h>0} \left[\frac{\phi\left[(Y_h - X'_h \beta)/\sigma\right]}{\sigma} \right] \tag{4}$$

Where Φ and ϕ represent the distribution function and the density function respectively.

Results
Descriptive statistics

Table 1 shows some socio-demographic characteristics of Togolese ISW households. The data indicates that overall, ISW aged 15 to 35 represent 48.4%. The following category is aged 35 to 60 (45.1%). People over 60 years of age represent only 6.4%. Most households had between 2 and 4 persons (56.9%). Nearly 70% of ISW are married, compared to 16% who are single. We also note that there are more widows than widowers. This result can be explained by two phenomena, namely higher male mortality and the age gap at first marriage. According to data from Togo's National Institute of Statistics and Economic and Demographic Studies (INSEED) [26], women's life expectancy at birth is 64.2 years compared to 56.4 years for men [27]. Similarly, women marry earlier than men; the age at first marriage for men is 25.0 years compared to 19.7 years for women [27].

Concerning education, the results show that most Togolese ISW (36%) have no educational level. 26.4% have primary school education, 34.5% secondary school education and only 3.1% have university education. Furthermore, Table 1 shows that 45.8% of women have no educational level compared to 21.9% of men. There are some gender-based disparities. The results show also that as the level of education rises, the gap between men and women increases. These disparities can be explained by the inequalities of retention between girls and boys in the school system. The low retention of girls can be explained by early pregnancies that increase their dropout rate compared to boys. In addition, some customary practices predispose girls to domestic work, which can increase their rate of failure and dropout compared to boys. The same customary practices explain the fact that girls most often drop out of school to be economically active in order to help the household when the need arises.

Table 1 Socio-demographic characteristics (%)

Characteristics	Urban			Rural			Total		
	Men	Women	All	Men	Women	All	Men	Women	All
Characteristics of household head									
Age									
15–35	56.8	52.3	54.0	41.4	41.4	41.4	49.1	47.9	48.4
35–60	40.4	43.6	42.4	48.9	48.1	48.5	44.7	45.4	45.1
More than 60 years	2.7	4.0	3.6	9.6	10.4	10.0	6.2	6.6	6.4
Educational level									
None	10.7	31.0	23.5	32.9	67.8	51.6	21.9	45.8	36.0
Primary	18.4	29.0	25.1	34.3	22.6	28.0	26.4	26.4	26.4
Secondary	59.3	38.1	45.9	32.3	9.5	20.1	45.8	26.6	34.5
University	11.5	1.9	5.4	0.4	0.1	0.3	6.0	1.2	3.1
Marital status									
Single	33.9	16.8	23.1	9.3	5.1	7.1	21.6	12.1	16.0
Married	60.7	66.2	64.2	84.5	70.3	76.9	72.6	67.8	69.8
Divorced or separated	3.9	7.5	6.2	3.6	6.3	5.1	3.7	7.0	5.7
Widow/widower	1.5	9.5	6.5	2.6	18.2	11.0	2.0	13.0	8.5
Household size									
Single	53.4	34.4	41.4	23.8	21.0	22.3	38.6	29.0	33.0
2 to 4	38.9	56.5	50.1	64.0	66.8	65.5	51.5	60.6	56.9
4 to 6	6.3	7.9	7.3	10.6	9.8	10.2	8.5	8.6	8.6
more than 6	1.2	1.2	1.2	1.6	2.5	2.1	1.4	1.7	1.6

Willingness to pay

Table 2 presents descriptive statistics of income and WTP. It shows that on average an ISW earns a monthly income of 59,726 FCFA (USD 108.6), or 1.71 times the guaranteed minimum wage (SMIG). Men earn a higher income (62,490.9 FCFA or USD 113.6) than women (57,076 FCFA or USD 103.8). Moreover, ISW in urban areas earn on average a higher income (72,734.6 FCFA, or USD 132.2) than those in rural areas (42,263.3 FCA or USD 76.8). However, overall, Togolese ISW are willing to pay 2569 FCFA (or USD 4.7) per month on average to be involved in MHI. This amount represents about 4.3% of their average monthly income. On average, men are willing to pay a higher premium (3168.9 FCFA or USD 5.8, which represents 5.1% of their average monthly income) than women (2077 FCFA or USD 3.8, which represents 3.6% of their average income). Similarly, ISW in urban areas are willing to pay on average a higher premium (2860 FCFA, or USD 5.2, which represents 3.9% of their income) than those living in rural areas (2116.4 FCFA or USD 3.8, which represents 5% of their income).

Table 2 also indicates that overall, WTP increases as we move from a lower quintile to an upper quintile. WTP increased from 1881.8 FCFA (or USD 3.4) in quintile 1 (the poorest quintile) to 3959.5 FCFA (or USD 7.2) in quintile 5 (the richest quintile). However, in terms of proportion, ISW in the poorest quintiles are willing to allocate more important part of their income to the premium than the richest quintiles. For example, ISW in quintile 1 are willing to allocate on average, 15% of their income to the MHI while those in quintile 5 are willing to allocate only 2.5% of their income. Furthermore, women are willing to allocate a lower part of their income (3.7%) than men (5.1%). Similarly, ISW in urban areas are willing to allocate a lower part of their income (3.9%) than those residing in rural areas (5%).

Table 3 summarizes the distribution of WTP by sex and location. Overall, 92.7% of Togolese ISW are interested in health insurance. This result reveals that there is a strong demand for health insurance by ISW. However, the majority of workers (47.2%) are willing to pay a maximum premium of 1226 FCFA (USD 2.2) per month, which is at least equal to the monthly premium of a worker in the formal sector who earns the guaranteed minimum wage (SMIG) per month. Furthermore, 45.43% of ISW are willing to pay more than the premium of an ISW earning more than the minimum wage, and more than 16% are willing to pay more than thrice the premium of an employee earning the SMIG.

Table 4 shows the distribution of willingness to pay by income quintile, taking into account gender and location.

Table 2 Descriptive statistics of income and WTP by quintile

	Income (in US Dollar)			WTP (in US Dollar)			Average WTP in percentage of average income
	Mean	Max	Min	Mean	Max	Min	
All households	108.6 (161.6)	3930.9	0.0	4.7 (7.7)	72.7	0.0	4.3
Quintile 1	22.8 (10.1)	36.4	0.0	3.4 (7.4)	72.7	0.0	15.0
Quintile 2	54.2 (6.4)	63.6	37.9	3.6 (5.6)	72.7	0.0	6.7
Quintile 3	81.9 (7.9)	90.9	65.5	4.3 (5.1)	29.1	0.0	5.2
Quintile 4	113.3 (10.3)	136.4	91.6	4.4 (5.1)	29.1	0.0	3.8
Quintile 5	283.8 (306.5)	3930.9	140.0	7.2 (11.9)	72.7	0.0	2.5
Men							
All men	113.6 (172.5)	3930.9	0.0	5.8 (9.7)	72.7	0.0	5.1
Quintile 1	23.6 (9.9)	36.4	0.0	5.0 (10.4)	72.7	0.0	21.3
Quintile 2	54.5 (6.5)	63.6	37.9	4.5 (5.3)	29.1	0.0	8.2
Quintile 3	82.7 (7.8)	90.9	65.5	5.0 (5.9)	29.1	0.0	6.0
Quintile 4	113.4 (10.5)	136.4	91.6	4.8 (5.4)	29.1	0.0	4.3
Quintile 5	273.2 (313)	3930.9	140.0	8.4 (14.9)	72.7	0.0	3.1
Women							
All women	103.8 (150.3)	2236.4	0.0	3.8 (5.4)	72.7	0.0	3.7
Quintile 1	22.2 (10.1)	36.4	0.0	2.2 (2.8)	15.3	0.0	9.7
Quintile 2	53.9 (6.3)	63.6	38.2	3.1 (5.7)	72.7	0.0	5.7
Quintile 3	81.0 (7.9)	90.9	65.5	3.8 (4.3)	15.3	0.0	4.6
Quintile 4	113.2 (10.1)	136.4	92.7	3.9 (4.9)	29.1	0.0	3.5
Quintile 5	297.7 (297.7)	2236.4	141.8	5.9 (7.0)	29.1	0.0	2.0
Urban							
All urban	132.2 (181.7)	3930.9	0.0	5.2 (7.9)	72.7	0.0	3.9
Quintile 1	25.2 (11.3)	36.4	0.0	2.3 (3.0)	15.3	0.0	8.9
Quintile 2	55.1 (6.0)	63.6	37.9	3.7 (4.8)	29.1	0.0	6.8
Quintile 3	82.5 (7.6)	90.9	65.5	4.6 (5.5)	29.1	0.0	5.6
Quintile 4	113.8 (10.2)	136.4	92.7	4.8 (5.3)	29.1	0.0	4.2
Quintile 5	276.6 (304.7)	3930.9	140.0	7.7 (11.9)	72.7	0.0	2.8
Rural							
All rural	76.8 (122.9)	2181.8	0.0	3.8 (7.4)	72.7	0.0	5.0
Quintile 1	22.2 (9.6)	36.4	0.0	3.8 (8.3)	72.7	0.0	17.2
Quintile 2	53.1 (6.7)	63.6	38.2	3.5 (6.5)	72.7	0.0	6.6
Quintile 3	80.7 (8.2)	90.9	65.5	3.6 (4.2)	15.3	0.0	4.5
Quintile 4	112.2 (10.4)	136.4	91.6	3.4 (4.5)	29.1	0.0	3.0
Quintile 5	313.0 (312.8)	2181.8	141.8	5.5 (12.0)	72.7	0.0	1.8

() Standard deviations

As shown in the Table 4, outside the poorest quintile where the proportion of women not interested in MHI (14.1%) is higher than that of men (6.7%), women are more interested in MHI than men, regardless of the income quintile considered. Similarly, a higher proportion of women are willing to pay less than the premium of a formal sector worker earning the SMIG, regardless of the income quintile (61.5%; 61.0%; 43.3%; 51.2% and 48.8% respectively, from the poorest quintiles to the richest quintiles). These proportions are 51.4%; 41.8%; 39.7%; 38.8% and 36.8% respectively for men. As one moves towards the higher WTP brackets, the proportion of men tends to increase and that of women to decrease, meaning that the number of men willing to pay grows higher than that of women in almost all income quintiles. This finding confirms that women are generally more interested in MHI than men but that men are willing to pay higher premiums than women regardless of income levels.

Table 3 Distribution of WTP by sex and location of residence

WTP (in US Dollars)	Urban (%)			Rural (%)			Total (%)		
	Men	Women	All	Men	Women	All	Men	Women	All
Not interested	6.9	6.5	6.6	9.1	7.9	8.5	8.0	6.9	7.3
Less than 2.2	36.7	47.4	43.8	45.4	58.8	52.4	40.9	51.3	47.2
2.2–3.8	21.9	20.0	20.7	22.2	20.4	21.2	22.0	20.2	20.9
3.8–7.6	8.7	9.0	8.9	10.0	4.6	7.2	9.3	7.5	8.2
7.6–19.1	23.7	16.1	18.6	13.0	8.1	10.5	18.5	13.4	15.4
More than 19.1	2.1	1.1	1.4	0.3	0.2	0.3	1.2	0.8	0.9

The analysis of WTP distribution by educational level (Table 5) shows that 90% of Togolese ISW with no level of education are interested in health insurance, compared to 94% of those with primary level education; and 93.8% of those with university level education.

Determinants of willingness to pay

Table 6 summarizes the results of the Tobit model. Column (1) shows the results of the whole sample; then an analysis by gender of the head of the household is presented in columns (2) and (3); finally, columns (4) and (5) summaries the results by location of residence. At a 5% level, Table 6 (column (1)) reveals that the sex of the household head, the household size, education, income and square income are the main determinants of the ISWs' willingness to pay for health insurance. The results indicate a negative correlation between sex (female) and WTP. We also found that when the household size is larger, the household head is willing to pay a higher premium. Otherwise, variables such as age, location, marital status of the head of household, number of children in the household, number of persons over 60 in the

household, and distance to the nearest health facility have no significant effect on WTP.

The comparison of results by gender indicates that for female-headed households, income is the only variable that significantly explains WTP; household size is significant only at a 10% threshold. On the other hand, for male-headed households, apart from income, education and household size have a significant and positive effect on WTP. There are also some differences depending on location. In urban areas, the sex of the household head has a negative and significant effect on WTP, and no significant effect in rural areas. Similarly, in urban areas, income, age, number of people over 60 years of age, and education have a positive and significant effect on WTP. On the other hand, only income and household size have a significant effect on WTP in rural areas.

Discussion

Our results show that men are willing to pay more than women and corroborate those of Dong et al. [28] who showed that in Burkina Faso (country bordering Togo), men were willing to pay a high amount for access to

Table 4 Distribution of WTP by income quintile (in %)

WTP in US dollars	Not interested		Less than 2.2		2.2–3.8		3.8–7.6		7.6–19.1		More than 19.1	
Income quintile												
	Men	Women	Men	Women	Men	Women	Men	Women	Men	Women	Men	Women
Very poor	6.7	14.1	51.4	61.5	24.8	15.6	1.9	3.0	15.2	5.9	0.0	0.0
Poor	8.2	5.2	41.8	61.0	23.3	19.9	8.2	5.6	17.8	8.2	0.7	0.0
Middle	6.9	9.0	39.7	43.3	23.7	24.2	9.9	11.2	18.3	12.4	1.5	0.0
Rich	8.2	5.3	38.8	51.2	17.0	21.8	15.0	7.1	20.4	14.1	0.7	0.6
Very rich	7.0	2.4	36. 8	48.8	23.2	16.1	9.2	5.4	21.1	23.8	2.7	3.6
Location												
	Urban	Rural	Urban	Rural	Urban	Rural	Urban	Rural	Urban	Rural	Urban	Rural
Very poor	13.6	4.8	31.8	56.6	40.9	20.5	0.0	2.4	13.6	15.7	0.0	0.0
Poor	7.0	9.3	42.2	41.3	21.1	25.3	7.0	9.3	21.1	14.7	1.4	0.0
Middle	6.3	7.3	36.5	42.6	23.8	23.5	7.9	11.8	22.2	14.7	3.2	0.0
Rich	6.2	10.6	35.8	42.4	18.5	15.1	12.3	18.2	27.2	12.1	0.0	1.5
Very rich	6.1	9.4	33.3	45.3	21.2	28.3	9.1	9.4	26.5	7.5	3.8	0.0

Table 5 Willingness to pay according to the level of education of the household head

WTP in US Dollars	Educational level			
	None (%)	Primary (%)	Secondary (%)	University (%)
Not interested	10.0	6.0	5.8	6.2
Less than 2.2	55.6	45.4	40.9	37.5
2.2–3.8	16.6	24.6	22.6	18.7
3.8–7.6	5.9	10.4	9.1	4.2
7.6–19.1	11.3	12.0	20.7	33.3
More than 19.1	0.6	1.5	0.9	0.0
Average WTP (in US dollars)	1.5	1.8	2.0	2.2

community insurance compared to women. Atake and Agbodji [12], Onwujekwe et al. [18] as well as Bärnighausen et al. [15] also arrived at the same conclusion. A possible explanation for this might be that women are poorer and more vulnerable than men in the informal sector. Indeed, Agbodji et al. [29], Djahini-Afawoubo [30], and Noglo [31] have shown that in Togo, women are more vulnerable and more affected by multidimensional poverty than men. Our results show that women in Togo have a low level of education, fewer job opportunities, less income, etc. compared to men. All these factors could explain the difference in willingness to pay between men and women. It is therefore important to take gender into account in extending mandatory health insurance, in order to ensure that in poor households, women's lack of access to resources and inequitable decision-making power does not hinder their participation in MHI. Our findings suggest that, in extending the MHI project to the informal sector workers, it is also necessary to consider the possibility of providing highly subsidized or free health insurance for women, as a way of limiting the impoverishment of female-headed households.

Another finding of our study is that income, square income, education and household size are the main determinants of ISWs' willingness to pay for health insurance. Income has a positive effect on WTP. This result corroborates our expectations. The demand theory predicts a positive elasticity income for most goods (except inferior goods). Previous studies have also found a similar result [15, 21, 32]. The sign of square income being negative suggests that the relation between income and WTP is not linear. For low income levels, WTP increases as income increases. But once a certain threshold is reached, when income increases, the household heads reduce the maximum premium amount they are willing to pay for health insurance. It is therefore likely that for incomes below the threshold, the household head considers that his household is more vulnerable to health care expenditures. In this regard, health insurance is valued and the household head agrees to pay a higher amount. On the other hand, when the income is above the threshold, the household head can

cope more easily with important health care expenditures without encountering financial difficulties. He then considers that his household is less vulnerable to health care expenditures and becomes more unwilling to pay. In other words, he substitutes the consumption of other goods such as foodstuff for the consumption of health insurance.

One of the most interesting results is that heads of households with a higher education are willing to pay a higher premium compared to those with other levels of education. We found that primary and middle school education have no significant effect on WTP. Bärnighausen et al. [15] also found that an educational level above middle school positively and significantly influences WTP. From the Togolese context, we can deduce the existence of an educational disparity in the WTP for health insurance. Hence, the more educated people are better informed or better able to process the available information on accessibility to health insurance and its consequences in terms of financial protection. There is therefore a need to adopt a communications strategy to mitigate the effect of education on health insurance.

As Table 6 shows, the larger the household size, the more willing a household head is to pay a higher premium amount. These results contradict those of De Allegri et al. [32] who found that household size was an obstacle to community health insurance coverage in Burkina Faso, citing the financial burden that health insurance would create for all household members. The same is true of the conclusions reached by Jehu-Appiah et al. [33] to the effect that large households in Ghana were less likely to be enrolled in a health insurance scheme. The positive effect of household size on WTP in Togo can be explained by the vulnerability of informal employment. Most people working in the informal sector are also the most vulnerable [34]. Thus, given the irregular nature of their income, large households in the informal sector would be the most vulnerable to health expenditures [12, 35]. Access to health insurance would reduce catastrophic health expenditures in these types of households, improve health status and increase the productivity of their members [34].

Table 6 Result of the Tobit model

Variables	(1) All	(2) Male	(3) Female	(4) Urban	(5) Rural
Willingness to pay for MHI (WTP)					
Age	−14.1	−48.7	21.3	175.6**	−88.8
	(53.5)	(112.2)	(47.8)	(88.8)	(71.4)
Age2	−0.1	0.2	−0.3	−2.7**	0.9
	(0.6)	(1.3)	(0.5)	(1.1)	(0.8)
Rural area	−227.2	−205.0	−46.6		
	(282.2)	(528.2)	(273.2)		
Education Primary	55.7	136.6	121.7	430.9	−444.6
	(298.6)	(610.2)	(271.2)	(402.5)	(445.5)
Secondary	423.1	821.0	77.1	596.1	344.6
	(308.4)	(596.7)	(291.4)	(393.9)	(505.2)
University	1,9***	2,4**	531.8	2,4***	−5,1
	(709.0)	(1,1)	(1,0)	(751.6)	(3,6)
Income	0.02***	0.03***	0.01***	0.02***	0.01**
	(0.0)	(0.0)	(0.0)	(0.0)	(0.0)
Income 2	−1.8e-08***	−4.0e-08***	−1.3e-08***	−2.2e-08***	−1.5e-08*
	(3.2e-09)	(9.5e-09)	(2.7e-09)	(3.6e-09)	(8.1e-09)
Distance to health center: 100 m to less than 1 km	47.5	−679.9	584.2*	233.9	−649.1
	(332.7)	(636.4)	(314.7)	(390.6)	(693.7)
1 km to 3 km	−215.5	−820.2	293.7	−43.4	−278.7
	(323.3)	(604.8)	(310.0)	(430.1)	(492.1)
3 km to 5 km	−632.9	−1280	32.65	−1071	−513.7
	(611.6)	(1042)	(650.0)	(951.4)	(804.8)
More than 5 km	77.5	−335.8	299.6	−826.1	−195.3
	(642.5)	(1207)	(608.8)	(4292)	(712.8)
Household size	261.5***	471.1**	154.9*	183.3	419.8***
	(97.9)	(193.7)	(91.6)	(124.6)	(157.5)
Number of old persons	−47.8	−323.9	−61.7	4018***	−1261*
	(643.4)	(1429)	(551.2)	(1350)	(725.4)
Number of children	−264.1	−586.8	−82.9	−71.8	−570.7*
	(231.5)	(462.8)	(211.9)	(324.0)	(327.8)
Marital status: Married	−155.3	−151.7	−264.8	−249.5	−21.9

Table 6 Result of the Tobit model (Continued)

Variables	(1) All	(2) Male	(3) Female	(4) Urban	(5) Rural
	(331.9)	(621.8)	(322.6)	(383.6)	(664.2)
Divorced or separated	13.8	1844	−681.0	519.5	−666.8
	(602.2)	(1497)	(509.2)	(771.6)	(993.2)
Widow/widower	−68.1	1267	−643.6	257.4	−446.9
	(514.1)	(1447)	(440.1)	(666.7)	(873.8)
Gender: female	−805.2***			−1022***	−458.3
	(245.1)			(308.9)	(401.2)
Constant	1953*	2018	477.5	−1699	3349**
	(1128)	(2213)	(1046)	(1711)	(1586)
Sigma					
	4281***	5414***	2979***	4240***	4214***
	(79.0)	(149.1)	(74.1)	(99.9)	(125.1)
Observations	1605	723	882	976	629

0 Standard errors; *** p < 0.01, ** p < 0.05, * p < 0.1

Our results also reveal that over 92% of ISW would like to have access to health insurance, like those in the formal sector do. The advantages of health insurance would explain this high rate of ISW willingness' to be insured [1, 8, 9]. Access to universal health insurance would enable all household members in the informal sector to access the health services they need without experiencing financial difficulties. Access to health services would also enable ISW, which accounts for about 30% of GDP, to be more productive and contribute more actively to family and community life. Our results suggest that one of the best ways to improve the well-being of the population and growth in Togo would be to extend mandatory health insurance to the informal sector. This proposal is supported by the fact that the lowest WTP indicated by informal sector workers is close to the premium of a formal sector worker earning the SMIG per month. These results suggest that health insurance for ISW is possible provided the State subsidizes the insurance of the formal and informal sector workers equally.

An important issue for policy makers is to know how much the state would need to subsidize the extension of MHI to ISW. To answer this question, we need information on income and the total number of informal sector households in the total population.

According to the National Institute of Statistics and Economic and Demographic Studies (INSEED), the total population of Togo in 2018 is estimated at 7,352,000 inhabitants or about 1,564,255 households. Knowing that the ISW represent 90.4% of the Togolese population, the ISW population can be estimated at 1,414,087 households.

ISW's average income has been updated using the Central Bank of West African States (BCEAO) price index. Since the average income can be sensitive to extreme values, the ISW are grouped into income quintile to minimize this effect. Table 7 presents the updated average income and average WTP per quintile as well as the share of each quintile in the total ISW households. According to Table 7, ISW in the first two quintiles (41.8%) earn a monthly income lower than the SMIG.

As a result they are not eligible for MHI. A strategy that fails to include them in the MHI would be inappropriate, for universal coverage purpose. Thereof, the state should include them in the MHI and entirely subsidize their premium.

Assuming that the state would subsidize the entire premium of ISW in the first two quintiles and 50% of the premium of the rest, the monthly amount that the state would need to subsidize can be calculated using the following equation:

$$S = \sum_{i=1}^{5} Q_i \times Income_i \times \lambda_i \qquad (5)$$

Where S is the monthly subsidy, $Income_i$, the updated average income of quintile i, λ_i, the share of the state contribution paid to quintile i, and Q_i, the total number of informal sector households in the quintile i. The annual subsidy can be then estimated by multiplying the monthly subsidy by 12. Based on eq. (5), the annual subsidy is estimated at 53,826,018,966 FCFA or 4.1% of the state current general budget and 96% of the health sector budget. This implies that the State should increase its total allocation towards health sector by 96% in order to be able to extend MHI to ISW. The budget allocated to the health sector currently represents only 4.2% of the State's overall budget. Even if the state increases the health sector budget by 96%, it will not be able to respect the Abuja recommendation that requires each African State to allocate at least 15% of their budget to health sector. Summarizing, the MHI can be extended to ISW provided the state subsidizes the MHI by 4.1% of its current budget.

However, it's important to emphasize the difficulty of Government to have reliable information on ISW income. Given that the state should fully cover the contribution of ISW with a monthly income below the SMIG, this can lead to free riding problem since some ISW would be encouraged to declare income below the SMIG in order to be entirely covered by the state. This involves designing differentiated health service packages according

Table 7 Distribution of WTP and income by quintile

	Share in the population (%)	Actualized Average Income (USD)			Actualized Average WTP (USD)		
		Men	Women	All	Men	Women	All
All households	100.0	131.8	120.4	126.0	6.7	4.4	5.4
quintile 1	20.2	27.3	25.7	26.5	5.0	2.5	4.0
quintile 2	21.6	63.3	62.5	62.9	4.5	3.6	4.2
quintile 3	19.9	95.9	93.9	95.0	5.0	4.4	5.0
quintile 4	19.2	131.6	131.4	131.5	4.8	4.6	5.1
quintile 5	19.1	316.9	345.3	329.2	8.4	6.8	8.4

to the amount of each ISW's premium, so that the higher the premium, the greater the number of health services included in the package. Such a measure would provide an incentive for high-income ISW to contribute significantly and thus guarantee the sustainability of the system.

Limitations of the study

This study has some limitations. The data used to measure the various indicators was declared by the respondents themselves and cannot be verified using other administrative sources. We furthermore used income as an indicator to understand households' living standards. However, it may have been more appropriate to use household consumption expenditure given that it is more difficult to measure the income of the self-employed, particularly the ISW, and that the respondents were most often reluctant to disclose their income. On the other hand, due to lack of information on household consumption expenditure, we had to use income as an indicator of the standard of living. Lastly, WTP must not be considered as an insurance premium as it is only an indication of the respondents' willingness to pay for a given benefits package.

Conclusion

The main objective of this paper was to assess the willingness of ISW to pay for MHI, and to analyze the determinants of WTP. We were thus able to analyze how MHI can be extended to ISW. We found that the extension of MHI to ISW is possible in Togo. It is clear from our findings that about 92% of ISW wish to be enrolled in MHI, like those in the formal sector. On average, ISW are willing to pay 2569 FCFA (USD 4.7), which is higher than the premium of a formal sector worker who earns twice the SMIG. 47.2% of ISW are willing to pay an amount that is less than or equal to the premium of an ISW earning the SMIG, while 45.4% are willing to pay a higher amount. Over 16% are willing to pay over three times as much as an employee earning the SMIG. Men are willing to pay on average a higher premium than women. Similarly, urban residents are willing to pay on average a higher amount than rural residents. The determinants of WTP were identified as: sex of the household head, household size, education and income. A number of economic policy recommendations emerged from our study, namely.

It is possible to extend health insurance to ISW, since over 92% are in favor of it, and since an ISW earns on average 59,726 FCFA (USD 108.59), which is 1.7 times the amount required to be enrolled in the MHI. Given that one must earn a salary that is at least equal to the SMIG in order to be enrolled in the MHI and that, on average, ISW agree to pay an amount that is higher than the premium of a formal sector employee who earns twice the SMIG, the extension of MHI to informal sector workers would not jeopardize the viability of MHI. However, for the sake of equity, the State should subsidize formal and informal sector workers equally to avoid creating double standards within the health insurance scheme. Currently, an employee's premium to MHI amounts to 7% of their gross salary. The employee contributes 3.5% of his salary and the Government pays the other half. In the case of ISW, the Government should therefore adopt the same subsidy policy by paying half the premium of each worker.

Our results shown that the annual subsidy is estimated at 53,826,018,966 FCFA or 4.1% of the State's current general budget or 96% of the health sector budget. This implies that the State should increase the budget allocated to the health sector by 96% in order to be able to extend MHI to ISW. With regard to tax revenues, the estimated annual subsidy represents about 8.1%. In the context of poverty and scarcity of resources, Togolese Government should develop resource mobilization strategies to fund the extension of the MHI to the ISW. For this purpose, Government could study the possibility to increase taxes on products such as tobacco, alcohol, airline tickets, financial transactions, etc. Some Asian countries such as the Philippines and India have successfully funded their universal health insurance system with high taxes on tobacco and alcohol [36, 37]. Moreover, Government could plead for donors funding. It is important to emphasize that resource mobilization and management, as well as health services delivery, would be effective only in a context of improved governance. [38]

Furthermore, the design of differentiated health service packages appear very important because it would provide an incentive for high-income ISW to contribute significantly and thus guarantee the sustainability of the system.

There is also a need to adopt a communications strategy to mitigate the effect of low level education on health insurance. With this regard, communication on ISWs' access to MHI and its advantages should be done in local language or mother tongue. Such a program could involve every ISW. All awareness raising tools and manuals should be translated into the local languages.

Abbreviations

CBMS: Community-Based Monitoring System; CNSS: National Social Security Fund; CRT: Pension Fund of Togo; DFID: Department for International Development; GDP: Gross Domestic Product; IDRC: International Development Research Center; INAM: National Institute of Health Insurance; ISW: Informal Sector Workers; MHI: Mandatory Health Insurance; OLS: Ordinary Least Squares; PEP: Partnership for Economic Policy; SMIG: guaranteed minimum wage; UK Aid: United Kingdom Aid; WTP: Willingness to Pay

Acknowledgements

The authors would like to acknowledge the Community-Based Monitoring System program of the Partnership for Economic Policy (PEP), the Department for International Development (DFID) and the International Development Research Centre (IDRC)-Canada.

Authors' contributions

DMDA developed the analytical approach, performed the statically analysis and wrote the first draft of the manuscript. EHA substantially contributed to the data analyses, interpretation of the data, and provided comments on all draft. Both authors approved the final manuscript.

Competing interests

The authors declare that they have no competing interests.

References

1. Arrow KJ. Uncertainty and the welfare economics of medical care. J Health Polit Polic. 2001. https://doi.org/10.1215/03616878-26-5-851.
2. Krugman P. Why markets can't cure healthcare. 2009. https://krugman.blogs.nytimes.com/2009/07/25/why-markets-cant-cure-healthcare/. Accessed 15 Jun 2018.Currie J, Madrian BC. Health, health insurance and the labor market. Handbook of labor economics. 1999; doi:https://doi.org/10.1016/S1573-4463(99)30041-9.
3. Currie J, Madrian BC. Health, health insurance and the labor market. Handbook of Labor Economics. 1999. https://doi.org/10.1016/S1573-4463(99)30041-9.
4. Chaudhuri A, Roy K. Changes in out-of-pocket payments for healthcare in Vietnam and its impact on equity in payments, 1992–2002. Health Policy. 2008. https://doi.org/10.1016/j.healthpol.
5. Xu K, Evans DB, Kawabata K, Zeramdini R, Klavus J, Murray CJL. Household catastrophic health expenditure: a multicountry analysis. Lancet. 2003. https://doi.org/10.1016/S0140-6736(03)13861-5.
6. Agyepong IA, Adjei S. Public social policy development and implementation: a case study of the Ghana National Health Insurance scheme. Health Policy Plann. 2008. https://doi.org/10.1093/heapol/czn002.
7. Chetty R, Looney A. Consumption smoothing and the welfare consequences of social insurance in developing economies. J Public Econ. 2006. https://doi.org/10.1016/j.jpubeco.2006.07.002.
8. Sackey FG, Amponsah PN. Willingness to accept capitation payment system under the Ghana National Health Insurance Policy: do income levels matter? Health Econ Rev. 2017. https://doi.org/10.1186/s13561-017-0175-1.
9. Atake EH, Amendah DD. Porous safety net: catastrophic health expenditure and its determinants among insured households in Togo. BMC Health Serv Res. 2018. https://doi.org/10.1186/s12913-018-2974-4.
10. Okungu V, Chuma J, Mulupi S, McIntyre D. Extending coverage to informal sector populations in Kenya: design preferences and implications for financing policy. BMC Health Serv Res. 2018. https://doi.org/10.1186/s12913-017-2805-z.
11. Mills A. Strategies to achieve universal coverage: are there lessons from middle income countries? 2007. http://researchonline.lshtm.ac.uk/id/eprint/7020. Accessed 15 Jun 2018.
12. Atake EH, Agbodji AE. Togolese informal sector workers' willingness to pay for access to social protection. DLSU B&E Review. 2017;27:97–106.
13. OMS. La situation du financement de la santé au Togo, in Conférence HHA des ministres de la Santé et des Finances de la région Africaine. 2012. http://afrolib.afro.who.int/documents/2012/Fr/Togo.pdf. Accessed 07 Feb 2018.
14. Bignandi. La protection sociale en santé au Togo. 2014. http://www.coopami.org/fr/coopami/formation%20coopami/2015/pdf/2015090306.pdf. Accessed 07 Feb 2018.
15. Bärnighausen T, Liu Y, Zhang X, Sauerborn R. Willingness to pay for social health insurance among informal sector workers in Wuhan, China: a contingent valuation study. BMC Health Serv Res. 2007. https://doi.org/10.1186/1472-6963-7-114.
16. Donfouet HPP, Makaudze E, Mahieu PA, Malin E. The determinants of the willingness-to-pay for community-based prepayment scheme in rural Cameroon. Int J Health Care Finance Econ. 2011. https://doi.org/10.1007/s10754-011-9097-3.
17. Dong H, Mugisha F, Gbangou A, Kouyate B, Sauerborn R. The feasibility of community-based health insurance in Burkina Faso. Health Policy. 2004. https://doi.org/10.1016/j.healthpol.2003.12.001.
18. Onwujekwe O, Okereke E, Onoka C, Uzochukwu B, Kirigia J, Petu A. Willingness to pay for community-based health insurance in Nigeria: do economic status and place of residence matter? Health Policy Plann. 2009. https://doi.org/10.1093/heapol/czp046.
19. Khan JA, Ahmed S. Impact of educational intervention on willingness-to-pay for health insurance: a study of informal sector workers in urban Bangladesh. Health Econ Rev. 2013. https://doi.org/10.1186/2191-1991-3-12.
20. Arrow K, Solow R, Portney PR, Leamer EE, Radner R, Schuman H. Report of the NOAA panel on contingent valuation. 1993. https://www.researchgate.net/profile/Edward_Leamer/publication/277297107_Kenneth_Arrow/links/572a241108ae2efbfdbc1959/Kenneth-Arrow.pdf. Accessed 15 June 2018.
21. N'Guessan CFJ. Le consentement des ménages ruraux à payer une prime d'assurance maladie en Côte d'Ivoire. Revue d'économie du développement. 2008. https://doi.org/10.3917/edd.221.0101.
22. Bejean S. De nouvelles théories en économie de la santé: fondements, oppositions et complémentarités. Politiques et management public. 1999;17:145–75.
23. Gertler P, Gaag JVD. The willingness to pay for medical care: evidence from two developing countries. 1990. http://documents.worldbank.org/curated/en/483411468740192932/The-willingness-to-pay-for-medical-care-evidence-from-two-developing-countries. Accessed 5 June 2018.
24. Cameron AC, Trivedi PK. Microeconometrics: methods and applications. 1st ed. Cambridge: Cambridge University press; 2005.
25. Tobin J. Estimation of relationships for limited dependent variables. Econometrica. 1958;26:24–36.
26. INSEED. Etat matrimonial et nuptialité. 2016. http://togo.unfpa.org/sites/default/files/pub-pdf/TOGO_RGPH4_ETAT%20MATRIMONIAL%20ET%20NUPTIALITE.pdf. Accessed 15 Jun 2018.
27. INSEED, Mortalité. 2016. http://www.stat-togo.org/contenu/pdf/pb/pb-mortalite-rgph4-tg-2010.pdf. Accessed 15 Jun 2018.
28. Dong H, Kouyate B, Snow R, Mugisha F, Sauerborn R. Gender's effect on willingness-to-pay for community-based insurance in Burkina Faso. Health Policy. 2003. https://doi.org/10.1016/S0168-8510(02)00144-6.
29. Agbodji AE, Batana YM, Ouedraogo D. Gender inequality in multidimensional welfare deprivation in West Africa: the case of Burkina Faso and Togo. Int J Soc Econ. 2015;42:980–1004.
30. Djahini-Afawoubo DM. Inégalités de Genre et Pauvreté Multidimensionnelle au Togo. Revue d'Economie Théorique et Appliquée. 2015;5:77–95.
31. Noglo YA, Afawubo K. The change in monetary inequality among households in Togo over 2011-2015: an illustration based on the decomposition of the Gini coefficient using the Shapley value approach. Econ Bull. 2017;37:2602–15.
32. De Allegri M, Sanon M, Bridges J, Sauerborn R. Understanding consumers' preferences and decision to enrol in community-based health insurance in rural West Africa. Health Policy. 2006. https://doi.org/10.1016/j.healthpol.2005.04.010.
33. Jehu-Appiah C, Aryeetey G, Spaan E, De Hoop T, Agyepong I, Baltussen R. Equity aspects of the National Health Insurance Scheme in Ghana: who is enrolling, who is not and why? Soc Sci Med 2011; https://doi.org/10.1016/j.socscimed.
34. Ahmad N, Aggarwal K. Health shock, catastrophic expenditure and its consequences on welfare of the household engaged in informal sector. J Public Health. 2017. https://doi.org/10.1007/s10389-017-0829-9.
35. Brinda EM, Andrés RA, Enemark U. Correlates of out-of-pocket and catastrophic health expenditures in Tanzania: results from a national household survey. BMC Int Health Hum Rights. 2014. https://doi.org/10.1186/1472-698X-14-5.
36. Reddy KS, Patel V, Jha P, Paul VK, Kumar AKS, Dandona L. Towards achievement of universal health care in India by 2020: a call to action. Lancet. 2011. https://doi.org/10.1016/S0140-6736(10)61960-5.
37. Madore A, Rosenberg J, Weintraub R. "Sin taxes" and health financing in the Philippines. 2015. https://www.globalhealthdelivery.org/case-collection/case-studies/asia-and-middle-east/sin-taxes-and-health-financing-in-the-philippines. Accessed 22 Aug 2018.
38. Atake EH. Sustaining Gains in Health Programs: Technical Efficiency and its Determinants in Malaria Programs in Sub-Saharan Africa. Appl Health Econ Health Policy. 2017. https://doi.org/10.1007/s40258-016-0294-6.

10

A survey-based design of a pricing system for psychotherapy

Beat Hulliger* and Martin Sterchi

Abstract

For admission to statutory health insurance, it is common in Switzerland that health care providers negotiate prices for health care services directly with health insurers. Once they agree upon a price, they must submit the resulting price to the Federal Office of Public Health (FOPH), which can then authorize it. Swiss law requires the prices in health care to be based on empirical data. There has been little research on how to derive such a price for health care from empirical data and which data should be used. Based on a collaboration with psychological psychotherapists in Switzerland, we have designed a pricing system. The empirical basis were two representative surveys: a survey about costs and earnings of psychotherapists, as well as a time-use survey for psychotherapy. This paper shows the methodology followed to establish an empirically based pricing system. The paper may serve as a practical guide for health service providers who want to develop a pricing system. Our approach offers a high degree of freedom because it involves the collection of the data and an explicit modelling phase. At the same time, it might be more resource intensive than other approaches that are based on existing data sources.

Keywords: Survey, Health insurance, Health care pricing, Tariff system, Regulation

JEL codes: C83, I13, I18

Introduction

The Swiss health care system comprises four main stakeholders. First, there are the resident citizens who are required to have statutory health insurance by law. Second, there are health care providers such as hospitals, medical practitioners and others. Third, private competing insurance companies provide statutory health insurance, as well as supplementary health insurance. The fourth important stakeholder, the government, regulates statutory health insurance. On a national level, most tasks with respect to health care are assumed by the Federal Office of Public Health (FOPH). FOPH authorizes the insurance premiums and oversees the scope of mandatory coverage of health services, among other things. In addition, the 26 cantons have a critical role since they are the main political entities responsible for health care in Switzerland. The cantons license insurance providers, organize the health care offered in hospitals and manage the subsidies for health care institutions, among other things [1].

In Switzerland, a fee-for-service scale called TARMED regulates the price of outpatient health care by medical doctors. It categorizes all the services of outpatient health care and contains a relative cost weight for each of these services. Based on this relative cost weight, the health insurance companies and health care providers negotiate the effective price for a service in every canton and on a yearly basis [1]. However, TARMED only applies to care providers with a medical degree. In particular, it regulates psychotherapeutic services offered by medical doctors with a psychiatric specialization. In recent years, the national government expanded the scope of statutory health insurance to include more non-medical care providers. The most recent expansion concerned the neuropsychologists. The national government officially recognized them as care providers in December 2016 [2]. This allows them to provide care independently and at their own account within the framework of statutory health insurance.

* Correspondence: beat.hulliger@fhnw.ch
Institute for Competitiveness and Communication, University of Applied Sciences and Arts Northwestern Switzerland (FHNW), Riggenbachstrasse 16, 4600 Olten, Switzerland

In 2012, the Federal Law on Psychological Professions (PsyG) became effective [3]. It defines the requirements for psychotherapists to obtain the psychotherapy practice license and in particular, it sets educational standards for psychological psychotherapists. This law serves as the basis for the extension of statutory health insurance to cover psychological psychotherapists. The Swiss Federal Health Insurance Act (KVG, Art. 43) defines that health care providers should negotiate the prices directly with the health insurers. The Swiss Federal Council only interferes if the negotiations do not succeed. In collaboration with three associations representing the psychological psychotherapists, a pricing system for psychotherapy, which will be the basis for the negotiations with the health insurers, was developed. During all stages of the process of designing the pricing system, a close collaboration of the research team with a project group that consisted of representatives from the three associations of psychotherapists, among them practicing psychotherapists, ensured proper alignment with the objectives of the project.

For a pricing system two elements are required: i) the tariff structure, which is a systematic nomenclature with the exact definitions of the services of psychotherapy including the units of measurement and ii) a relative price scale for each position of the tariff structure. The price scale is expressed in terms of tax points and is set in such a way that one tax point corresponds to approximately one Swiss Franc. The challenges for establishing a pricing system are manifold. First, the services must be mapped correctly and coherently onto the tariff structure. Second, the tariff structure must be sufficiently precise and detailed such that psychotherapists can clearly and unambiguously assign their time spent to the appropriate position in the tariff structure. Likewise, the tariff structure must be sufficiently general in order to fulfil the requirements of all types of psychotherapists (e.g. general psychotherapy vs. emergency psychotherapy). Nevertheless, the tariff structure should be simple enough such that it can be applied in practice without too much effort. Finally, yet importantly, the pricing system must allow an efficient practitioner to achieve a fair income. In other words, a psychotherapist satisfying some predetermined share of therapy-related (billable) activities must be able to cover all their costs and earn a fair income. However, the question of what a fair income for a psychotherapist is will be the subject of negotiations between the stakeholders.

Apart from a vast body of literature about systems based on diagnosis related groups (DRG) (e.g. [4]), there is little published literature on designing pricing systems for statutory health care. However, the Swiss regulatory body outlines some principles for designing such a pricing system. First and foremost, statutory health insurance must be non-profit [1]. Accordingly, the Health Insurance Ordinance (KVV, Art. 59c, 1b) states that the price can only cover the costs necessary for an efficient service provision. Furthermore, it defines that the underlying costs need to be disclosed (KVV, Art. 59c, 1a). In other words, the pricing system needs to be transparent and it must be based in some way on empirical data. However, it does not define how the empirical data should be collected and how it should be used in designing a pricing system.

In this paper, we propose a pricing system for psychotherapy that relies upon the results of a representative survey about the costs and earnings of psychotherapists, as well as a representative time-use survey. This paper may serve as a pragmatic guide for other health care providers attempting to establish a pricing system in health care. We present the methodological choices faced and the rationale for decisions made. Due to confidentiality agreements with the three associations representing the psychotherapists, we cannot reveal any specific results of our approach. Nevertheless, the description of the approach should help to stimulate the discussion about the methods of establishing a tariff system.

This paper is organized as follows. Section Methods explains how the tariff structure was developed and describes the design, execution, data preparation and analysis of the costs and earnings survey and of the time-use survey. Section Results presents the results and explains how we used the empirical results to establish a pricing model for the computation of the final price for psychotherapy services. Section Discussion discusses some problems and possible extensions of our approach. Finally, Section Conclusion concludes.

Methods

Tariff structure

Before a price can be established, the goods to be priced must be clearly defined. In the case of psychotherapy, the goods are services. The systematic nomenclature of psychotherapy services is the tariff structure. It represents the different health care services offered by psychotherapists in a structured way such that they can be aggregated into categories of services. For every service, the mode of delivering the service is determined. A psychotherapy session, for example, can be held as a face-to-face meeting, but also by phone or even online. In addition, a psychotherapy session involving a group or the parents of the patient is different from a one-on-one session, first because the work of the psychotherapist is different and secondly because the amount charged for the psychotherapy session may be split up among the patients of the group session. Furthermore, for some services such as the evaluation of psychological test results there is no physical presence of the patient necessary. The tariff structure precisely describes every service and defines the billable unit. A psychotherapy service is either priced overall, or, as in other service-oriented tariffs, the service is priced per time used. The elements in the tariff structure are based on 5 min-units, i.e. the smallest billable unit are 5 min of a service. However, some services such as writing a formalized report for the health insurers are priced overall and are thus reimbursed with a flat rate price.

The project team developed a first version of a tariff structure in several rounds of discussion. Qualitative interviews with several psychological psychotherapists helped to structure the tariff. For the further development of the tariff structure, a workshop with psychotherapists was organised in order to establish a better understanding of the domain and of the different services of psychotherapy. The participating psychotherapists were from different fields such as general psychotherapy, psychotherapy for children and adolescents, psychotherapy for elderly people, and emergency psychotherapy. The goal of the workshop was to find out, which services need to be taken into account and whether or not the proposed tariff structure was covering the needs of various types of psychotherapy in a useful way. In order to have a concentrated discussion, four fictional cases of psychotherapy were submitted to the participants. The cases were meant to capture many facets of psychotherapy and were sent to the participants prior to the workshop. The fictional cases also covered typical situations such as a patient not showing up for a meeting, an emergency meeting or a psychotherapy session in special conditions such as accompanying patients when using public transport. After the integration of the outcomes of the workshop, a next version of the tariff structure was developed. This version was used in a pilot study with ten volunteering psychotherapists. The participants reported all their activities during one week as if the tariff structure was already in place. The tariff structure was further adapted by taking the outcome of the pilot study into account. Thus, the tariff structure evolved in five feedback loops. This included adding and removing positions or simply clarifying certain positions. The elements of the tariff structure served as the basis for the time-use survey.

Survey about costs and earnings

A major issue for the survey on costs and earnings is that psychotherapists in Switzerland work in different economic models [5]. While many psychotherapists work independently and at their own account, there are psychotherapists who are working on behalf of a psychiatrist or a general practitioner (GP). In that case, the medical doctor (psychiatrist or GP) is the responsible therapist and thus the treatment is eligible for coverage through statutory health insurance under TARMED.

This model of psychotherapy is called delegated psychotherapy. Furthermore, there are psychotherapists who are employed by an in- or outpatient facility for mental health care, which bills psychotherapy costs under a special tariff. Finally, a considerable number of psychotherapists exhibit some combination of the aforementioned models and assume further activities such as academic teaching. As a result, most of the psychotherapists' independent work is part-time. Hence, the survey needed to account for those different economic models. For example, a psychotherapist who works independently and at their own account while, at the same time, is also employed by a psychiatrist needs to be able to capture their costs and earnings for the different models separately. Another complication is that some psychotherapists work in multiple practices and keep separate accounts.

A pilot survey clearly showed that the respondents cannot be asked for detailed accounts of all these activities separately. The questionnaire, although implemented in an online tool, was too complex. Therefore, we redesigned the questionnaire in order to define the most important independent primary practice with respect to costs and earnings. In other words, a participant working in more than one practice must only report the costs and earnings of the practice in which they worked the most during the survey period. Finally, several psychotherapists may work together in a group practice and thus share the costs. In that case, participants were asked to only report their share of the costs.

The survey focused on the costs and earnings of psychotherapists in 2014. Of particular interest are the costs and earnings of the psychotherapists who work independently and at their own account since this economic model resembles the future of psychotherapy the most. Nevertheless, the survey also captured the costs and earnings of delegated psychotherapists. This procedure has two advantages. First, it allows us to compare the independently working psychotherapists with the delegated psychotherapists. Secondly, it triggered participants working in both models to separate costs and earnings of the different models and therefore enforced consistent answers. However, the inclusion of delegated psychotherapists involved a delicate filtering scheme at the beginning of the questionnaire. The filtering prioritized the independent economic model as long as the psychotherapist worked at least 8 h per week in this model. Psychotherapists working less than 8 h per week as independent psychotherapists were still questioned about costs and earnings as delegated psychotherapists as long as the workload in this model accounted for at least 8 h per week. For all other psychotherapists, no questions about costs and earnings were asked.

Next, the questionnaire contained some general questions about the working model, including forms of collaboration, facilities, number of employees and sub-contractors. We also asked participants if their practice was set up in 2014 or if it was shut down during the course of 2014 in order to determine non-representative observations.

As for the costs, we asked participants to report their acquisitions as well as their operational costs. The positions are listed in Table 1. Certain positions were further divided; for example, salaries were broken down into net income, social security contributions, pension fund contributions and insurance premiums. Positions that were unclear were explained with examples. Moreover, participants had the option to specify further costs manually in the form of free text input. In order to check the consistency and plausibility of the reported costs, we asked participants to indicate their earnings as well. Earnings were subdivided based on who paid for the treatment. Hence, the main categories were private patients/supplementary health insurance, accident insurance and disability insurance, among others.

In addition to costs and earnings, the survey asked participants to specify the average workload in the primary practice in hours per week and work weeks per year. This information was necessary to compute the average level of capacity utilization for every participant. This was crucial since most of the participants work part-time as psychotherapists and hence, in most cases,

the reported costs and earnings correspond to a part-time workload. For example, a participant working only one day as an independent psychotherapist was supposed to indicate only the costs related to this work-load. Consequently, the responses were standardized in the processing phase (see Section Processing of survey results) in order to represent the costs of a full time employment.

The population of interest are all psychological psychotherapists in Switzerland with a federal license. Since the register of FOPH containing all relevant psychotherapists was not operational at the time of the survey, the address databases of the three associations of psychological psychotherapists involved in the project were used as sampling frame. The information about the practice license was used to delimit the members of the associations who should participate in the survey. However, there is a number of psychotherapists who are federally licensed but are not a member of an association [5]. The population coverage by the members of the associations was estimated to be at least 87%. Hence, the sampling frame was restricted to the members of the associations with a psychotherapy license. The sampling frame contained $N = 4297$ psychotherapists (Table 2). Since a considerable non-response must be expected in such a time consuming survey, the sample was exhaustive, i.e. the full population was surveyed. This resulted in a sufficiently large net sample size of 1336 observations before data processing, whereof 466 observations correspond to psychotherapists who work, at least partially, as independent psychotherapists.

The survey was administered with the software *Questback* that allowed participants to enter their data online. The questionnaire was available in German and French. The survey allowed participants to report their answers within a period of 3 weeks. They received an information letter and an invitation by e-mail and they were able to contact the survey team via a generic e-mail address. After 2 weeks, a reminder with full support of the psychotherapy associations was sent out and the fieldwork was extended by 2 weeks to allow more participants to finish the data entry. At the end of the questionnaire about the costs and earnings, survey participants were asked to choose one out of three subsequent weeks to participate in the time-use survey. The participants were

Table 1 Overview of cost positions that participants of the survey had to answer

Acquisitions
Furnishing
Electrical equipment
Telecommunication devices (including computers)
Vehicles
Therapy-related acquisitions
Psychological test material and other acquisitions
Operational costs
Lease costs
Transportation expenses
Staff costs
Salaries
Training costs
Interest
Telecommunication
Office supplies
Insurance fees
Marketing and accounting expenditures
Therapy-related costs (books, tests, etc.)

Table 2 Size of sampling frame and number of completed questionnaires

Sampling frame (N)	4297
Completed questionnaires (total)	1336
Independent psychotherapists	466
After processing	355

advised to choose a week that is representative of their typical workload.

Time-use survey

The design of a time-use survey involves a substantial amount of methodological considerations about the mode of the survey, the coding scheme and follow-up probes [6]. The mode of the time-use survey was similar to that used for the survey about the costs and earnings. Hence, the time-use survey was conducted online with the software *Questback*. The advantage of the online mode compared to more traditional paper and pencil approaches or approaches involving *Microsoft Excel* was more control at the input stage, more coherent reporting and more control for the survey managers about the response behavior. The participants reported their activities on a daily basis during a week including the weekend. One reason why weekends were included was because some psychotherapists are part of an emergency service and thus, they might report activities on weekends as well. Furthermore, it is common for psychotherapists to see patients on Saturdays. We notified participants by e-mail before the start of the week they had chosen at the end of the costs and earnings survey. Every morning during the survey period, an e-mail with the link to the survey was sent to the participants in order to motivate them to report their activities promptly.

In order to conduct a clear and meaningful time-use survey, we needed to provide a comprehensive list of possible activities of psychotherapists, i.e. a coding scheme, from which the participants could choose. Generally, the list of activities reflected the elements of the tariff structure. However, it was necessary to add further elements in order to cover the range of possible activities completely. For example, we included activities such as work breaks, the waiting time in-between patients and administration and organization of the practice. Finally, with 'other activities' we were able to capture any other activities that could not be assigned to an activity of the list. Overall, participants could choose from a list of 25 activities. We asked participants to report their activities chronologically and provided 40 possible entries per day. However, reported activities and their order could be revised at any time. To avoid typing errors participants could select their answers from a drop-down menu. In addition to the activity coding, the time spent on every activity was required. The time unit was 5 min as for the tariff. Again, participants were able to choose from a drop-down menu of time periods starting with 5 min and ending at 600 min. Furthermore, we asked participants to indicate the mode of work, the mode of communication and whether the activity reported corresponded to an emergency or not. For the

mode of work, participants could choose between independent work, work resulting from an employment by a psychiatrist, i.e. delegated psychotherapy, or activities in a mental health care facility. The possible modes of communication were face-to-face, by phone or online.

In addition to the activities, we asked participants to specify the start and end time of the respective workday, which allowed us to check whether the reported activities were consistent with the total daily work time or not.

Of the 551 psychotherapists who agreed to participate in the time-use survey, 321 completed the questionnaire.

Processing of survey results

Survey data typically contains missing values and outliers and is inconsistent in many different ways. Therefore, the data must be processed before starting with the analysis. In the paragraphs that follow, the performed processing of the costs and earnings data is explained in detail. At the end of this section, we briefly describe the processing of the results of the time-use survey.

Implausible observations in the survey about the cost and earnings were discarded. One source to assess the plausibility of an observation was the participant's comments. For example, observations were dropped if the participant specified that the indicated costs and earnings were not representative for their usual work situation. Furthermore, observations were discarded if either all costs or all operational costs were missing. Observations with missing earnings were not discarded although in those cases the cross-checks between costs and earnings were not possible. Discarding observations due to non-reporting of earnings would have reduced the sample size dramatically. It seems that a majority of the participants experienced difficulties indicating their proper earnings.

Based on common accounting principles, we transformed reported values for acquisitions into amortization values, which represent the yearly cost of an acquisition. The current linear depreciation rates of the Swiss tax authorities for business entities were used as amortization rates [7]. For example, if a psychotherapist acquires a computer for 3000 Swiss francs, the corresponding amortization rate is 20%.[1] Hence, the psychotherapist needs to take into account yearly costs of 600 Swiss francs for the acquisition of the computer. Critics might argue that the survey should ask participants to report amortization values instead of acquisition values. However, in order not to increase the complexity of the survey any further, only the acquisition values were collected.

Imputation of missing lease costs and salaries was necessary because of the importance of these two positions. They turned out to be the most substantial cost drivers of independent psychotherapy. As for the lease costs, the survey contained different questions depending on whether a psychotherapist owns the rooms for the practice or only rents them. In the latter case, the participants were asked to indicate the lease costs (on a yearly basis) as well as the supplementary costs such as costs for heating and electricity. However, if the participants own the rooms for their practice, they were asked to declare the imputed rental value, a concept used in the computation of taxes in Switzerland. The supplementary costs were added either to the lease costs or to the imputed rental value in order to get the gross rental costs per year. If the resulting gross rental cost was less than 2000 Swiss francs, we assumed that the participant erroneously indicated the monthly cost instead of the yearly cost. In those cases, we multiplied the amount by 12 in order to impute yearly costs. With regard to the salaries, a number of participants did not indicate their salary but all their other costs and earnings. In that case, the difference between earnings and costs was imputed as a proxy of their salary. Furthermore, some participants indicated zero costs for positions that, by definition, cannot be zero. For example, every psychotherapist who works independently must exhibit costs arising from social security contributions. Therefore, such zero values were set to missing values in order not to distort the statistical computations (Section Statistical analysis) with zeros that are in fact missing values.

Finally, as discussed above, comparability of costs requires standardizing all the observations related to a part-time workload. For this purpose, the capacity utilization level was determined for every participant. Based on the average workload in the primary practice expressed in hours per week and weeks per year, the average workload per year in hours could be determined for every participant in the sample. Following the recommendations of the professional associations [8], observations with at least 1824 h per year were considered a full time workload. The workload of observations with less than 1824 h per year was determined proportionally. A psychotherapist working, for example, 900 h per year exhibits a workload of 49%. The capacity utilization level was used to standardize all costs except for the amortization values of the acquisitions and the gross rental costs. The rationale for excluding the amortization values from the standardization process is that at least part of these costs are fixed, in other words, they do not vary with the capacity utilization level. For example, psychotherapists acquire office furniture regardless of whether they work one or five days a week. Moreover, a comparison of the gross rental costs with the capacity utilization levels showed that for some observations rental costs are disproportionately high. This implies that in some cases, the capacity of a practice might not be used

efficiently. Therefore, the amortization values of the acquisitions and the gross rental costs were standardised using factors that are smaller than the corresponding capacity utilization levels. This ensured that acquisition costs and gross rental costs were not overstated. As can be seen in Table 2, the final sample after processing contained 355 observations.

As for the time-use survey, we first imputed the time for mandatory work breaks based on Swiss law since work breaks were in many cases not reported properly. Hence, for every 4 h of work, we imputed a break of 15 min. Based on those imputed values and all the other activities reported by the participants, we were able to compute the total workload for each participating psychotherapist. We then discarded observations with a workload of less than 8 h per week because we considered such a workload as not representative. The final sample contained 187 observations. Finally, we aggregated the time for every activity over all participants and divided the sum per activity by the overall number of hours worked, thus arriving at a weighted proportion where the weight is proportional to the total work time per participant. As a result, we found a percentage for every activity that is likely to represent a psychotherapist's typical workday. As a hypothetical example, we might have found that a psychotherapist typically spends 10% of their time on the administration and organization of their practice, 70% on psychotherapy sessions, and so forth.

We carried out the processing of the data, as well as the statistical computations (Section Statistical analysis) in R [9].

Statistical analysis

In order to use the survey results for designing the pricing system, we needed to calculate average costs and earnings for every position that are a good representation of a typical psychotherapy practice. An obvious choice for summarizing data is the arithmetic mean. However, using the arithmetic mean in our case would have serious drawbacks due to the characteristics of the data. First of all, the data contains outliers that tend to inflate the arithmetic mean. This is especially problematic if outliers are the result of measurement error, i.e. misreported costs or earnings. Secondly, the data contains many observations that are zero and thus exhibit characteristics of a semi-continuous distribution with a peak at zero. Furthermore, we decided that observations should be weighted according to the capacity utilization level. In other words, we consider participants with a high capacity utilization level as more representative for a typical psychotherapist's practice than those with a low capacity utilization level. For all those reasons, we decided to summarize the data by using a trimmed, weighted mean that accounts for zero-inflated variables with the weights being the capacity utilization level.

Our concerns about selection bias were mitigated as the responding sample corresponded well with the population shares of the available covariates. Thus, no additional poststratification weights were applied. Potential selection bias may arise as the result of two scenarios. First, psychotherapists with a low income may have higher non-response rates than the rest of the psychotherapists due to stress. Secondly, psychotherapists who desire to change their working conditions may have lower non-response rates than the rest of the psychotherapists. Both scenarios can lead to a bias in average costs. We could imagine similar effects if highly efficient psychotherapists exhibit a low non-response, and/or inefficient psychotherapists exhibit a high non-response. The sample structure of respondents gives no clear indication of bias in one direction or the other. The discussion of the survey results with practitioners and the project team has shown that our results are credible.

Trimming of extreme observations is a commonly used robustification method. It relies on the assumption that the bulk of the data has a normal or near-normal distribution and that a few outliers occur on both sides of the main distribution. If the data has a semi-continuous distribution with one discrete mass (in our case the zero observations), then this assumption does not hold anymore. One way to treat outliers is to separate the discrete part before trimming is applied and add the discrete value with its appropriate weight after trimming. In addition, we often need to compute a weighted estimator. A detailed description of our estimation procedure is provided in the appendix. In the section that follows, we will show how the statistical results of the costs and earnings survey were combined with the results from the time-use survey in order to compute the price of psychotherapeutic care.

Results

The key elements for the computation of the price are the results from the survey about the costs and earnings and the time-use survey. However, the survey results represent the current situation of psychotherapists whereas the price must be based on costs and a time-use that represent the future work situation of psychotherapists under the new tariff system. Hence, it was crucial to transform and adjust the survey results into a pricing system that models the future situation of psychotherapists appropriately. This included: i) omitting certain costs reported in the survey, ii) adding costs not contained in the survey and iii) deviating from the survey results in some cases. Similar to the time-use survey, the primary task was to define which activities are covered under statutory health insurance. A more

detailed account of the steps necessary is given in the following paragraphs and Fig. 1 illustrates the model.

First of all, a careful analysis of every cost position was conducted in order to determine the total cost that is admissible under statutory health insurance. For every cost position, we defined whether it should be included in the computation or not. The transportation expenses illustrate this point. They were included in the survey in order to have a comprehensive set of costs but were not considered in the final pricing model. Including the transportation expenses in the computation of the price for psychotherapy services would be hard to justify in negotiations since having a car, for example, is not necessary to practice psychotherapy and the costs thereof should not be billed to patients. In a second step, certain cost positions, which were not considered in the survey, were added. For example, under a statutory health insurance scheme a professional billing software is required, which the survey did not account for. Hence, based on the standards applied by medical practitioners we added yearly costs for a billing system. Finally, some of the survey results were implausible or not applicable for other reasons and, therefore, we decided to deviate from the survey results. Most importantly, we did not consider the net income as expressed in the survey results. As mentioned above, the pricing system should represent the future work situation of psychotherapists in Switzerland. Therefore, the pricing system was set up such that the net income could be entered manually as an external parameter. The benefit of this approach is that the pricing system is sufficiently flexible, especially if we consider that the net income may be the most controversial cost element discussed in negotiations between the health care providers and health insurers due to its relative importance. Another example where we were deviating from the survey results are the pension fund contributions. The resulting average value of pension fund contributions in the survey was considered too low compared with professional standards in Switzerland. Therefore, based on the net income and the prevailing contribution rates in Switzerland, the pension fund contributions were recalculated. It is important to note that for all deviations from the survey results a clear argumentation and well-documented external sources were provided to the project partners. After adding, removing and modifying some cost positions, the remaining costs were added to yield the total yearly cost that is needed for an efficient full time psychotherapist and thus should be covered by statutory health insurance.

Secondly, we determined for every activity in the time-use survey whether it is relevant for statutory health insurance or not. For example, the health insurers do not cover the waiting time in-between patients. Thus,

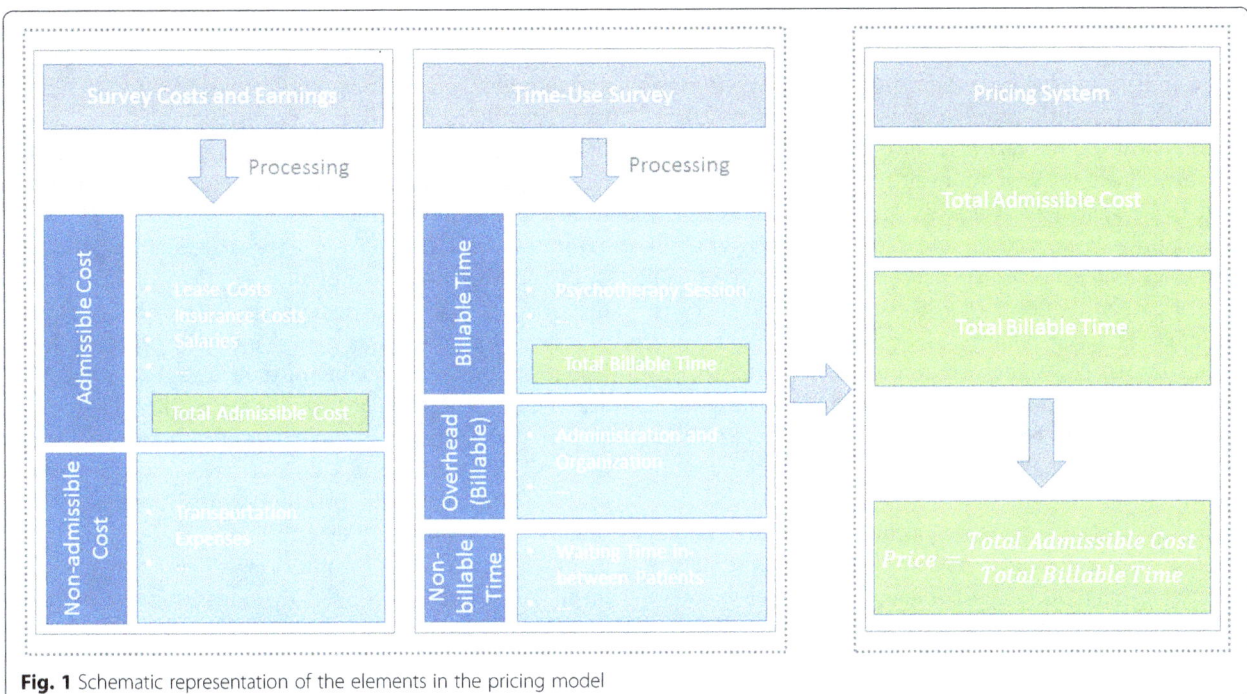

Fig. 1 Schematic representation of the elements in the pricing model

the percentage share of waiting time in-between patients is not relevant for statutory health insurance. In addition, for all activities that are relevant for statutory health insurance, we specified whether the activity is directly billable to patients or forms part of the overhead. For example, the administration and organization of the practice is obviously a necessary task in any medical practice and should be covered by the practice's income. However, it is not directly billable to patients and hence, the activity is part of the overhead and its costs are spread proportionately over all the billable activities. Furthermore, activities such as the mandatory work breaks as well as activities that are compensated by a flat rate price are excluded from the billable time. The result of the steps mentioned in this paragraph is a list of necessary activities for psychotherapy that are either directly or indirectly billable. The time shares of these necessary activities are restandardized to add up to 1. This last step is crucial because we want to pass on the total cost of a full time psychotherapist to the billable part of a full time workload. Restandardizing the time shares makes sure that we do not underestimate the billable part of the workload. One final important step is the definition of the disposable weekly work time. In Switzerland, it is common to work for 42 h per week. However, since mandatory work breaks are not part of the list of directly or indirectly billable activities, the time for the mandatory work breaks is subtracted from the 42 h. Furthermore, a weekly constant for further education, which is compulsory by law (PsyG, Art. 27, b) is also subtracted from the weekly normal work time.

This reduces the average disposable weekly work time to 37.7 h.

Finally, we had to set the costs and the work time on equal footing. The costs admissible under statutory health insurance were calculated on a yearly basis. Thus, they must be divided by the number of weeks worked per year (43 weeks[2]) in order to compare them with the weekly work time. Then, weekly costs admissible under statutory health insurance are divided by the billable time share of the disposable weekly work time. The result is the cost per minute. As was mentioned above, psychotherapy services are billed based on 5-min units. Hence, the cost per minute multiplied by 5 is the price for any type of psychotherapeutic activity that can be billed. The computation of the price can be summarized with the following formula:

$$Price = \frac{Total\ admissible\ cost\ (Swiss\ francs)}{Total\ billable\ work\ time\ per\ week\ (Min.)} \times 5$$

As in TARMED, the price for all services is the same. To give an example, assume that weekly costs admissible under statutory health insurance are 5000 Swiss francs and further assume that the time share of billable activities is 80% which corresponds to 1810 min per week. In that case, it results a price of 13.81 Swiss francs per 5 min. It is crucial that the costs admissible under statutory health insurance are only divided by the time share of billable activities. This way we implicitly pass on overhead activities such as the administration and organization to the price.

A complete pricing system for psychotherapy, or more generally for health care, requires additional specifications. Firstly, the flat rate prices for services such as writing formalized reports for health insurance companies need to be specified. Secondly, some mark-up over the regular price is needed for emergencies, which is common in pricing schemes in health care. Finally, the travel time of psychotherapists to visit patients should be compensated. This last point is particularly important since, in our approach, transportation expenses are not included in the admissible cost. Most of these additional specifications can be based on existing regulations in TARMED with some adjustments for the special case of psychotherapy.

The calculations for the pricing model are implemented in a *Microsoft Excel* worksheet such that the parameters can be entered manually (e.g. net income) and, at the same time, the basic input from the surveys remains separated from the pricing model.

Discussion

The results of this study show that it is possible to build a pricing system for psychotherapy based on the results of a survey about the costs and earnings and a time-use survey. However, as we have seen above, the design of the pricing system involves methodological decisions on many different levels. As there exists relatively little research in this field, many of those decisions were based on the domain knowledge of the project group that actively followed the progress of this study. In many other cases, we were able to base our decisions on principles that are already implemented in the Swiss health care system. For example, we decided that further education should not have an effect on the price a psychotherapist can charge. The reason for that is to conform to TARMED. It specifies a unique price for every service in outpatient health care regardless of individual attributes of the medical practitioner performing the service such as further education or experience.

Moreover, our approach might suffer from limitations that are commonly known in health care systems. One such problem might be moral hazard [10]. Psychotherapists might have an incentive to advise patients to seek more hours of therapy than is necessary. Currently, Swiss health care authorities address this problem as follows: a psychiatrist is free to mandate 40 sessions of therapy that are covered by statutory health insurance. If more therapy sessions are necessary, the psychiatrist must write a report for the attention of the health insurance company of the patient. The latter then decides whether it covers more than 40 sessions of therapy or not. It is therefore likely that such a rule will also apply

to psychotherapists once they are admitted to statutory health insurance. In addition, health insurers supervise and monitor the efficiency and expenditures of health care providers. Therefore, a psychotherapist who would have an extraordinary cost or therapy structure would have to justify this and, ultimately, could be excluded from the health insurance system.

Another limitation of our approach might be the lack of considering treatment quality. A pricing system where the price of a treatment depends on its quality can be beneficial for patients as it may incentivize psychotherapists to improve the quality of their care. However, there are certain problems with treatment quality. First of all, one of the premises of the Swiss health care system is that medical practitioners do not have to guarantee the success of a treatment. In other words, medical practitioners are reimbursed regardless of whether the treatment was successful or not as long as care was provided in all conscience. Secondly, the measurement of treatment quality is in itself a challenging endeavor and there exist different approaches [11]. One approach, for example, is based on assessing the outcome of a treatment. While the measuring of outcomes is already hard for many physical diseases, it may become impossible for the various forms of mental disease. Although treatment quality is difficult to determine, psychotherapists are usually involved in supervision processes where either they supervise the work of a colleague or they receive advice from a colleague about their own cases. Furthermore, as mentioned above, minimal further education is required by law. Hence, two mechanisms already in place have the aim of ensuring quality of treatment.

Conclusion

The purpose of this paper was to outline the process of designing a pricing system in health care. The different steps are explained through the example of psychological psychotherapy in Switzerland. According to Swiss regulation, the proposal of a pricing system needs to be based on a transparent empirical data basis. Hence, this paper set out to combine the results of two surveys in order to design a pricing system. A survey about the costs and earnings of psychotherapists helped to determine the essential costs incurred when practicing psychotherapy, while a time-use survey served as the basis for learning what share of the work time is directly billable. Dividing the relevant total cost by the billable time resulted in the price for psychotherapy. Together with the tariff structure, this price builds the core of the pricing system.

Overall, this paper shows that it is possible to design a pricing system for health care based on survey results. However, the design involves many methodological decisions that often require a sound knowledge of the concrete domain studied. This can be achieved by conducting, for example, workshops with the practitioners or pilot studies. Moreover, the pricing system crucially relies on the validity of the survey results. Hence, a comprehensive and sound design of the surveys is critical for the whole project. In addition, the pricing system is always just a model of the reality and certain factors such as false incentives or quality of treatment cannot be directly built into the pricing system but must be addressed in a more general way accounting for common principles of the whole health care system.

As was previously mentioned, it is not possible to present numeric results due to confidentiality agreements. This is a major limitation of this paper. Future research should assess the procedure that is proposed in this paper and hopefully can present numeric results.

Endnotes

[1]An amortization rate of 20% implies that the computer is used for 5 years.

[2]This roughly corresponds to the 1824 h that we assumed in Section Processing of survey results.

Appendix

Let the data be x_i $(i = 1, ..., n)$ with weights w_i $(i = 1, ..., n)$, denote the sample by S and let Z denote the set of the indices of the observations with a value of 0, i.e. $Z = \{i \mid x_i = 0\}$. Estimate the proportion of the observations with a value of 0 in the population with $p_z = \sum_{i \in Z} w_i / \sum_{i \in S} w_i$. To simplify the treatment assume that $\sum_{i \in S} w_i = n$. Let the trimmed mean of the non-zero observations be m_{tnz}. Note that for the trimmed mean with weighted data the weighted quantiles must be calculated and the weights for $i \in Z$ must be set to 0 before calculating m_{tnz}, the trimmed weighted mean of the non-zero observations. Assuming x_l and x_h denote the lower and upper trimming quantiles, then $n_t = \sum_{S \setminus Z} w_i \ 1\{x_l \leq x_i \leq x_h\}$ denotes the number of non-trimmed observations (or, more generally, the sum of the weights of the non-trimmed observations).

The estimator for the population mean is

$$m_t = p_z \cdot 0 + (1 - p_z) \cdot m_{tnz}.$$

The variance estimator must take into account the variability of p_z and m_{tnz}. Under the assumption that the two estimators are independent the variance can be estimated as

$$v(m_t) = v(1 - p_z)v(m_{tnz}) + (1 - pz)^2 v(m_{tnz}) + m_{tnz}^2 v(1 - p_z),$$

and, assuming simple random sampling and negligible finite population correction, $v(1 - p_z) = p_z(1 - p_z)/n$.

The variance $v(m_{tnz})$ is more difficult to estimate. Generally, the variance of the winsorised mean is used to estimate the variance of the trimmed mean because the two estimators are asymptotically equivalent. The winsorized mean is calculated by setting the extreme observations to the trimming quantiles x_l and x_h. Suppose $x'_i, i \notin Z$ are the winsorized values and n_t is the sum of the weights in the non-trimmed part. Then the winsorised mean is $m_{wnz} = \sum_{i \notin Z} x'_i w_i / \sum_{i \notin Z} w_i$. Thus the winsorised mean is the weighted mean of the new values $x'_i, i \notin Z$. A variance estimator for the winsorised mean is

$$v(m_{tnz}) = v(m_{wnz}) = \frac{1}{n_t(n_t - 1)} \sum_{i \notin Z} w_i (x'_i - m_{wnz})^2.$$

Applying the formulas outlined above results in a trimmed, weighted mean and the corresponding variance estimator. For a discussion on the estimation of the variance of a trimmed mean, see also [12].

Abbreviations

DRG: Diagnosis related groups; FOPH: Federal Office of Public Health; GP: General practitioner; KVG: Swiss Federal Health Insurance Act; KVV: Health Insurance Ordinance; PsyG: Federal Law on Psychological Professions

Acknowledgements

We are grateful for the contributions of the user project leader Heinz Marty and the core team from the psychotherapy associations. The views and opinions expressed in this paper are those of the authors and do not necessarily reflect those of the funding institutions.

Funding

This study was funded by 'Föderation der Schweizer Psychologinnen und Psychologen' (FSP), 'Schweizerischer Berufsverband für Angewandte Psychologie' (SBAP), 'Assoziation Schweizer Psychotherapeutinnen und Psychotherapeuten' (ASP) and by the University of Applied Sciences and Arts Northwestern Switzerland (FHNW), School of Business.

Authors' contributions

BH supervised the study and was responsible for the design and the execution of the survey. MS conducted the data analysis. Both authors contributed equally to the creation of the manuscript. All authors read and approved the final manuscript.

Competing interests

The authors declare that they have no competing interests. All the funding institutions support the publication of this article. This study was conducted according to scientific criteria and none of the funding institutions had an influence on the outcome of the study.

References

1. Camenzind P. The Swiss health care system, 2015. In: Mossialos E, Wenzl M, Osborn R, Sarnak D, editors. International profiles of health care systems. New York: the Commonwealth Fund; 2016. p. 161–9.
2. Swiss Federal Council: Anerkennung neuer Leistungserbringer. Medienmitteilungen des Bundesrats. https://www.admin.ch/gov/de/start/dokumentation/medienmitteilungen/bundesrat.msg-id-64875.html. Accessed 06 March 2018.

3.   Swiss Federal Council: Der Bundesrat setzt das Psychologieberufegesetz in Kraft. Medienmitteilungen des Bundesrats. https://www.admin.ch/gov/de/start/dokumentation/medienmitteilungen/bundesrat.msg-id-48161.html. Accessed 06 March 2018.

4.   Vogl M. Assessing DRG cost accounting with respect to resource allocation and tariff calculation: the case of Germany. Heal Econ Rev. 2012;2:15.

5.   Stettler P, Stocker D, Gardiol L, Bischof S, Künzi K. Strukturerhebung zur psychologischen Psychotherapie in der Schweiz 2012. Bern: BASS; 2013.

6.   Stinson LL. Measuring how people spend their time: a time-use survey design. Monthly Labor Review. 1999;122:12–9.

7.   Swiss Federal Tax Administration: Merkblatt A 1995 – Gechäftliche Betriebe. Fachinformationen. https://www.estv.admin.ch/estv/de/home/direkte-bundessteuer/direkte-bundessteuer/fachinformationen/merkblaetter.html. Accessed 06 March 2018.

8.   Kaufmännischer Verband Schweiz: Jahresarbeitszeit. http://www.kfmv.ch/data/docs/de_CH-1996/5256/dok-Jahresarbeitszeit.pdf. Accessed 06 March 2018.

9.   R_Core_Team: R: A language and environment for statistical computing. R Foundation for Statistical Computing. https://www.R-project.org/. Accessed 06 March 2018.

10. Zweifel P, Manning WG. Moral hazard and consumer incentives in health care. In: Culyer AJ, Newhouse JP, editors. Handbook of health economics. Amsterdam: Elsevier; 2000. Chapter 8.

11. Chung KC, Shauver MJ. Measuring quality in healthcare and its implications for pay-for-performance initiatives. Hand Clin. 2009. https://doi.org/10.1016/j.hcl.2008.09.001.

12. Capéraà P, Rivest LP. On the variance of the trimmed mean. Statistics and Probability Letters. 1995;22:79–85.

11

Technical efficiency of selected hospitals in Eastern Ethiopia

Murad Ali[1], Megersa Debela[1]*(iD) and Tewfik Bamud[2]

Abstract

This study examines the relative technical efficiency of 12 hospitals in Eastern Ethiopia. Using six-year-round panel data for the period between 2007/08 and 2012/13, this study examines the technical efficiency, total factor productivity, and determinants of the technical inefficiency of hospitals. Data envelopment analysis (DEA) and DEA- based Malmquist productivity index used to estimate relative technical efficiency, scale efficiency, and total factor productivity index of hospitals. Tobit model used to examine the determinants of the technical inefficiency of hospitals. The DEA Variable Returns to Scale (VRS) estimate indicated that 6 (50%), 5 (42%), 3 (25%), 3 (25%), 4 (33%), and 3 (25%) of the hospitals were technically inefficient while 9 (75%), 9 (75%), 7 (58%), 7 (58%), 7 (58%) and 8 (67%) of hospitals were scale inefficient between 2007/08 and 2012/13, respectively. On average, Malmquist Total Factor Productivity (MTFP) of the hospitals decreased by 3.6% over the panel period. The Tobit model shows that teaching hospital is less efficiency than other hospitals. The Tobit regression model further shows that medical doctor to total staff ratio, the proportion of outpatient visit to inpatient days, and the proportion of inpatients treated per medical doctor were negatively related with technical inefficiency of hospitals. Hence, policy interventions that help utilize excess capacity of hospitals, increase doctor to other staff ratio, and standardize number of inpatients treated per doctor would contribute to the improvement of the technical efficiency of hospitals.

Keywords: Technical inefficiency, DEA, Scale efficiency, Hospitals, Malmquist total factor productivity

Background

The health care system of many countries in Sub-Saharan Africa including Ethiopia faces resource constraints to provide quality health services to the people. The shortage of health care resources may be related to poor economic performance, rapid population growth, and a decline in public spending. Moreover, in Sub-Saharan Africa, communicable, maternal, nutritional, and new borne diseases continue to dominate and putting stress on the already scarce health care resources of these countries [1].

Hospitals consume a larger proportion of the total public health budget. Even though the percentage vary from country to country, hospitals in Sub-Saharan African countries consume a larger proportion of public health care resources. The situation in Ethiopia is like other Sub-Saharan countries. Hence, the efficiency of

hospitals need to be given due attention as the budget they consume is enormous.

It is recognized that improved efficiency is one of the main goals of health systems [2]. Health policy makers in Africa have also stressed the need to utilize the scarce health sector resources efficiently [3]. A growing number of countries in Africa have undertaken health facility efficiency study to guide the development of interventions to reduce wastage of scarce health system resources.

Data Envelopment Analysis (DEA) has been used to analyze technical efficiency of hospitals in several Sub-Saharan African countries. Different studies have used different inputs and outputs to measure efficiency. For instance, studies conducted in Eritrea [4], Botswana [5], Benin [6] and Burkina Faso [7] are among the few. Most of the studies focused on measuring the first stage of efficiency analysis. Few studies conducted the second stage analysis to examine the determinants of technical (in) efficiency using panel data. This study uses panel data for six-year-round (that is between 2007/08 to

* Correspondence: mdebela4@gmail.com
[1]Department of Economics, Haramaya University, College of Business and Economics, Dire Dawa, Ethiopia

2012/13) data for each hospital. Panel data enables analysis hospitals productivity changes. The benefit of having multiple observations (panel data) on the same units allows controlling for unobserved heterogeneous characteristics of hospitals. And thus, facilitate causal inference [8]. The second stage analysis involves converting the DEA efficiency score into inefficiency score and running regression against some factors. In this regard, [9] analyzed technical efficiency and productivity in South Africa using panel data.

In the case of Ethiopia, few studies have been conducted to examine the efficiency of hospitals. A study by [10] examined technical efficiency of the health centers in Ethiopia. Other study in Ethiopia is by [11] which used Stochastic Frontier Approach (SFA) to analysis the technical efficiency of 8 selected public hospitals. These few studies focused on the first stage of efficiency analysis. Therefore, this study seeks to analyze the technical efficiency and productivity of hospitals in eastern Ethiopia. This study also examines factors that determine the inefficiency of hospitals. The findings will deepen understanding of the extent of inefficiency and its causes in eastern Ethiopia. In the rest of the paper, methods and materials, result and discussions, and conclusion and recommendations are presented.

Methods

This study was conducted on selected hospitals in eastern Ethiopia. The selected hospitals are from Eastern Hararghe (Oromia region), Harari region, Somali region, and Dire Dawa administration council. The included hospitals are both public and private. Panel data were collected from 12 hospitals for the period 2007/08 to 2012/13. The inputs include beds, health staff and drug supplies while the outputs include outpatient visits, inpatient days, and surgery.

Method of data analysis
Data envelopment analysis (DEA)
Data envelopment analysis (DEA) involves the use of linear programming methods to construct a nonparametric piece-wise surface (or frontier) over the data [12]. DEA is based upon a comparative analysis of observed producers to their counterparts [13]. First, [14] coined DEA which had an input-oriented model with constant return to scale (CRS). Subsequently, variable returns to scale (VRS) model was also developed and introduced to the DEA literature by [15]. Furthermore, chance-constrained efficiency analysis was also integrated [16] to the DEA model.

CRS vs. VRS models The assumption of CRS may not be feasible due to the presence of imperfect competition, government regulations, and constraints on finance that force firms to run at suboptimal scale [12]. For this reason, [15] developed a variable return to scale (VRS) which enables to capture the magnitude of scale effect. Linear programming model of VRS is like the CRS with some modification.

The mathematical relationship between VRS and CRS efficiency measurements is given by $TE_{CRS} = TE_{VRS}$ (SE) [12]. "SE" denotes scale efficiency. This means that CRS technical efficiency of a firm can be decomposed into pure technical efficiency and scale efficiency (SE).

Malmquist productivity index It is the measure of the relationship between the outputs of a hospital and the inputs used to produce those outputs. Productivity increase is manifested by rise in output per health worker hour and/or the use of more and/ or better health technology. In general, a productivity index is defined as the ratio of an output quantity index to an input quantity index, i.e. $P_t = \frac{Y_t}{X_t}$; Where: Pt is a productivity index; time t = 0..., T; Y_t is an output quantity index and X_t is an input quantity index. Each index represents accumulated growth from period 0 to period t.

The DEA-based Malmquist Productivity Index (MPI) is often opted to study efficiency and productivity changes over a given period. The model is preferred for several reasons: it does not require information on the prices of inputs and outputs rather on quantities of inputs and outputs; imposition of functional form of production technology is not required; it easily accommodates multiple hospital inputs and outputs; and it can be broken down into the constituent sources of productivity change - i.e. efficiency changes and technological changes [17].

Malmquist-DEA is applied to panel data to calculate indices of changes in Total Factor Productivity (TFP), technology, technical efficiency, and scale efficiency. The Malmquist Productivity Index (MPI) takes a value of more than one for productivity growth, a value of one for stagnation and a value of less than one for productivity decline. The output-oriented MPI is defined as the geometric mean of two periods' productivity indices, subsequently broken down into various sources of productivity change [18].

Specification of the DEA model
The DEA model adopted is based on [19–21]; and many other model specifications that are applied in the health sector.

The constant returns to scale (CRS) model
The efficiency score of decision-making units that employs multiple input and output is defined as:

$$Effeciency = \frac{weighted\ sum\ of\ hospital\ outputs}{weighted\ sum\ of\ hospital\ inpunts} \quad (1)$$

Following [14], if there are n hospitals, each with m hospital inputs and s hospital outputs, the relative efficiency score of a given hospital P is obtained by solving the following model:

$$Efficiency_P = Max \frac{\sum_{r=1}^{s} U_r Y_{rp}}{\sum_{i=1}^{m} V_i X_{ip}}$$

$$s.t: \frac{\sum_{r=1}^{s} U_r Y_{rj}}{\sum_{r=1}^{m} V_i X_{ij}} \leq 1; \ j = 1; 2; ...; n$$

$$U_r,\ V_i > 0; \forall_r, \forall_i; r = 1; 2; ..s; i = 1; 2; ..m \quad (2)$$

Where:

x_{ij} = the amount of health system input i utilized by the jth hospital;

y_{rj} = the amount of health system output r produced by the jth hospital;

u_r = weight given to health system output r;

v_i = weight given to input i.

The functional programming model of equation (2) can be converted to a linear programming model by introducing the following constraint:

$$\sum_{i=1}^{m} V_i X_{ip} = 1$$

Thus, the relative efficiency score of hospital p can be obtained by solving the following equation:

$$Max\ Efficiency_P = Max_{u, v_i} \sum_{r=1}^{s} U_r Y_{rp}$$

$$S.t: \sum_{r=1}^{s} U_r Y_{rj} - \sum_{i=1}^{m} V_i X_{ij} \leq 0; \forall_i$$

$$\sum V_i X_{ip} = 1$$

$$U_r, V_i > 0; \forall_r, \forall_i \quad (3)$$

The first constraint implies that all hospitals are on or below the frontiers while the second constraint implies that the weighted sum of inputs for the hospital equals one.

The variable returns to scale (VRS) model

To separate the technical and scale efficiency scores, variable returns to scale (VRS) model is considered. In variable returns to scale, the data are enveloped more closely than the CRS model. The main advantage of the VRS model is that it enables an inefficient firm to be relatively compared to efficient hospitals of the same size only. Therefore, the relative efficiency score of hospital p can be obtained by solving the following equation:

$$Max\ Effeciency_P = Max_{u, v_i} \sum_{r=1}^{s} U_r Y_{rp} + U_0$$

$$S.t: \sum_{r=1}^{s} U_r Y_{rj} - \sum_{i=1}^{m} V_i X_{ij} + U_0 \leq 0; \forall_i$$

$$\sum V_i X_{ip} = 1$$

$$U_r, V_i > 0; \forall_r, \forall_i \quad (4)$$

Where:

U_0 = is the convexity constraint and its sign determines the returns to scale. If $U_0 < 0$ it indicates increasing returns to scale, if $U_0 > 0$ it is decreasing returns to scale and if $U_0 = 0$ it is constant returns to scale. The other notations are as given in the case of CRS model.

DEA like Malmquist model

The DEA like Malmquist model is used to obtain the DEA efficiency scores of all the sample periods observations. The model applies for panel data and calculates indices of total factor productivity (TFP) change, technological change, technical efficiency change and scale efficiency change. The output based Malmquist productivity change index of [18] is specified as follows:

$$M_0\left(y^{t+1}, x^{t+1}, y^t, x^t\right) = \left[\frac{D_0^t(x^{t+1}, y^{t+1})}{D_0^t(x^t, y^t)} X \frac{D_{0^{t+1}}(x^{t+1}, y^{t+1})}{D_{0^{t+1}}(x^t, y^t)}\right]^{\frac{1}{2}} \quad (5)$$

Where:

M_0 = measures productivity of the production point (x^{t+1}, y^{t+1}) relative to the production point (x^t, y^t);

$D_0^t(x^{t+1}, y^{t+1})$ = represents the distance from the period $t + 1$ observation to the period t technology; and

$D_0^t(x^t, y^t)$ = represents the distance from period t observation to the period $t + 1$ technology.

If the value of M_0 is greater than one, it shows the existence of positive total factor productivity from period t to period $t + 1$ while a value less than one indicates a decline in total factor productivity. Further decomposition of equation (5) provides measures of efficiency change and technical change separately.

$$M_0\left(y^{t+1}, x^{t+1}, y^t, x^t\right) = \frac{D_0^t(x^{t+1}, y^{t+1})}{D_0^t(x^t, y^t)} x$$
$$\left[\frac{D_0^t(x^{t+1}, y^{t+1})}{D_0^t(x^t, y^t)} X \frac{D_{0^{t+1}}(x^{t+1}, y^{t+1})}{D_{0^{t+1}}(x^t, y^t)}\right]^{\frac{1}{2}} \quad (6)$$

The first term measures efficiency change while the second term measures technical change in the two periods. An improvement of efficiency occurs from period t to period $t + 1$ if the ratio is greater than 1 (one). The output-oriented DEA model was estimated for CRS DEA and VRS DEA models.

Selection of input and output variables

The ultimate measure of output is an improvement in the quantity and quality of life. However, practical difficulties limit the use of outcomes approach [22]. Hence, hospital output is measured as an array of intermediate output (health services) that improves health status [23]. In this study, we included three output and three inputs based on the literature on health sector technical efficiency [4, 9, 24]. The outputs include outpatient department visit, inpatient days, and number of surgery. The inputs include total health staff, cost of drug supply, and capital input proxied by total beds.

Specification of the regression model

The DEA efficiency scores will be analyzed by regressing them against some characteristics of the hospitals to examine how these factors affect the (in) efficiency of hospitals. The censored Tobit model was used since the dependent variable is censored at zero from below. Like the studies of [19] and [25], in this study also the DEA scores are transformed into inefficiency scores using the following formula:

$$Inefficiency\ score = \left(\frac{1}{DEA\ score}\right) - 1 \qquad (7)$$

The model is specified in the following form:

$y_i^* = \beta_i X_i + u_i;$

$y_i = y_i^*\ if\ y_i^* > 0;\ and$

$y_i = 0\ if\ y_i^* \leq 0$

Where:

$u_i \sim N\ (0, \delta^2);$

y_i = the observed inefficiency score;

β_i = a Kx 1 vector of unknown parameters; and

X_i = a $Kx1$ vector of explanatory variables.

Therefore, the empirical regression model is specified as:

$$\begin{aligned} INEFF = \alpha_0 &+ \beta_1 L\ size + \beta_2 BOR \\ &+ \beta_3 Teacstat + \beta_4 dcstaf \\ &+ \beta_5 opinpdays + \beta_6 impdoc + \varepsilon_i \qquad (8) \end{aligned}$$

The variables in the model are defined as follows:

INEFF: inefficiency scores.

Size: The natural logarithm of numbers of bed is taken as a proxy to measure hospitals' size.

BOR: It is the ratio number of inpatient days multiplied by 100 and divided by the available hospital beds multiplied by number of days in a year.

Teachstat: It is teaching status dummy variable. It is 1 if it is teaching hospital and 0 other wise.

Docstaff: This variable is measured by dividing the total number of medical doctors by the total staff of the hospital.

Opinpdays: It is the outpatient visits as a proportion of inpatient days.

Impdoc: It is the proportion of inpatients per medical doctor.

α_0, β_1, β_2, β_3, β_4, β_5, and β_6, are coefficients to be estimated and ε_i is the random disturbance term.

These variables used in the second stage (that is econometric analysis). We converted the efficiency results into inefficiency score using equation eight (8). Thus, we used this inefficiency score as dependent variable and run it against the above defined independent variables. Some of the determinants of the hospital facility technical efficiency include average length of stay, outpatient visit as proportion of the inpatient days, bed occupancy rate, doctors to staff ratio, teaching status of the hospital, proportion of inpatients per medical doctor, and bed size [9, 26, 27]).

The data

Regional bureaus of health collect data on inputs and outputs and other health related data. The study was conducted based on the data obtained from these bureaus of health of each respective region (Oromia, Harari, Dire Dawa Administrative City Council, and Somali) in Eastern Ethiopia. The study used panel data of six year-round starting from 2007/08 to 2012/13 for each hospital. Having this panel data enables us analysis hospitals productivity changes overtime and allows us to control for unobserved heterogeneous characteristics of hospitals.

Result and discussions

Results of the study

Basic characteristics of hospitals

All (that is 12) hospitals in the Eastern Ethiopia are included in the study, except one for which the data was incomplete. The data collected covers the time between 2007/08 and 2012/13. Table 1 summarizes the basic characteristics of all hospitals and their respective average yearly inputs for the study period. Among the hospitals, eight were publicly owned while four were privately owned. In Harari region, 5 hospitals were selected for the analysis. Among the hospitals, Hiwot Fana, Jugal, Police and Army were public hospitals while Yimaj hospital was privately owned. From Dire Dawa, five hospitals were included: Dilchora and France hospital were public hospitals whereas Bilal, Yemariamwork and ART hospitals were privately owned. The other public hospitals considered in the analysis were Bisidimo and Karamara hospitals from East Hararghe zone of Oromia and Somali regions respectively. Regarding their year of

Table 1 Basic characteristics of hospitals and average yearly inputs 2007/2008–2012/2013

Name of hospital	Establishment	Staff			Average			
		Health	Administrative	Total	Salary	Drug	Recurrent	Bed
France	1911	14	23	37	591,637	381,532	414,248	68
Hiwot Fana	1941	225	196	421	6,406,047	1,765,662	6,278,350	204
Jegol	1951	151	112	263	3,495,719	831,116	3,899,048	118
Dilchora	1951	184	77	262	7,646,767	2,600,874	8,027,770	85
Karamara	1956	214	140	354	7,608,026	1,401,988	2,045,428	193
Bisidimo	1958	56	137	194	280,200	1,100,000	317,410	116
Police	1965	69	72	141	2,222,641	484,050	1,083,953	82
Army	1975	73	77	150	2,519,660	593,810	1,327,650	97
Yemariamwork*	2007	15	12	28	550,832	580,028	651,801	29
ART*	2007	20	5	25	1,914,318	560,297	1,168,419	28
Yimaj*	2006	45	10	55	982,006	113,572	3,877,606	54
Bilal*	2000	43	50	93	1,576,075	3,470,000	2,840,759	40

Source: own computation

establishment, France and Hiwot Fana hospitals were among the oldest hospitals where as ART and Yemariamwork were the youngest.

Taking the average for the study period, Hiwot Fana hospital had the highest total staff which is 421 (196 administrative and 225 health staff) followed by Karamara, whereas ART had the lowest total staffs (5 administrative and 20 health staff) followed by Yemariamwork hospital.

Regarding the average yearly expenditure on salary, Dilchora hospital incurred the highest followed by Karamara hospital. The lowest expenditure on salary was incurred by Bisidimo. With respect to expenditure on drug, Bilal incurred the highest while Yimaj incurred the lowest. On the other hand, the average for yearly recurrent expenditure of the hospitals revealed that Dilchora hospital incurred the highest followed by Hiwot Fana. The lowest recorded was for Bisidimo followed by France.

The average number of bed for the study period revealed that Hiwot Fana had the highest number of bed followed by Karamara and Jugal. The lowest recorded was for ART followed by Yemariamwork hospital.

In this study, three major outputs of hospitals were considered for technical efficiency evaluation of hospitals. These three outputs were total yearly outpatient visit, total yearly inpatient days and total surgery performed in the respective hospitals. From Table 2, we can see that Dilchora had the highest average total

outpatient visit followed by Hiwot Fana and Karamara hospitals. The lowest was recorded by Yemariamwork followed by ART and Yimaj.

When we consider the total average yearly inpatient days, Dilchora had the highest average yearly inpatient days followed by Hiwot Fana and Karamara. The lowest was for ART followed by Yemariamwork and Bisidimo. About surgery, Dilchora had the highest total average yearly surgery followed by Jugal and Karamara. On the other hand, the lowest was recorded for ART followed by Yemariamwork and Police.

Table 3 shows that in the sampling period (2007/08 to 2012/13), the average yearly output of the hospitals were 19,015 outpatient visits, 12,630 inpatient days and 750 number of surgeries, whereas the average yearly input of the total health staff, number of beds and expenditure on drugs was 92, 93, and birr 1,156,910, respectively.

Overall, the public hospitals on average accounted for about 24,712, 999 and 16,431 outpatient visit, number of surgeries and inpatient days, respectively. Regarding inputs, on average over the sample period public hospitals accounted for about 123, 120 and 1,144,879 numbers of health staff, bed, and amount of birr of drug expenditure, respectively. From the above data, we can see that the share of the public in terms of average outputs and inputs is higher than the private hospitals except in drug expenditure.

Table 2 Hospitals average outputs 2007/2008–2012/2013

Name	France	Hiwotfana	Jegol	Dilchora	Karamara	Bisidimo	Police	Army	Yemariamwork	ART	Yimaj	Bilal
Outpatient visits	8740	35,424	26,191	64,272	28,484	7488	14,579	12,518	5602	5797	6832	12,256
Inpatient days	6308	26,520	13,789	44,233	24,122	3914	7207	5354	1979	1384	7914	8838
Surgery	193	949	1356	3825	1008	31	149	184	102	72	443	393

Source: various reports of hospitals and own computation

Table 3 Means of outputs and inputs of the hospitals based on their ownership

No		Variable	Mean			Maximum		Minimum	
			All	Public	Private	Public	Private	Public	Private
I. Outputs	1	Outpatient visit	19,016	24,712	7622	64,273	12,256	7488	5602
	2	Surgery	751	1000	253	3825	443	149	73
	3	Inpatient days	12,631	16,431	5029	44,234	8839	3914	1384
II. Inputs	1	Health Staff	93	124	31	225	45	14	16
	2	Capital Input (Beds)	93	121	38	204	55	68	28
	3	Drug Supplies	1,156,911	1,144,879	1,180,974	2,600,874	3,470,000	381,532	113,572

Source: own computation

Technical and scale efficiency

To separate the technical and scale efficiency in the health service production process which is often nonlinear, it is appropriate to assume output oriented variable returns to scale BCC model. Hence for this study we estimate the efficiency of hospitals assuming the variable returns to scale BCC model [21].

Tables 4 and 5 presents individual hospital's technical and scale efficiency for the year 2007/08 to 2012/13. It reveals that in year 2007/08 and 2008/09 out of 12 hospitals 3 (25%) registered a constant return to scale technical efficiency (CRSTE) score of 100%. Therefore, 9 (75%) of hospitals in both 2007/08 and 2008/09 period has been run inefficiently given the assumption of constant return to scale.

On the other hand, 6 (50%) hospitals in the year 2007/08 and 7 (58.33%) of hospitals in the year 2008/09 registered a variable return to scale technical efficiency

(VRSTE) score of 100%. Moreover, out of 12 hospitals, 3 hospitals (25%) in the year 2007/08 and 3 hospitals (25%) in the year 2008/09 were scale efficient. Regarding returns to scale, 3 (25%) of hospitals in the year 2007/08 and 3 (25%) of hospitals in the year 2008/09 manifested increasing returns to scale, respectively. Moreover, 6 (50%) and 6 (50%) of hospitals manifested decreasing returns to scale in the respective periods.

Individual hospitals' technical and scale efficiency for the year 2009/10 and 2010/11 indicated that out of 12 hospitals, 5 (41.67%) registered a constant return to scale technical efficiency (CRSTE) score of 100%, whereas in the year 2010/11 again 5 (41.67%) hospitals registered a constant return to scale technical efficiency (CRSTE) score of 100%. Therefore, 7 (58.33%) of hospitals in the year 2009/10 and 7 (58.33%) of hospitals in the year 2010/11 were inefficient given the assumption of constant return to scale.

Table 4 Hospital's technical and scale efficiency for 2007/08 to 2009/10

Hospitals	2007/08				2008/09				2009/10			
	CRSTE	VRSTE	Scale	RTS	CRSTE	VRSTE	Scale	RTS	CRSTE	VRSTE	Scale	RTS
France	0.52	0.72	0.72	DRS	0.71	0.86	0.83	DRS	0.57	0.81	0.70	DRS
Hiwot Fana	0.54	0.55	0.99	DRS	0.55	0.59	0.93	DRS	0.86	0.88	0.98	DRS
Jegol	0.85	0.90	0.94	DRS	1.00	1.00	1.00	CRS	1.00	1.00	1.00	CRS
Dilchora	0.76	0.77	0.99	DRS	0.75	0.78	0.96	DRS	0.97	1.00	0.97	DRS
Karamara	0.98	1.00	0.98	IRS	0.39	1.00	0.39	IRS	0.58	1.00	0.58	IRS
Bisidimo	1.00	1.00	1.00	CRS	0.78	1.00	0.78	DRS	1.00	1.00	1.00	CRS
Police	0.85	1.00	0.85	IRS	0.83	1.00	0.83	IRS	0.70	1.00	0.70	IRS
Army	1.00	1.00	1.00	CRS	0.89	1.00	0.89	DRS	1.00	1.00	1.00	CRS
Yemariamwork	0.26	0.31	0.84	DRS	1.00	1.00	1.00	CRS	1.00	1.00	1.00	CRS
ART	0.62	0.70	0.88	IRS	0.19	0.24	0.77	DRS	0.47	0.52	0.92	DRS
Yimaj	0.96	1.00	0.96	DRS	0.73	0.82	0.89	IRS	1.00	1.00	1.00	CRS
Bilal	1.00	1.00	1.00		1.00	1.00	1.00	CRS	0.83	1.00	0.83	DRS
Mean	0.78	0.83	0.93		0.73	0.86	0.86		0.83	0.93	0.89	
SD	0.24	0.22	0.09		0.25	0.23	0.17		0.20	0.15	0.15	
Min	0.26	0.31	0.72		0.19	0.24	0.39		0.47	0.52	0.58	
Max	1.00	1.00	1.00		1.00	1.00	1.00		1.00	1.00	1.00	

Source: Own computation

Table 5 Hospital's technical and scale efficiency in 2010/11 to 2012/13

Hospitals	Hospitals efficiency 2010/11				Hospitals efficiency 2011/12				Hospitals efficiency 2012/13			
	CRSTE	VRSTE	Scale	RTS	CRSTE	VRSTE	Scale	RTS	CRSTE	VRSTE	Scale	RTS
France	0.71	0.71	0.99	DRS	0.72	1.00	0.72	DRS	0.79	1.00	0.79	DRS
Hiwot Fana	0.71	0.71	0.99	DRS	0.53	0.54	0.99	DRS	0.56	0.62	0.90	DRS
Jegol	1.00	1.00	1.00	CRS	1.00	1.00	1.00	CRS	1.00	1.00	1.00	CRS
Dilchora	1.00	1.00	1.00	CRS	0.80	0.80	0.99	DRS	0.67	0.69	0.97	DRS
Karamara	0.52	1.00	0.52	IRS	0.64	1.00	0.64	IRS	0.66	1.00	0.66	IRS
Bisidimo	0.75	1.00	0.75	DRS	0.86	1.00	0.86	DRS	0.82	1.00	0.82	DRS
Police	1.00	1.00	1.00	CRS	1.00	1.00	1.00	CRS	1.00	1.00	1.00	CRS
Army	0.85	1.00	0.85	DRS	1.00	1.00	1.00	CRS	0.75	1.00	0.75	DRS
Yemariamwork	1.00	1.00	1.00	CRS	1.00	1.00	1.00	CRS	1.00	1.00	1.00	CRS
ART	0.52	0.54	0.97	DRS	0.58	0.64	0.91	DRS	0.50	0.65	0.77	DRS
Yimaj	1.00	1.00	1.00	CRS	1.00	1.00	1.00	CRS	1.00	1.00	1.00	CRS
Bilal	0.88	1.00	0.88	DRS	0.54	0.67	0.81	DRS	0.73	1.00	0.73	DRS
Mean	0.83	0.91	0.91		0.80	0.89	0.91		0.79	0.91	0.87	
SD	0.18	0.16	0.15		0.20	0.18	0.13		0.18	0.16	0.13	
Min	0.52	0.54	0.52		0.53	0.54	0.64		0.50	0.62	0.66	
Max	1.00	1.00	1.00		1.00	1.00	1.00		1.00	1.00	1.00	

Source: Own computation

On the other hand, 9 (75%) of hospitals in both periods registered a VRS technical efficiency score of 100%. Moreover, 5 hospitals (41.67%) were scale efficient in both periods. Regarding returns to scale, 2 (16.67%) of hospitals and 1 (8.33%) of hospitals manifested increasing returns to scale in the respective periods. However, 5 (41.67%) of hospitals and 6 (50%) of hospitals manifested decreasing returns to scale in the respective periods.

Individual hospitals' technical and scale efficiency for the year 2011/12 and 2012/13 showed that out of 12 hospitals, 5 (41.67%) of the hospitals in 2011/12 and 4 (33.33%) in 2012/13 registered a constant return to scale technical efficiency (CRSTE) score of 100%, respectively. Therefore, given the assumption of constant return to scale in the year 2011/12 7 (58.33%), and in the year 2012/13, 8 (66.67%) of hospitals run inefficiently.

On the other hand, 8 (66.7%) and 9 (75%) of hospitals in the respective periods registered a variable return to scale technical efficiency (VRSTE) score of 100%. Moreover, 5 (42%) and 4 (33%) of hospitals were scale efficient in respective periods. Regarding returns to scale, 1 (8.3%) of the hospitals in both periods manifested increasing returns to scale whereas 6 (50%) of the hospitals in 2011/12 and 7 (58%) in 2012/13 manifested decreasing returns to scale.

The average scale efficiency score was 93%, 86%, 89%, 91%, 91%, 87% in the respective years between 2007/08 and 2012/13. The average VRSTE scores of hospitals in Eastern Ethiopia stood at 91, 89, 91, 83, 86 and 93% respectively.

The required change in input and output to make inefficient hospitals efficient

Table 6 shows the required change in input reduction or output increase to make inefficient hospitals efficient for the study period. For example, in the year 2012/13, if inefficient hospitals were concerned with the output side, the inefficient hospitals would have increased outpatient visit by 3554, inpatient days by 1837 and surgery by 770 to become efficient. If hospitals were concerned with the level of inputs, the inefficient hospitals should have decreased their bed by 93 to be efficient. Specifically, Bisidimo hospital should increase outpatient by 3554 while army and police hospitals should also increase inpatient days by 511 and 1326, respectively. Moreover, army and police hospitals should also have increased the number of surgery operated by 365 and 404, respectively in 2012/13. This is if hospitals are concerned with output side. If the hospitals are concerned with level of input, Army, Police, and Bisidimo Hospitals should have reduced their bed size by 29, 7 and 57, respectively to be efficient.

Malmquist Total Factor Productivity (MITFP) change

The study analyzed the differences in productivity over time based on Malmquist Total Factor Productivity (MTFP) index taking the year 2007/08 as the technology reference (see Table 7). Table 7 presents the Malmquist index summary of annual geometric means. In the last row (last column), we observe that on average MTFP decreased slightly by 3.6% over period 2007/08-2012/13.

Table 6 The Required Change in input and output to Make Inefficient Hospitals Efficient

	Year	Values	Output			Input		
			Outpatient visit	Impatient days	Surgery	Bed	Drug expenditure	Health staff
Required Change in input and output for all Hospitals for study period	2007/08	Total	8424	26,291	2711	77	1,007,946	70
		Mean	702	2191	226	6	83,995	6
	2008/09	Total	11,310	15,599	5186	72	1,872,247	16
		Mean	942	1300	432	6	156,021	1
	2009/10	Total	0	8659	38	130	626,184	57
		Mean	0	722	3	11	52,182	5
	2010/11	Total	3656	3256	0	118	0	15
		Mean	305	271	0	10	0	1
	2011/12	Total	6979	8142	877	170	689,659	14
		Mean	582	678	73	14	57,472	1
	2012/13	Total	3554	1837	770	95	0	0
		Mean	296	153	64	8	0	0
Total			33,923	63,783	9581	662	4,196,035	172
Mean			471	886	133	9	58,278	2

Source: Own computation

On average, the deterioration in MTFP was due to technical change rather than efficiency change. Hospital efficiency was increased by 1.2%, technical change decreased by 4.7%. The efficiency change was attributed to an increase in pure efficiency of 2.4% and a decline in scale efficiency of 1.2%.

MTFP change was 1.034in 2012/13. This shows that hospital productivity grew by 3.4% in 2012/13 compared to the reference year 2007/08. MTFP change was the highest in 2012/13 (MTFP = 1.034) and the lowest was in 2010/11 (0.907).

Table 8 provides a summary of the annual geometric mean values of the Malmquist Productivity Index (MPI) and its components for each hospital. Five (42%) out of 12 hospitals had MPI score greater than one, indicating growth in productivity. The hospitals include Karamara, Jugal, Bilal, France and Yemariamwork and their respective score is 0.6, 0.6, 7.7, 1.9 and 21.1%. The productivity growth in France was attributed to technical change only. Meanwhile, the productivity growth in Karamara, Jugal and Bilal was due to improvements in efficiency

only. However, productivity change in Yemariamwork is due to both efficiency and technical change.

On the other hand, 7 (58%) out of the 12 hospitals had Malmquist index score of less than one, indicating deterioration in productivity. Overtime productivity regression in Yimaj, Dilchora, Army and Bisidimo hospitals was due to deterioration in technical progress. However, productivity regression in the case of Police, ART and Hiwot Fana hospitals was due to decline in efficiency and technical progress.

Pure efficiency change In Table 8, it is showed that 5 hospitals had an average pure efficiency change (PECH) score of greater than one. Hospitals registering a pure technical efficiency increase included Karamara (6.7%), Army (2.5%), Jugal (2.2%), Bisidimo (13.5%), and Bilal (7.4%). On the other hand, ART, France, Yemariamwork, Yimaj, Dilchora and Hiwot Fana hospitals registered a PECH score of one, indicating no change in efficiency at those hospitals between 2007/08 and 2012/13. However, Police hospital experienced a decline in PECH by 2.2%.

Table 7 Malmquist index summary of geometric annual means (Output oriented)

Year	Efficiency change [A = (C*D)]	TE change [B]	PE change [C]	SE change [D = (A/C)]	MITFP change [E = A*B]
2008/09	0.923	1.01	1.036	0.891	0.932
2009/10	1.23	0.791	1.123	1.096	0.973
2010/11	1.01	0.898	0.99	1.02	0.907
2011/12	0.938	1.044	0.949	0.988	0.979
2012/13	0.988	1.047	1.031	0.958	1.034
Mean	1.012	0.953	1.024	0.988	0.964

Source: Own computation

Table 8 Malmquist Index Summary of firm means

Year	Efficiency change [A = (C*D)]	TE change [B]	PE change [C]	SE change [D = (A/C)]	MITFP change [E = A*B]
Karamara	1.06	0.95	1.07	1.00	1.01
Army	1.01	0.96	1.03	0.98	0.97
Jugal	1.03	0.97	1.02	1.01	1.01
Police	0.98	0.98	0.98	1.00	0.95
ART	0.93	0.90	1.00	0.93	0.84
France	1.00	1.02	1.00	1.00	1.02
Yemariyam work	1.03	1.17	1.00	1.03	1.21
Yimaj	1.00	0.97	1.00	1.00	0.97
Dilchora	1.00	0.79	1.00	1.00	0.79
Bisidimo	1.12	0.85	1.14	0.99	0.95
Bilal	1.10	0.98	1.07	1.03	1.08
Hiwot Fana	0.91	0.95	1.00	0.91	0.86
Mean	1.01	0.95	1.02	0.99	0.96

Source: Own computation

The average PECH score for the entire sample was 1.024 during the study period, implying that PECH reduced efficiency by 4.2%.

Scale efficiency change Scale efficiency change (SECH) is expressed as a value less than, equal to, or greater than one if a hospital scale of production contributes negatively, not at all, or positively, respectively, to productivity change [28]. The scale of production in Jugal, Yemariamwork and Bilal contributed positively to TFP change by a factor of 1.2, 3.2 and 2.6%, respectively.

France, Yimaj and Dilchora hospitals had a scale efficiency index value of one (1) meaning that those hospitals' scale of production did not contribute to MTFP change. On the other hand, the SECH score for 5 hospitals was less than one (1) indicating that the scale of production in Karamara, ART, Army, Police and Hiwot Fana hospitals contributed negatively to productivity change by 0.5, 7.3, 1.8, 0.3 and 9%, respectively. The average SECH score for the entire sample was 0.988 indicating that the scale of production on average reduced efficiency change by 1.2%.

Technical change Ten hospitals (83%) registered technical change (TECH) of less than one indicating a decline in technical progress. The lack of technological progress in Karamara, Army, Jugal, Police, ART, Yimaj, Dilchora, Bisidimo, Bilal, and Hiwot Fana led to decrease in TFP (Total Factor Productivity) of 5.3, 3.8, 2.7, 2.3, 9.6, 2.8, 21.3, 2.2, 5.6 and 5.4%, respectively. France and Yemariamwork hospitals registered technical progress between the period t and t+1 of 1.9 and 17.3%, respectively.

Tobit regression model results
In this study, we used random effect Tobit model. The panel data is for 6 periods running from 2007/08 to 2012/13. To analyze the determinants of inefficiency of hospitals, the technical efficiency score of hospitals was converted to inefficiency score of hospitals. Subsequently, the inefficiency score was used as a dependent variable and regressed against hypothesized determinants (Size, Teachstat, BOR, Dcstaf, Opvinpdays and impdoc) using a censored Tobit model. Table 9, indicates that among the explanatory variables included in the analysis, four of them (Teachstat, Dcstaff, Opinpdays, impdoc) were found statistically significant while the remaining two were insignificant.

Teaching status (**Teachstat**) of the hospital is positively related with inefficiency score at 5% level of significance. This implies that being a teaching hospital reduces the expected efficiency score by 3.03.

The proportion of **Dcstaff** (medical doctors to the total staff) is negatively related with inefficiency and

Table 9 Summary of the Censored-Tobit regression analysis

Explanatory variables	Coefficient	Std. Err	Z
Lsize	−1.715701	2.451574	−0.7
Teachstat	3.034462**	1.340485	2.26
BOR	−0.0065286	0.0048885	−1.34
Dcstaf	−26.65755*	7.197905	−3.70
Opvinpdays	−0.3298481***	0.1885694	−1.75
Impdoc	−4.807009*	1.479342	−3.25
Constant	23.71757	6.968924	3.4

observations 72; 29 left-censored observations at Ineff ≥ 0; 43 uncensored observations

0 right-censored observations chi2 (7) = 28.87 Prob > chi2 0.0002

*$p \leq 0.01$ ** $p \leq 0.05$*** $p \leq 0.1$

statistically significant at one (1) % level of significance. This implies that for a one unit increase in Dcstaff (medical doctors to the total staff ratio); there is a 3.75 unit decrease in inefficiency score.

The coefficient for Opinpdays (outpatient visits to inpatient days ratio) has a negative sign that is consistent with our a priori expectation and significant at 10% level of significance. A one unit increase in the ratio of outpatient visit to inpatient days would lead to a decrease in hospital expected inefficiency score by 1.75.

The coefficient of the **Impdoc** (proportion of inpatients treated per medical doctor) is negatively related to inefficiency score and statistically significant at one percent level of significance. It shows that the number of inpatients per medical doctor has negative relationship with inefficiency score. This implies that a one percent increase in the ratio of inpatient per doctor would drop the predicted value of inefficiency score by 3.25%.

Discussions
Technical and scale efficiency of the hospitals
The average Variable Returns to Scale Technical Efficiency (VRSTE) scores of hospitals in Eastern Ethiopia were 91, 89, 91, 83, 86 and 93% during the period, respectively. This finding implies that if run efficiently the hospitals could have produced 9, 11, 9, 17, 14 and 7% more output (outpatient department visit, impatient days and number of surgery) for the same volume of inputs. The average VRSTE of hospitals in Eastern Ethiopia exhibit similarity with hospitals in Northern and Western Cape Provinces (82–82.8%) [29], Kwazulu Natal province of South Africa (90.6%) [30], and Kenya (84%) [31]. On the other hand, the average VRSTE scores were higher than those of Angola (65.8–67.5%) [8], Ghana (61%) [21], Zambia (67%) [32], Benin (63.3–85.8%) [9] and Namibia (62.7–74.3%) [33]. But it is lower than those for Uganda (90.2–97.3%) [34].

The average scale efficiency scores were 93%, 86%, 89%, 91%, 91%, 87% in the respective years between 2007/08 and 2012/13. These average scale efficiency scores were within the range of those for Angola (81–89%) [35], Kenya (90%) [31], and South Africa (Eastern, Northern and Western Cape Provinces) (82.5–90%) [29]. However, it is higher than those for Benin (41.9–73.6%) [6], Ghana (81%) [21], Namibia (73.2–83.7%) [33], and Zambia (80%) [32]. Moreover, the average scale efficiency scores for Botswana were lower than those of Kwazulu-Natal Province of South Africa (95.3%) [30], and Uganda (97.5%) [34].

The required change in input and output to make inefficient hospitals efficient
Table 6 shows the required change in input reduction or output increase to make inefficient hospitals efficient for

the study period. In this vein, if inefficient hospitals were concerned with the output side, the inefficient hospitals would have increased outpatient visit, inpatient days and surgery to become efficient. If hospitals were concerned with the level of inputs, the inefficient hospitals should have decreased their bed to be efficient.

Accordingly, the finding suggest that for hospitals with outputs that fall short of DEA targets, health policymakers could improve efficiency by improving access to and utilization of underutilized maternal and neonatal health and other services that has been underutilized. This may call for a multi-pronged strategy involving: Utilizing health promotion strategies and techniques such as: social mobilization, advocacy; social marketing; information, education, and communication (IEC); regulation and legislation; partnerships and alliances with public, private, non-governmental organization and civil society: and inter-sectoral action to address determinants of health to improve the use of underutilized health services [36].

It is also possible to provide access to universal health services through pooled pre-paid contribution collected based on ability to pay through the tax based funding [37]. The other alternative, if it is not possible to solve the inefficiency problem through the improved utilization of hospital health services, is to transfer the excess health staff, beds and drugs to health clinics, health posts and other health stations located in remote areas. However, an efficiency analysis of these lower level health facilities should guide this.

Total factor productivity change
The average MTFP of 0.964 for hospitals in eastern Ethiopia was comparable to those obtained in China inland of 0.985 [38], Greece of 0.986–0.988 [39], Ireland country of 0.977 [40], South Africa of 0.879 [19], and Taiwan 0.788 [41]. Unlike hospitals in Eastern Ethiopia, several countries hospitals had an average MTFP score greater than one signifying productivity growth. Portugal had 1.042 [42] Ireland regional hospitals had 1.028 [43], India district hospital had 1.235 [28], Angola municipal hospital had 1.045 [35] and China coastal hospitals had 1.121 [38].

Technical progress registered by hospitals may have been the result of applying better techniques with regard to both physical and human capital which allowed greater output with health system inputs held constant. This improvement could also have resulted from increases in motivation and/or skill of the health workforce.

Technical progress (or regression) depends on different factors. These factors may include: the availability of appropriate health technology which require minimum skill with accompanying inputs and institutional changes. The existence of close cooperation of health policy makers and the hospital management is also essential. Moreover, it is also important to equip the relevant health workforce so that they will be able to use the new technology efficiently [44].

Determinants of inefficiency of hospitals

Random effect Tobit model showed that teaching status of the hospital (Teachstat), medical doctor total staff ratio (Dcstaff), outpatient visits to inpatient days ratio (Opinpdays), and proportion of inpatients treated per medical doctor (impdoc) significantly determine the hospitals inefficiency in the study area.

Accordingly, the fact that teaching status of the hospital (**Teachstat**) has hospital is positively effect on inefficiency score of the hospital implies that being a teaching hospital reduces the expected efficiency. This might be related to the focus that these teaching hospitals are given in terms of materials and other necessary inputs. These teaching hospitals offer specialized services that attract patients. The hospital that provides both health services and training are less efficient than other hospitals. This finding may explain that teaching hospitals are a place where knowledge, skills, and experience are obtained through practical training, learning, and demonstration in the hospital. Doing these learning and teaching alongside with provision of the health services may complicate and adds to inefficiency of the hospitals. This is may be because of teaching hospitals may not get focused on the activities as they care for both the academics and health services provision. Moreover, teaching hospitals care much the training, education, skills, that their staffs and students must acquire from the hospital.

The fact that the proportion of medical doctors to the total staff (**Dcstaff**) negatively related to inefficiency implies that for an increase in ratio of medical doctors to the total staff there is a decrease in inefficiency score of hospitals. In the hospital, medical doctors are the staffs that have the highest level of education and training, and this may positively increase the efficiencies of the hospital. It may also be related to the spillover effect of the doctors to the other staffs. Additionally, this might be related to the improvement that might occur in facilitating service delivery associated with increasing of doctors as their quantity is few in developing country compared to the number of patient each serve. In contrast to this result, a study conducted in West Bengal in India by [45] discovered that doctor staff ratio negatively affected the technical efficiency of hospitals.

The negative relation between outpatient visits to inpatient day ratio (Opinpdays) and hospital inefficiency score indicates that an increase in the ratio of outpatient visit to inpatient days would lead to a decrease in hospital expected inefficiency score of hospitals. This result also agrees with the result obtained by [4] in the study of determinants of technical efficiency of hospitals in Eritrea. Similarly, [19] also discovered the same result in the case of determinants of technical efficiency of hospitals in South Africa.

The proportion of inpatients treated per medical doctor (**Impdoc**) is negatively related to inefficiency score of hospitals. This shows that the number of inpatients per medical doctor has negative relationship with inefficiency score. This implies that an increase in the ratio of inpatient per doctor would drop the predicted value of inefficiency score of hospitals. This finding may explain that there is a need to efficiently use available doctors and hospitals that provide health services. By doing so, efficiency and standard ratio of inpatients to the doctors can be maintained.

Conclusion and recommendation

This study attempts to analysis technical efficiency of hospitals in eastern Ethiopia. To achieve the objective of the study DEA, MTFP, and Tobit model are used. The DEA used to estimate the efficiency score of hospitals, MTFP used to analyses productivity change of hospitals and Tobit model used to analysis factors that determine inefficiency of hospitals.

Estimate of DEA indicates that under a VRS assumption, 6 (50%), 5 (42%), 3 (25%), 3 (25%), 4 (33%) and 3 (25%), while under a CRS assumption, 9 (75%), 9 (75%), 8 (67%), 7 (58%), 7 (58%) and 8 (67%) of the 12 hospitals were run inefficiently between 2007/08 and 2012/13. The results also indicate that 9 (75%), 9 (75%), 7 (58%), 7 (53%), 7 (58%) and 8 (67%) of the 12 hospitals were scale inefficient between 2007/08 and 2012/13. The estimate of the MTFP indicates that among the 12 hospitals, 7 (58%) experienced MTFP deterioration over the six years. The Tobit model indicates that teaching hospital is less efficient than other hospitals. The Tobit regression model further indicates that medical doctor to total staff ratio, the proportion of outpatient visit to inpatient days, and the proportion of inpatients treated per medical doctor were negatively related with technical inefficiency of hospitals.

Based on the findings, the following policy recommendations are forwarded. Further improvements can be made in the hospitals' efficiency by taking the following policy measures.

➢ Hospitals should monitor their services delivery efficiency and need to identify inputs that are underutilized. This may help hospitals identify which input need to increase or decrease or transfer to other health services facilities so that the use of underutilized health sector services will be promoted.

➢ Hospitals should monitor their services delivery efficiency and need to identify output that fall short of targets. This may help hospitals identify which output/services need to increase or decrease so that they may deliver better services. In this regard, it is crucial to institutionalize efficiency monitoring of health facilities within health management information system. This can be implemented by either having section with in structure of each hospital that study the efficiency or regularly hiring study agent. By doing so hospitals may maintain their pure efficiency, scale efficiency and/or technical efficiency and thereby total factor productivity in delivering the service would increase.

➢ Policy interventions that increase utilization of underutilized hospital outpatient health services and reduce the average length of stay, increase doctor to other staff ratio and the number of inpatients treated per doctor would contribute to improve the technical efficiency of hospitals. This may be achieved by provision of the capacity building like training for the staff members of the hospitals on efficient resource utilization and service delivery. Increasing the health staffs that considers the population of the study area and standard of the health staff to patient ratio may help improve the efficiency of the hospitals. This can be achieved through hiring additional health staffs, and upgrading the capacity of the existing staffs through provision of on job training.

Abbreviations
CRS: Constant return to scale; CRSTE: Constant return to scale technical efficiency; DEA: Data envelopment analysis; MITFP: Malmquist Total Factor Productivity; MPI: Malmquist Productivity Index; SFA: Stochastic Frontier Approach; TFP: Total factor productivity; VRS: Variable returns to scale; VRSTE: Variable return to scale technical efficiency

Acknowledgements
We are immensely grateful to the East Hararghe Zone, Harari Region, and Dire Dawa city council Hospitals for their cooperation in data collection. We are also thankful to Haramaya University for facilitating coordination for data collection for the study.

Funding
Haramaya University fund the study. The role of the Haramaya University provided fund for data collection. The design of the study and collection, analysis, and interpretation of data and writing of the manuscript are solely the role of the authors.

Authors' contributions
MA, MD and TB were equally involved in the literature review, data analysis, interpretation of the results, and drafting of the manuscript. Three of authors read and approved the final manuscript.

Competing interests
The authors declare that they have no competing interests.

Author details
[1]Department of Economics, Haramaya University, College of Business and Economics, Dire Dawa, Ethiopia. [2]Department of Economics, Hawasa University, College of Business and Economics, Awasa, Ethiopia.

References
1. World Bank. The World Bank Annual Report 2013. Washington, DC: 2013.
2. WHO. The World health report 2000 : health systems : improving performance. 2000.
3. Lambo E, Sambo LG. Health sector reform in sub-Saharan Africa: a synthesis of country experiences. East Afr Med J. 2003;80(6):S1–20.
4. Kirigia JM, Asbu EZ. Technical and scale efficiency of public community hospitals in Eritrea: an exploratory study. Health Econ Rev. 2013;3(1):6.
5. Tlotlego N, Nonvignon J, Sambo LG, Asbu EZ, Kirigia JM. Assessment of productivity of hospitals in Botswana: a DEA application. Int Arch Med. 2010;3(1):27.
6. Kirigia JM, Mensah OA, Mwikisa CN, Asbu EZ, Emrouznejad A, Makoudode P, Hounnankan A. Technical efficiency of zone hospitals in Benin. Afr Health Monit. 2010;12:30–9.
7. Marschall P, Flessa S. Assessing the efficiency of rural health centres in Burkina Faso: an application of Data Envelopment Analysis. J Public Health. 2009;17(2):87–95.
8. Wooldridge MJ. Introductory Econometrics: A Modern Approach. USA: South-Western College Publishing; 2009.
9. Zere E, Mcintyre D, Addison T. Technical efficiency and productivity of public sector hospitals in three South African provinces. S Afr J Econ. 2001; 69(2):336–58.
10. Tamiru B. Technical efficiency of public health centers: the case of Addis Ababa and selected health centers of Oromia. 2002.
11. Getachew A. Technical efficiency of selected public hospitals in Ethiopia. 2002.
12. Coelli TJ, Rao DS, O'Donnell CJ, Battese GE. An introduction to efficiency and productivity analysis. Springer Science & Business Media; 2005.
13. Greene WH. The econometric approach to efficiency analysis. The measurement of productive efficiency and productivity growth. 2008;1:92–250.
14. Charnes A, Cooper WW, Rhodes E. Measuring the efficiency of decision making units. Eur J Oper Res. 1978;2(6):429–44.
15. Banker RD, Charnes A, Cooper WW. Some models for estimating technical and scale inefficiencies in data envelopment analysis. Manag Sci. 1984;30(9): 1078–92.
16. Land KC, Lovell CA, Thore S. Chance-constrained data envelopment analysis. Manag Decis Econ. 1993;14(6):541–54.
17. Grifell-Tatjé E, Lovell CK. The sources of productivity change in Spanish banking. Eur J Oper Res. 1997;98(2):364–80.
18. Färe R, Grosskopf S, Norris M, Zhang Z. Productivity growth, technical progress, and efficiency change in industrialized countries. Am Econ Rev. 1994:66-83.
19. Eyob Z. Hospital efficiency in Sub-Sahara Africa: evidence from South Africa. 2000.
20. Talluri S. Data envelopment analysis: models and extensions. Decision Line. 2000;31(3):8–11.
21. Osei D, George M, d'Almeida S, Kirigia J, Mensah A, Kainyu L. Technical efficiency of public district hospitals and health centres in Ghana: a pilot study. Cost Eff Resour Alloc. 2005;3:9.
22. Clewer A, Perkins D. Economics for health care management. 1998.
23. Grosskopf S, Valdmanis V. Measuring hospital performance: A non-parametric approach. J Health Econ. 1987;6(2):89–107.
24. Kirigia JM, Emrouznejad A, Gama Vaz R, Bastiene H, Padayachy J. A comparative assessment of performance and productivity of health centres in Seychelles. Int J Product Perform Manag. 2007;57(1):72–92.
25. Linna M, Hakkinen U. Determinates of cost efficiency of finish hospital: a comparison of DEA and SFA. 1997.
26. Rosko M, Chilingerian J, Zinn J, Aaronson W. The effects of ownership, operating environment, and strategic choices on nursing efficiency. Med Care. 1995;1001–1021.
27. Valdmanis V. Sensitivity analysis for DEA models: An empirical example using public vs. NFP hospitals. J Public Econ. 1992;48(2):185–205.

28. Kirigia J, Lambo E, Sambo L. Are public hospitals in Kwazulu-Natal province of South Africa technically efficient? Afr J Health Sci. 2000;7(3–4):25–32.

29. Felix M. Investigating health system performance: An application of data envelopment analysis to Zambian hospitals. BMC Health Services Research. 2007; 7(58).

30. Zere E, Mbeeli T, Shangula K, Mandlhate C, Mutirua K, Tjivambi B, et al. Technical efficiency of district hospitals: evidence from Namibia using data envelopment analysis. Cost Eff Resour Alloc. 2006;4:5.

31. Yawe B, Kavuma S. Technical efficiency in the presence of desirable and undesirable outputs: a case study of selected district referral hospitals in Uganda. Health Policy Dev. 2008;6(1):237–53.

32. Kirigia JM, Emrouznejad A, Cassoma B, Asbu EZ, Barry S. A performance assessment method for hospitals: the case of Municipal Hospitals in Angola. J Med Syst. 2008;509–19.

33. World Health Organization (WHO). Milestones in health promotion statements from global conferences. Geneva: 2009.

34. World Health Organization (WHO). Primary health care: now more than ever. Geneva: 2008.

35. Ng YC. The productive efficiency of the health care sector of China. Rev Reg Stud. 2008;38(3):381.

36. Dash U. Evaluating the comparative performance of district head quarters hospitals, 2002–07: a non-parametric Malmquist approach. Mumbai: Indira Gandhi Institute of Development Research (IGIDR); 2009.

37. Zere E, Mcintyre D, Addison T. Technical efficiency and productivity of public sector hospitals in three South African provinces. S Afr J Econ. 2001; 69(2):336–58.

38. Karagiannis R, Velentzas K. Productivity and quality changes in Greek public hospitals. Oper Res. 2012;12(1):69-81.

39. Ouellette P, Vierstraete V. Technological change and efficiency in the presence of quasi-fixed inputs: A DEA application to the hospital sector. Eur J Oper Res. 2004;154(3):755–63.

40. Chang SJ, Hsiao HC, Huang LH, Chang H. Taiwan quality indicator project and hospital productivity growth. Omega. 2011;39(1):14–22.

41. Barros CP, De Menezes AG, Peypoch N, Solonandrasana B, Vieira JC. An analysis of hospital efficiency and productivity growth using the Luenberger indicator. Health Care Manag Sci. 2008;11(4):373–81.

42. Gannon B. Technical efficiency and total factor productivity growth of hospitals in Ireland. Data Envelop Anal Perform Manag. 2004;125.

43. Killick T. Policy economics: a textbook for applied economics on developing countries. London: Heinemann; 1981.

44. Arijita D, Bandyopadhyay S, Ghose A. Measurement and determinants of public hospital efficiency in West Bengal, India. J Asian Public Policy. 2014; 231–244.

45. Kirigia JM, Emrouznejad A, Sambo LG. Measurement of technical efficiency of public hospitals in Kenya: using data envelopment analysis. J Med Syst. 2002;26(1):39–45.

12

Public release of hospital quality data for referral practices in Germany

Martin Emmert[1]* ⓘ, Nina Meszmer[1], Lisa Jablonski[1], Lena Zinth[1], Oliver Schöffski[1] and Fatemeh Taheri-Zadeh[2]

Abstract

Objective: To evaluate the impact of different dissemination channels on the awareness and usage of hospital performance reports among referring physicians, as well as the usefulness of such reports from the referring physicians' perspective.

Data sources/Study setting: Primary data collected from a survey with 277 referring physicians (response rate = 26.2%) in Nuremberg, Germany (03–06/2016).

Study design: Cluster-randomised controlled trial at the practice level. Physician practices were randomly assigned to one of two conditions: (1) physicians in the control arm could become aware of the performance reports via mass media channels (Mass Media, n^{pr}_{MM}=132, n^{ph}_{MM}=147); (2) physicians in the intervention arm also received a printed version of the report via mail (Mass and Special Media, n^{pr}_{MSM}=117; n^{ph}_{MSM}=130).

Principal findings: Overall, 68% of respondents recalled hospital performance reports and 21% used them for referral decisions. Physicians from the Mass and Special Media group were more likely to be aware of the performance reports (OR 4.16; 95% CI 2.16–8.00, $p < .001$) but not more likely to be influenced when referring patients into hospitals (OR 1.73; 95% CI 0.72–4.12, $p > .05$). On a 1 (very good) to 6 (insufficient) scale, the usefulness of the performance reports was rated 3.67 (±1.40). Aggregated presentation formats were rated more helpful than detailed hospital quality information.

Conclusions: Hospital quality reports have limited impact on referral practices. To increase the latter, concerns raised by referring physicians must be given more weight. Those principally refer to the underlying data, the design of the reports, and the lack of important information.

Keywords: Public reporting, Hospital quality, Patient referral, Patient counselling, Public health

Background

The aim of public reporting is to improve healthcare quality by both stimulating quality improvement on the provider level ("Improvement Through Changes in Care") and also by helping patients and other consumers select the "right" provider ("Improvement Through Selection") [1]. While the published literature has confirmed the potential for public reporting to induce changes in clinical practice [2–5], little to no impact on the selection of

* Correspondence: Martin.Emmert@fau.de
[1]School of Business and Economics, Health Services Management, University of Erlangen-Nuremberg, Lange Gasse 20 90403 Nuremberg, Nuremberg, Germany

healthcare providers has been demonstrated [2, 3]. So far, most of the literature has addressed whether patients use publicly reported quality information to search for and to select health care providers [6–10]. However, less information is available regarding whether public reporting plays a role from the physicians' perspectives for referring patients to hospitals.

The available international literature suggests a limited impact of publicly reported quality information on the hospital referral behavior of physicians. For example, surveys of cardiologists in Pennsylvania in 1996 [11] and New York in 1997 [12] have revealed that even though most cardiologists were aware of cardiac surgery report cards, the impact of these on their hospital referral behavior was limited. Two decades later, despite an almost universal awareness of cardiac surgeon report cards, their impact on referral practices still remains limited [13]. Also, recent evidence from France [14] and the Netherlands [15] backs up those findings. The issue of whether and how physicians use publicly reported hospital quality information for referring patients to hospitals in Germany has yet to be addressed. In addition, there is still a gap in international research in evaluating the effectiveness of different dissemination channels [16] and presentation formats [17, 18] to maximize the impact of performance reports. Therefore, this study explores the impact of different dissemination channels on the awareness and usage of a hospital performance reporting initiative, namely the *Nuremberg hospital quality reporting system (NHQRS)*, among referring physicians, as well as the usefulness of such reports from the referring physicians' perspective. The latter publicly reported about the quality of care of hospitals for 14 clinical procedures in the region of Nuremberg (Bavaria, Germany) between January and April 2016.

New contribution

To the best of our knowledge, no evidence regarding the impact of public reporting on hospital referrals in the German healthcare setting has been published. Some survey results show that quality performance information does not play an important role for hospital referrals [19–21] but no study has yet addressed the impact of a public reporting intervention on referral behavior. When looking at this from an international perspective, research is necessary to evaluate the effectiveness of different dissemination channels in order to maximize the impact of performance reports [16]. In this context, Gombeski and colleagues have developed a model that illustrates the interaction of factors and channels influencing the referral decision. It shows that information about a referral organization/physician flows to physicians through interpersonal media (e.g., met physician at events, social event), mass media (e.g., television, newspapers), or special media (e.g., direct mail, brochures) [22]. We therefore hypothesize that a combination of such dissemination channels will increase awareness compared with a single approach. Barr and colleagues have further raised the question whether greater awareness of public reports will result in more willingness by physicians to use these reports in decision making about patient care [16]. Based on this, we investigate whether an increased level of awareness will also result in a greater willingness to use the NHQRS for referring patients to hospitals. Finally, studies have shown that less complex information displays should be employed to increase the comprehensibility and usage of report cards [17, 23]. So far, most research has focused on patients as

the target group of report cards. Given evidence from a recently published systematic review, no research has addressed whether physicians also prefer simplified information displays for hospital referrals [17]. We thus evaluate the usefulness of different quality presentation formats (e.g., ordering providers, presenting composite measures, different amounts of quality information) from the physicians' perspective for referral practices.

As follows, three major research questions guided this study:

1. To what extent do physicians become aware and make use of publicly reported hospital quality reports when referring patients to hospitals?
2. Does a combined mass and special media dissemination approach (i.e., newspaper and direct mailing) lead to higher awareness and usage results compared with a single mass media dissemination approach (i.e., newspaper)?
3. What are physicians' attitudes and perceptions of the performance reports in general and of different presentation formats in particular?

Methods

The Nuremberg hospital quality reporting system (NHQRS)

The NHQRS was developed by the authors of this investigation in cooperation with a local newspaper (Nürnberger Zeitung) with the aim of publicly reporting about the quality of hospitals in a region 50 km around Nuremberg, located in the south of Germany. In 2016, the estimated population for Nuremberg, where the Nürnberger Zeitung is mainly distributed, was estimated to be 529,047. Quality results were published on a weekly basis every Saturday in the local newspaper (Nürnberger Zeitung; daily print circulation approx. 2016: 33,000) and on corresponding online media websites (e.g., Facebook, nordbayern) between January 2nd and April 9th 2016. [Number of fans of the Facebook page of the Nürnberger Zeitung 01/2016: 53,047 fans; Number of followers on Twitter 12/2016: 59,740.] The public reporting intervention encompassed quality results for 14 clinical procedures, such as gallbladder resection, artificial hip replacement, and percutaneous coronary intervention. Those procedures were chosen based on the availability of clinical performance data as well as on the number of cases in Germany.

Four different *data sources* were used to determine hospital quality: (1) The German external quality assurance: hospital treatment for selected interventions is documented for each patient based on a set of in-house related quality indicators. Currently, the assurance system comprises 400 quality indicators within 30 different clinical areas [24]. Besides other objectives, these data can be used for public reporting purposes [19, 23, 25];

[For the special purpose of the NHQRS, all available publicly reported quality indicators with a defined reference range were used.] (2) Insurance claims data (Allgemeine Ortskrankenkasse): these data allow for an assessment of hospital quality based on routine data which enable a long-term perspective after hospital discharge (e.g., up to 365 days in prostate cancer treatment) [26]. [Here, all publicly reported quality indicators were used; see [26] for further statistical information regarding the underlying ranking procedure.] (3) The number of cases treated in 2014, as well as (4) patient satisfaction. The latter was derived from a patient satisfaction survey administered by two German statutory health insurances (AOK, BARMER GEK) and one hospital report card provider (the Weisse Liste). So far, roughly 2,000,000 patients have answered the Patients' Experience Questionnaire (PEQ) [27, 28].

Based on those data, we developed *three different presentation formats* to display different levels of hospital quality information. For example, a patient might be less interested in very detailed quality information in contrast to referring physicians or hospital management. Of these, two versions were published in the newspaper. They included one short overall ranking, whereby all hospitals were ranked into 3–5 performance groups without presenting any quality information (Version 1), as well as one alphabetical overview showing a composite score for each of the four data sources (Version 2) (see above). For developing version 1, we assigned a higher weight to medical quality and assigned hospitals to 3–5 different performance groups according to medical quality results (i.e., based on the the German external quality assurance data and insurance claims data). For example, hospitals with better than average results in both analysis were assigned to the first performance group. In constrast, those with lower than average results were assigned to the last performance group. Afterwards, the ordering within each performance group was based on the number of cases (i.e., below average, average, above average) and patient satisfaction scores. Besides this, one detailed presentation format was published online showing the results for each hospital on a quality-indicator based level (Version 3) (See Additional file 1).

Study design

Our study was designed as a cluster-randomized controlled trial at the physician practice level. Based on previously published literature discussing different information dissemination models [16, 22], we randomly assigned referring physicians (n^{pr}=789, n^{ph}=1057; where n^{pr}, n^{ph} denote the total number of practices and physicians in the region 25 km around Nuremberg, respectively) either to the control group ("Mass Media"; n^{pr}_{MM}=381, n^{ph}_{MM}=527) or

the intervention group ("Mass and Special Media"; n=408, n^{ph}_{MSM} =530) using a software-generated random number table. While mass media are defined as channels of communication aimed at the public with no opportunity for immediate feedback (e.g., newspapers, television, radio), special media are defined as highly focused communication channels designed for specific audiences with no immediate feedback (e.g., direct mail, brochures, books) [22]. Thus, physicians from the Mass Media group did not receive any additional information but could become aware of the NHQRS via the newspaper or other mass media channels. In contrast, physicians from the Mass and Special Media group also received a printed version of the newspaper article via mail.

We surveyed all referring physicians in the region 25 km around Nuremberg between March and June 2016. Thereby, we contacted referring physicians from six clinical areas 2 months after the publication of the results for the relevant clinical procedure. The physicians included both general practitioners and specialists (i.e., orthopedists, gastroenterologists, urologists, gynecologists, cardiologists). In a first step, physicians with an online available email address were contacted via email which contained a link to participate online (in a web-based survey), while the remaining physicians were contacted via regular mail and received a printed version of the survey (see Additional file 2 for the survey instrument). The cover letter contained some information about the NHQRS, the study and its purpose. After 1 week, a first reminder was sent out, followed by a second reminder a week later. The questionnaire was piloted by 25 individuals to ensure the comprehensibility of the wording and internal validity; final adjustments were made accordingly. The online survey was designed using Questback's internet-based EFS survey software and was also pre-tested. As an incentive, we held draws for one of four Amazon vouchers with a value of €150 each.

Data analysis

The applied survey contained both scaled-survey questions as well as open-ended text questions. We thus used a mixed-method approach by analyzing quantitative as well as qualitative data [29]. Quantitative results are presented as both means and standard deviations for continuous variables and as numbers and percentages for categorical variables. We performed comparisons between two groups by using a Chi-square test (two-sided) for categorical variables and a Mann-Whitney U test for continuous nonparametric variables. In addition, generalized estimating equation (GEE) models were performed to identify the main predictors associated with awareness and usage of the NHQRS by considering demographic (age, gender), professional (medical discipline, practice type, performing the publicly reported procedure), and study-related (e.g., Mass Media vs. Mass and Special Media group) characteristics. The generalized estimating equations are used for analyzing data from clustered randomized controlled trials on the individual level by accounting for the structure of the correlations within clusters [30–32]. The structure of GEE is like generalized linear models (GLM) defined by

$$(E(Y)) = \beta_0 + \beta_1 X_1 + \beta_2 X_2 + \cdots + \beta_k X_k$$

where Y denotes the response variables awareness respectively usage and $X_1, X_2, \cdots, X_k$ denote the independent variables.

Due to the binary form of the response variable Y (i.e., awareness/usage), we applied the logit function $g(p) = \log\left(\frac{p}{1-p}\right)$ as the link.

The QIC- and QICC-statistic were applied as the goodness-of-fit and model-selection criterion for our GEE based models [33]. All statistical analyses were conducted using SPSS version 23.0 (IBM Corp. Released 2012. IBM SPSS Statistics for Windows, Armonk, NY: IBM Corp.). Observed differences were identified as statistically significant if $p < .05$, and highly significant if $p < .001$.

Besides, qualitative analysis techniques were used to evaluate all open-ended text comments. We created a posteriori codebook by using small sets of between five and 10 reviews. Two evaluators coded independently and discussed the discrepancies. The codebook was updated in an iterative process until no new codes were identified. Some main categories were split into major and minor themes based on a directed qualitative content analysis method [34–36]. Finally, qualitative results were converted into quantitative data [37]. To ensure accuracy of coding, one author checked the qualitative approach by second-level coding.

Results

Our final study sample consisted of 277 respondents who completed the survey (overall response rate = 26.2%). The mean age was 54.67 (±8.47) years, 31.8% of the respondents were female and slightly more than half of the respondents were specialists (54.5%) (Table 1). The Mass Media group consisted of 147 physicians (response rate = 27.9%; $n^{pr}_{MM} = 132$, $n^{ph}_{MM} = 147$) and the Mass and Special Media group was comprised of 130 physicians (response rate = 24.5%; $n^{pr}_{MSM} = 117$; $n^{ph}_{MSM} = 130$), respectively. As shown, no statistically significant differences between both study groups in terms of age, gender, medical discipline, and practice type ($p > .05$ each) could be detected, thereby demonstrating an effective randomization process.

Table 1 Overview of the study sample (p value was calculated using chi-square test)

Characteristics	Study sample (n^{ph}=277)	Mass media (n^{ph}_{MM}=147)	Mass and special media (n^{ph}_{MSM}=130)	p
Age				
18 to 44 years	12.3%	16.0%	8.5%	.358
45 to 49 years	16.1%	16.0%	16.2%	
50 to 54 years	19.1%	18.5%	19.7%	
55 to 59 years	22.0%	22.7%	21.4%	
60 to 64 years	16.9%	12.6%	21.4%	
65 years and older	13.6%	14.3%	12.8%	
Gender				
Male	68.2%	67.3%	69.2%	.737
Female	31.8%	32.7%	30.8%	
Medical discipline				
General practitioner	45.5%	44.9%	46.2%	.834
Specialist	54.5%	55.1%	53.8%	
Practice type				
Single physician practice	43.0%	45.2%	40.7%	.747
Multiple physician practice	45.0%	42.7%	47.5%	
Medical care unit	12.0%	12.1%	11.9%	

Study design

Cluster-randomised controlled trial at the practice level. Physician practices were randomly assigned to one of two conditions: (1) physicians in the control arm could become aware of the performance reports via mass media channels; (2) physicians in the intervention arm also received a printed version of the report via mail.

Awareness of the NHQRS

Awareness of the NHQRS was reported by 177 (68.3%) respondents. As presented in Table 2, there were no statistically significant differences regarding age, gender, medical discipline, whether or not performing the publicly reported procedure, the communication measure as well as the time of the survey ($p > .05$ each). In contrast, physicians who work in any form of multiple physician practices (74.8% vs. 58.7%, $p < .05$), or those from the Mass and Special Media group were shown to have significantly higher awareness levels of the NHQRS (83.2% vs. 54.5%, $p < .001$).

The regression model based on generalized estimating equations on the physician level showed that demographic and professional characteristics were not associated with awareness of the NHQRS. However, the dissemination channel of the quality information was shown to be significantly associated with awareness of

Table 2 Descriptive analysis and GEE based regression model predicting awareness of NHQRS

Parameter	Description (Overall 68.3%)	Regression analysis					
		Regression coefficient	Standard error	Odds ratio	95%-Wald CI lower bound	95%-Wald CI upper bound	p-value
Age		−0.020	0.105	0.98	0.80	1.21	0.851
Gender							
Male	71.3%						
Female	62.4%	−0.312	0.341	0.73	0.38	1.43	0.359
Medical discipline							
General practitioner	63.6%						
Specialist	72.3%	0.613	0.788	1.85	0.39	8.65	0.437
Practice type							
Single physician	58.7%*						
Practice otherwise	74.8%	0.474	0.332	1.61	0.84	3.08	0.153
Performing publicly reported procedure							
No	69.2%						
Yes	69.7%	−0.316	0.468	0.73	0.29	1.82	0.500
Dissemination channel							
Mass Media	54.5%**						
Mass and Special Media	83.2%	1.425	0.334	4.16	2.16	8.00	<0.001
Communication measure (survey)							
Email	69.8%						
Mail	67.6%	−0.341	0.368	0.71	0.35	1.46	0.354
Time of survey							
Before the last published report	63.6%						
After the last published report	72.3%	−0.208	0.803	0.81	0.17	3.92	0.795
Constant	–	0.244	0.547	1.28	0.44	3.73	0.655

The first expression of the variable is regarded as the reference group
Age considered as a continuous variable in the model
QIC = 259.68, QICC = 260.07
*$p < 0.05$ (using chi-square test)
**$p < 0.001$ (using chi-square test)

the reporting system; the odds of being aware of the performance reports is 4.2 times greater for physicians from the Mass and Special Media group compared with those from the Mass Media group, all other variables of the model being held constant (OR 4.16; 95% CI 2.16–8.00, $p < .001$).

Impact of the NHQRS on referral practices

Overall, every fifth physician (20.6%) stated that he/she had been influenced by the NHQRS when referring patients to hospitals (Table 3). The results indicate no statistically significant differences regarding age, gender, practice type, whether or not performing the publicly reported procedure, and the communication measure of the survey ($p > .05$ each). In contrast, general practitioner (33.3% vs. 10.8%, $p < .001$), those who were surveyed after the last published report (31.5% vs. 9.1%, $p < .05$), or those from

the Mass and Special Media group were shown to have significantly higher impact levels of the NHQRS (26.0% vs. 13.2%, $p < .05$). More specifically, almost every sixth physician stated that NHQRS had had an impact either in a positive or negative direction (15.0% vs. 14.9%).

The regression results could not reveal any demographic and professional characteristics to be associated with impact of the NHQRS on hospital referrals. Here, the dissemination channel of the quality information could not be shown to be a significant predictor of impact on hospital referrals (OR 1.73; 95% CI 0.72–4.12, $p > .05$).

Based on a paper of Brown and colleagues [13], we performed another regression model without considering the time of the survey (i.e., before or after the last published report). In line with the findings above, the dissemination channel of the quality information could not be shown to be a significant predictor of impact on

Table 3 Descriptive analysis and GEE based regression model predicting impact of NHQRS on hospital referrals

Parameter	Description (Overall 20.6%)	Regression analysis					
		Regression coefficient	Standard error	Odds ratio	95%-Wald CI lower bound	95%-Wald CI upper bound	p-value
Age		−0.184	0.142	0.83	0.63	1.77	0.196
Gender							
Male	17.7%						
Female	26.8%	0.072	0.429	1.08	0.46	2.49	0.866
Medical discipline							
General practitioner	33.3%**						
Specialist	10.8%	−0.721	0.899	0.49	0.08	2.83	0.422
Practice type							
Single physician practice	19.1%						
Otherwise	20.6%	0.339	0.431	1.40	0.60	3.27	0.431
Performing publicly reported procedure							
No	24.2%						
Yes	11.5%	0.048	0.734	1.05	0.25	4.42	0.948
Dissemination channel							
Mass Media	13.2%*						
Mass and Special Media	26.0%	0.546	0.443	1.73	0.72	4.12	0.219
Communication measure (survey)							
Email	15.3%						
Mail	23.1%	0.684	0.515	1.98	0.72	5.43	0.184
Time of survey							
Before the last published report	31.5%*						
After the last published report	9.1%	−1.155	0.880	0.32	0.06	1.10	0.189
Constant	–	−1.216	0.712	0.296	0.07	1.20	0.088

The first expression of the variable is regarded as the reference group
Age considered as a continuous variable in the model
QIC = 158.83, QICC = 158.98
*$p < 0.05$ (using chi-square test)
**$p < 0.001$ (using chi-square test)

hospital referrals (OR 1.88; 95% CI 0.80–4.39, $p > .05$). However, we could detect significantly lower odds for specialists compared with general practitioner (OR 0.20; 95% CI 0.07–0.58, $p < .05$).

The usefulness of the NHQRS

Based on the German school grading system (1 = very good to 6 = insufficient), the NHQRS was rated 3.67 (±1.40) (Table 4). More specifically, an assessment of the trustworthiness, helpfulness, credibility, and informative value indicates slightly less favorable results in these areas. On a 1 (not trustworthy etc. at all) to 5 (very trustworthy etc.) scale, the results vary between 2.49 (±1.16) for helpfulness and 2.85 (±1.08) for credibility, respectively. Therefore, the more detailed versions of the reporting formats were rated as less helpful (version 1: 2.69 ± 1.34; version 2: 2.43 ± 1.24; version 3: 2.35 ± 1.27). The future impact on referral practices was

shown to be highest for the overall ranking result (2.29 ± 1.33), and lowest for the second version that presented hospitals in alphabetical order along with the overall performance scores for all four data sources (2.11 ± 1.18), respectively. It is interesting to note that general practitioners gave significantly better ratings than specialists regarding all issues ($p < .05$ each). We also analyzed rating results between both study groups according to the dissemination channel of the information but did not detect any significant differences (not presented here).

Critical analysis of the NHQRS

In total, 68 open-ended text answers were analyzed which comprised 147 critical statements about the usefulness of the NHQRS (Table 5). Most frequently, referring physicians criticized the underlying data ($n = 38$), particularly with respect to the appropriateness of the

Table 4 The usefulness of the NHQRS (p value was calculated using Mann-Whitney U)

Rating	Overall (n^{ph}=277)	General practitioner (n^{ph}=126)	Specialist (n^{ph}=151)	p
Overall rating[a]	3.67 (1.40)	3.37 (1.37)	3.92 (1.38)	.002
Detailed rating categories[b]				
Trustworthiness[b]	2.68 (1.08)	2.89 (0.99)	2.50 (1.12)	.003
Helpfulness[b]	2.49 (1.16)	2.77 (1.15)	2.25 (1.12)	<.001
Credibility[b]	2.85 (1.08)	3.03 (1.03)	2.69 (1.10)	.009
Informative value[b]	2.65 (1.14)	2.87 (1.14)	2.47 (1.11)	.004
Version 1 (overall ranking, 3–5 performance groups)				
Helpfulness[b]	2.69 (1.34)	3.05 (1.30)	2.38 (1.29)	<.001
Likely impact on future referral practice[b]	2.29 (1.33)	2.66 (1.31)	1.98 (1.26)	<.001
Version 2 (alphabetical order; categorical overall performance)				
Helpfulness[b]	2.43 (1.24)	2.66 (1.21)	2.23 (1.23)	.004
Likely impact on future referral practice[b]	2.11 (1.18)	2.38 (1.19)	1.88 (1.13)	<.001
Version 3 (alphabetical order; detailed quality indicator-based information)				
Helpfulness[b]	2.35 (1.27)	2.64 (1.30)	2.10 (1.20)	.001
Likely impact on future referral practice[b]	2.22 (1.25)	2.56 (1.29)	1.92 (1.13)	<.001

[a]German school-based rating system; 1 to 6 scale (1 = very good; 2 = good; 3 = satisfactory; 4 = sufficient; 5 = deficient; 6 = insufficient)
[b]1 to 5 scale (1 = not trustworthy etc. at all; 5 = very trustworthy etc.)

data used concerning claims (n = 9) and the risk of manipulation of the data (n = 6). Furthermore, 21 comments were related to the design of the ranking, such as the placement of explanatory information (n = 6), type size (n = 3), order of hospitals (n = 2) or the traffic light color-based design used in version 1 (n = 2). Twenty comments contained statements that important quality information was missing. For example, urologists stated that aspects such as mortality or complications within 30 days after surgery were included, but not relevant patient-reported outcome measures (e.g., continence success, potency success). Furthermore, others raised the importance of integrating the satisfaction of the referring physicians.

Discussion

Our results show that by publishing hospital quality information only in the mass media, almost six out of 10 physicians (55%) became aware of the NHQRS; this is mainly in line with findings from the US. For example, Schneider and Epstein showed that after publishing the Consumer Guide to Coronary Artery Bypass Graft (CABG) Surgery in Pennsylvania four times, 82% of cardiologists surveyed were aware of the data [11]. Two decades later, an almost universal awareness among cardiologists had been reached (94%) [13]. It is important to mention that the era of public reporting in Germany has just begun to develop. Even though the German Federal Joint Committee states that "To date, no other country in the world has a similar, nationwide procedure requiring documentation and online disclosure of health care quality performance in inpatient

settings" [38], the awareness of such quality information still remains low in Germany. A survey showed that only 39% of physicians are aware of corresponding hospital quality reports and 11% of internet websites on which the information is publicly disclosed [21]. In contrast to previous evidence, we did not find any statistically significant differences regarding age [11]. We observed, however, significantly higher awareness among those who work in any form of multiple physician practices or those from the Mass and Special Media group.

We were able to show that the dissemination channel of the quality information matters. By sending a printed copy of the article via mail to the physicians' practices we were able to significantly increase the awareness level by almost 30 percentage points. This has major implications for health policymakers with respect to achieving a rapid and broad awareness of hospital quality information among physicians. As mentioned above, the Consumer Guide to CABG surgery had been published four times in Pennsylvania starting in 1992 before Schneider and Epstein determined the awareness level to be 82% [11]. We could slightly exceed this awareness level in the first year of the NHQRS (here, 83.2% of physicians reported awareness) by combining mass and special media dissemination channels.

Every fifth physician (20.5%) stated that he/she had been influenced by the NHQRS when referring patients to hospitals, which is in line with international evidence. For example, in the study conducted by Schneider and Epstein, only 13% of the cardiologists surveyed responded that the Consumer Guide ratings had a moderate or substantial impact on their referral [11]. Hannan

Table 5 Results of the qualitative analysis regarding criticism from the physicians' perspective

Topic of the criticism	N	Examples
Flaws of underlying data (e.g., timeliness, risk-adjustment, validity, risk of manipulation)	38	• "The number of cases based on insurance claims data is not sufficiently large" • "Individual data are too often manipulated"
Design (e.g., type size, placement of information, rank order, traffic light colors)	21	• "The alphabetical order is not helpful" • "Tables with insurance claims data include terms far too complex"
Missing of further quality information (e.g., PROMs, satisfaction of referring physicians)	20	• "Access to hospitals is not included" • "You should survey referring physicians"
Impact of the public reporting initiative (e.g., risk of misinformation, short-term impact)	11	• "Experience shows that such actions cause uncertainty for patients" • "The effect is of limited duration"
Methodology for deriving the quality scores (e.g., weighting of quality information)	10	• "The methodical approach to deal with this issue does not reflect reality" • "The data were not assessed accurately"
Publication media (e.g., daily newspaper inappropriate)	10	• "I do not use quality information provided by a newspaper" • "I believe that the newspaper NZ is not the appropriate media to publish scientific data"
Other factors more relevant (e.g., own experience, patient preference, distance)	10	• "I rely on results which I can see on patients and patients' experiences myself" • "Personal experiences are more important"
Hospital related issues (e.g., ownership structure)	8	• "No consideration of multi-morbid patients, which are treated in small hospitals - > bad grade of large hospitals" • "Regarding the fact that "private hospitals" treat very highly selected patients (e.g. no risk patients), it is difficult to compare the number of cases and statistical analysis regarding mortality with local community hospitals"
Transparency (e.g., funding, methodology, conflict of interests)	5	• "Was there any relationship with the newspaper? (conflict of interests)?" • "I don't know about the significance of the criteria, the transparency is questionable"
Ranking does not match physicians' experience	4	• "Based on daily practice some hospitals are overrated" • "I was treated in hospitals which are rated as under-performer and I was extremely satisfied"
Structural changes in hospitals	3	• "Structures are changing quickly" • "Since 2013/2014 several surgeons have been changing hospitals (retirement, other hospital!)"
Scope of the public reporting initiative	3	• "A smaller number of hospitals would be easier to recognize" • "I cautiously read the Focus hospital ranking which contains also the remaining hospitals in Germany"
Subjectivity of the ranking	2	• "In my opinion such rankings are usually created by persons who have no or less insight in daily routines of a hospital. As a result subjective opinions/impressions are included" • "Shouldn't there be more newspapers or institutes to conduct such a ranking?"
No specific reasons stated	2	• "Rankings seem generally suspicious to me" • "Rankings are very meaningful for the majority of the population. Whether rankings present the exact condition of hospitals is questionable"

et al. showed slightly higher impact scores; in their study, 6% of the cardiologists surveyed responded that the New York CABG surgery reports had affected their referrals to surgeons "very much", and 32% "somewhat". In addition, only 22% stated that they routinely discussed the information in the cardiac report with their patients [12]. Two decades later, Brown et al. surveyed cardiologists in New York and showed that still, only 25% reported that the reports had a moderate or substantial influence on referral decisions, and 29% stated that they had discussed the report cards with patients [13]. Available studies from Europe have also demonstrated the limited impact of public reporting on referral behavior. For example, Ferrua et al. surveyed 503 self-employed general practitioners in private practice in France. They showed that approximately 14% of the practitioners had already used publicly available comparative indicators to influence hospital choices for their patients [14]. Similar results have also been shown in the Netherlands. For example, in a study by Ketelaar et al. only 12% of physicians surveyed reported that they had used comparative performance information when selecting a hospital [15].

It furthermore seems that the positive and negative impact of hospital performance reports are alike. In our study, almost every sixth physician stated that performance reports had had an impact either in a positive (15.0%) or negative (14.9%) direction. This confirms evidence from the US showing that 35% of physician rating website users reported selecting a physician based on good ratings, while 37% had avoided a physician with bad ratings. Slightly in contrast, two studies from Germany showed higher impact results in a positive direction for both hospitals [39] and physicians [9]. The higher impact results might be due to different survey samples. In contrast to our study, in which health care providers were surveyed, the mentioned studies have focused on the general population. Barr and colleagues have further raised the question concerning whether a greater awareness of public reports will result in more willingness by physicians to use those reports [16]. Based on our findings, the impact among physicians from the Mass and Special Media group, for whom statistically greater awareness levels were presented, could be shown to be significantly greater. However, the regression results could not prove the dissemination channel of the quality information to be a significant predictor of impact on hospital referrals.

Overall, the physicians surveyed gave a slightly less favorable rating regarding the value of the performance reports for making hospital referrals (mean 3.67 on a 1 = very good to 6 = insufficient scale), thus confirming international findings. For example, Hannan et al. surveyed 450 cardiologists in New York to determine the value of the CABG surgery outcomes for all hospitals in New York. Here, the average rating was 2.40 on a 1 (not at all useful) to 5 (extremely useful) scale. In addition, 84% of the respondents rated the report to be between "not at all useful" and "somewhat useful" [12]. We also found that general practitioners gave significantly more favorable ratings than specialists. Specialists probably do not feel the need for such information due to their more focused clinical areas. These individuals might feel more capable of overseeing possible hospitals for inpatient treatment while assessing the quality of them. In this regard, Epstein examined referral patterns to cardiac surgeons to assess whether public reporting added information to what referring physicians already knew [40]. As a result, he showed that CABG patients were significantly less likely to be treated by high-mortality surgeons and more likely to be treated by low-mortality surgeons even without the report cards. He concludes that

referring specialists appear to have been knowledgeable about the relative performance of cardiac surgeons on their own without the need to use report cards. However, this finding is true for a medical intervention that is typically cared for by specialists and not general practitioners, who deal with a broader range of patients and diseases. General practitioners might need knowledge about treatment options for a greater variety of clinical areas, and thus they might see a greater benefit in publicly reported quality data.

Previous evidence has demonstrated that less complex information displays should be favored to increase the comprehensibility and usage of performance report cards among patients and other consumers [17, 23]. We initially hypothesized that this might not be true for referring physicians who are more likely to be interested in detailed hospital quality information. However, we determined that the most aggregated presentation format (overall composite measure based ranking, 3–5 performance groups) was rated the most helpful for referral decisions. This seems to be somewhat surprising; especially since only every fourth physician surveyed (27.3%) rated this presentation format as confidential. On the other hand, every second physician (50.5%) found it useful to present hospitals in different performance groups as we did. In contrast to other quality reporting initiatives, which publicly report only top-performing hospitals (e.g., The US 100 top hospitals, the US News hospital ranking, the German FOCUS Ärzteliste), we decided to present both high- and low-performing hospitals what was assessed as positive by approximately 70% of all physicians. Again, the presentation of hospital quality information on a quality-indicator based level in alphabetical order was rated as least helpful. Interestingly, only one of three physicians (34.5%) thought that such a detailed level was necessary to assess the quality of hospitals. Therefore, those who thought it was necessary gave a more favorable rating that those who did not (3.19 vs. 1.82; $p < .001$). Consequently, our findings supplement the results from a recently published systematic review [17] by demonstrating that the majority of referring physicians also seem to prefer simplified information displays.

Given these findings and the effort which has been put into further developing report cards in health care over the last two decades [41, 42], one might contemplate the reasons for the still limited impact. One major hurdle seems to be that physicians do not trust the publicly reported quality information and thus do not use it [12, 16, 43, 44]. Despite the incorporation of the best available hospital quality data in Germany, referring physicians in our study raised several concerns which need to be addressed. In line with international evidence, publicly reported data in Germany do not seem to include all relevant quality information [11, 13]. Exclusively focusing on clinical metrics (e.g., mortality or complications), the number of cases, or patient satisfaction does not suffice when making referral decisions. But, patient-reported outcome measures, which provide information that is relevant from a patient's perspective, were missing. For example, in prostate cancer treatment, aspects such as continence and potency success are also important for patients undergoing prostatectomy surgery. Others wish further information such as the satisfaction of referring physicians or the case mix of the patients in each hospital. Others mentioned that some included quality metrics were even inappropriate to determine the quality of hospitals [13], and thus would be misleading for patients who are searching for a hospital.

There are some limitations that have to be taken into account when interpreting the results of our study. First, we achieved a response rate of 26%. This means that we cannot ensure representativeness for all referring practitioners in the region (nonresponse bias). Nevertheless, our response rate is within the range of studies with a similar approach [13, 45, 46]. Besides, literature has suggested that there is no consistent relationship between nonresponse rates and nonresponse bias [47]. Second, our results focus on the short-term impact of public reporting. We estimated the results regarding the awareness, usage, and impact 2 months after the public reporting intervention. Thus, we were not able to determine the long-term effect of the intervention as reported in other studies [11–13]. Furthermore, the findings about the impact of the NHQRS were calculated based on the responses of the surveyed referring physicians. Those results might differ from studies applying an experimental design under real conditions when analyzing empirical data regarding the impact, such as the numbers of cases per year. Finally, hospital quality information was published mainly in one regional newspaper. The publication in further newspapers might have led to higher awareness results.

Conclusions

Despite all the efforts that have been undertaken to further develop public reporting [41, 42], its impact on hospital referrals is still limited. Based on our results, much has to be done if we want quality reporting initiatives to be more meaningful from the referring physician's perspective. One the one hand, this is partly due to the low awareness levels concerning publicly available hospital quality information. In this regard, the dissemination channel of the quality information matters; for a rapid and broad awareness to be reached, a singular mass media approach does not seem to be appropriate. On the other hand, we assume that the limited impact of hospital quality reports is much more likely due to the fact that referring physicians do not trust the published information and thus do not make use of it [44].

Implications for health policymakers

Before putting even greater effort into promoting publicly available quality information, health policymakers should rather address the concerns raised by referring physicians. These concerns mainly refer to different issues regarding the underlying data, the design of reporting initiatives, and the lack of important quality information. As stated by Mukamel and colleagues, "Quality report cards are only as good as the measures they include" [10]. Otherwise, many resources will be spent without significantly increasing the impact and benefit of reporting systems.

Acknowledgements
Not applicable.

Funding
This study was partly financed by the Hans Frisch Foundation at the Friedrich Alexander University of Erlangen, Nuremberg.

Authors' contributions
ME participated in the study design, methods, collection of the data, quantitative analysis and interpretation of data, and contributed to the manuscript. NM participated in the study design, methods, collection of the data, interpretation of data, and contributed to the manuscript. LJ and LZ participated in the collection of the data, interpretation of data, and contributed to the manuscript. OS participated in the study design, interpretation of data, and contributed to the manuscript. OS participated in the study design, interpretation of data, and contributed to the manuscript. FTZ participated in the methods, quantitative analysis and interpretation of data, and contributed to the manuscript. All authors reviewed and approved the final manuscript.

Competing interests
The authors were responsible for the development of the Nuremberg hospital quality reporting system (NHQRS) but declare that there is no competing interest.

Author details
[1]School of Business and Economics, Health Services Management, University of Erlangen-Nuremberg, Lange Gasse 20 90403 Nuremberg, Nuremberg, Germany. [2]Media, Information and Design Department of Information and Communication, University of Applied Sciences and Arts, Hannover, Germany.

References
1. Berwick DM, James B, Coye MJ. Connections between quality measurement and improvement. Med Care. 2003;41:I30–8.
2. Fung CH, Lim YW, Mattke S, Damberg C, Shekelle PG. Systematic review. The evidence that publishing patient care performance data improves quality of care. Annals of the Internal Medicine. 2008;148:111–23.
3. Totten AM, Wagner J, Tiwari A, O'Haire C, Griffin J, Walker M. Closing the quality gap: revisiting the state of the science (vol. 5: public reporting as a quality improvement strategy). Evid Rep Technol Assess (Full Rep). 2012; (208.5):1–645.
4. Schlesinger M, Grob R, Shaller D. Using Patient-Reported Information to Improve Clinical Practice. Health Ser Res. 2015:2116–54.

5.   Emmert M, Meszmer N, Sander U. Do Health Care Providers Use Online Patient Ratings to Improve the Quality of Care? Results From an Online-Based Cross-Sectional Study. J Med Internet Res. 2016;18:e254.
6.   Hibbard JH, Greene J, Daniel D. What is quality anyway? Performance reports that clearly communicate to consumers the meaning of quality of care. Med Care Res Rev. 2010;67:275–93.
7.   Hibbard JH, Peters E. Supporting informed consumer health care decisions. Data presentation approaches that fa-cilitate the use of information in choice. Annual Rev pub Health. 2003;24:413–33.
8.   Castle NG. The Nursing Home Compare report card. Consumers' use and understanding. J Aging Soc Pol. 2009;21:187–208.
9.   Emmert M, Meier F, Pisch F, Sander U. Physician choice making and characteristics associated with using physician-rating websites: cross-sectional study. J Med Internet Res. 2013;15:e187.
10. Mukamel DB, Weimer DL, Zwanziger J, Gorthy S-FH, Mushlin AI. Quality report cards, selection of cardiac surgeons, and racial disparities: a study of the publication of the New York State Cardiac Surgery Reports. Inquiry 2004–2005, 41:435-446.
11. Schneider EC, Epstein AM. Influence of cardiac-surgery performance reports on referral practices and access to care. A survey of cardiovascular specialists. N Engl J Med. 1996;335:251–6.
12. Hannan EL, Stone CC, Biddle TL, De Buono BA. Public release of cardiac surgery outcomes data in New York. What do New York state cardiologists think of it? Am Heart J. 1997;134:55–61.
13. Brown DL, Epstein AM, Schneider EC. Influence of cardiac surgeon report cards on patient referral by cardiologists in New York state after 20 years of public reporting. *Circulation*. Cardiovasc Qual Outcomes. 2013;6:643–8.
14. Ferrua M, Sicotte C, Lalloue B, Minvielle E. Comparative Quality Indicators for Hospital Choice: Do General Practitioners Care? PLoS One. 2016;11:e0147296.
15. Ketelaar NA, Faber MJ, Elwyn G, Westert GP, Braspenning JC. Comparative performance information plays no role in the referral behaviour of GPs. BMC Fam Pract. 2014;15:146.
16. Barr JK, Bernard SL, Sofaer S, Giannotti TE, Lenfestey NF, Miranda DJ. Physicians' views on public reporting of hospital quality data. Med Care Res Rev. 2008;65:655–73.
17. Kurtzman ET, Greene J. Effective presentation of health care performance information for consumer decision making: A systematic review. Patient Educ Couns. 2016;99:36–43.
18. Emmert M, Schlesinger M. Hospital Quality Reporting in the United States: Does Report Card Design and Incorporation of Patient Narrative Comments Affect Hospital Choice? Health Serv Res. 2016;52(3):933–58.
19. Geraedts M, Schwartze D, Molzahn T. Hospital quality reports in Germany: patient and physician opinion of the reported quality indicators. BMC Health Ser Res. 2007;7:157.
20. Hermeling P, W De C, Geraedts M. Informationsbedarf niedergelassener Ärzte bei Ein- und Überweisungen. Gesundheitswesen (Bundesverband der Ärzte des Öffentlichen Gesundheitsdienstes (Germany)). 2013;75:448–55.
21. Hermeling P, Geraedts M. Kennen und nutzen Ärzte den strukturierten Qualitätsbericht? Gesundheitswesen. 2013;75:155–9.
22. Gombeski WR, Carroll PA, Lester JA. Influencing decision-making of referring physicians. J Health Care Mark. 1990;10:56–60.
23. Sander U, Emmert M, Dickel J, Meszmer N, Kolb B. Information presentation features and comprehensibility of hospital report cards: design analysis and online survey among users. J Med Int Res. 2015;17:e68.
24. AQUA-Institut: German Hospital Quality Report 2014; Commissioned by Federal Joint Committee. Göttingen. 2015. [https://www.sqg.de/sqg/upload/CONTENT/Qualitaetsberichte/2014/AQUA-Qualitaetsreport-2014.pdf]. Accessed 17 Sept 2017.
25. AQUA-Institut: German Hospital Quality Report 2013; Commissioned by Federal Joint Committee. Göttingen. 2014. [https://sqg.de/upload/CONTENT/EN/Quality-Report/AQUA-German-Hospital-Quality-Report-2013.pdf]. Accessed 17 Sept 2017.
26. Wissenschaftliches Instituts der AOK (WidO): Qualitätssicherung mit Routinedaten [http://www.qualitaetssicherung-mit-routinedaten.de/]. Accessed 17 Sept 2017.

27. Gehrlach C, Altenhöner T, Schwappach D. Der Patients' Experience Questionnaire: Patientenerfahrungen vergleichbar machen. Gütersloh: Bertelsmann Foundation; 2009.
28. Weisse Liste gemeinnützige GmbH: Versichertenbefragung mit dem Patients' Experience Questionnaire (PEQ) [https://weisse-liste.de/de/service/ueber-krankenhaussuche/versichertenbefragung/]. Accessed 17 Sept 2017.
29. Bishop FL, Holmes MM. Mixed Methods in CAM Research: A Systematic Review of Studies Published in 2012. Evidence-based complementary and alternative medicine: eCAM. 2013;2013:187365.
30. Chuang J-H, Hripcsak G, Heitjan DF. Design and analysis of controlled trials in naturally clustered environments. Implications for medical informatics. J Am Med Inform Assoc. 2002;9:230–8.
31. Zeger SL, Liang KY. Longitudinal data analysis for discrete and continuous outcomes. Biometrics. 1986;42:121–30.
32. Peters TJ, Richards SH, Bankhead CR, Ades AE, JAC S. Comparison of methods for analysing cluster randomized trials. An example involving a factorial design. Int J Epidemiol. 2003;32:840–6.
33. Pan W. Akaike's information criterion in generalized estimating equations. Biometrics. 2001;57:120–5.
34. Goff SL, Mazor KM, Gagne SJ, Corey KC, Blake DR. Vaccine counseling: a content analysis of patient-physician discussions regarding human papilloma virus vaccine. Vaccine. 2011;29:7343–9.
35. Lagu T, Goff SL, Hannon NS, Shatz A, Lindenauer PK. A mixed-methods analysis of patient reviews of hospital care in England: implications for public reporting of health care quality data in the United States. Jt Comm J Qual Patient Saf. 2013;39:7–15.
36. Hsieh H-F, Shannon SE. Three approaches to qualitative content analysis. Qual Health Res. 2005;15:1277–88.
37. Fetters MD, Curry LA, Creswell JW. Achieving integration in mixed methods designs-principles and practices. Health Serv Res. 2013;48:2134–56.
38. Federal Joint Committee: External Quality Assurance. Public Reporting of Hospital Quality Performance [https://www.g-ba.de/institution/themenschwerpunkte/qualitaetssicherung/qualitaetsdaten/qualitaetsbericht/]. Accessed 17 Sept 2017.
39. Emmert M, Hessemer S, Meszmer N, Sander U. Do German hospital report cards have the potential to improve the quality of care? Health policy (Amsterdam, Netherlands). 2014;118:386–95.
40. Epstein AJ. Effects of report cards on referral patterns to cardiac surgeons. J Health Econ. 2010;29:718–31.
41. Lagu T, Hannon NS, Rothberg MB, Lindenauer PK. Patients' evaluations of health care providers in the era of social networking: an analysis of physician-rating websites. J Gen Intern Med. 2010;25:942–6.
42. Damberg CL, McNamara P. Postscript: research agenda to guide the next generation of public reports for consumers. M Care Res Rev. 2014;71:97S–107S.
43. Marshall MN, Hiscock J, Sibbald B. Attitudes to the public release of comparative information on the quality of general practice care: qualitative study. BMJ. 2002;325:1278.
44. Mukamel DB, Mushlin AI: The impact of quality report cards on choice of physicians, hospitals, and HMOs. A mid-course evaluation. Joint Comm J Qual Improv 2001, 27:20-27.
45. Drolet BC, Christopher DA, Fischer SA. Residents' response to duty-hour regulations–a follow-up national survey. New England J Med. 2012;366:e35.
46. The Commonwealth Fund: New international survey: One quarter of U.S. primary care doctors say their practices are not prepared to manage sickest patients; 84% not prepared for severly mentally ill patients [http://www.commonwealthfund.org/~/media/files/news/news-releases/2015/dec/ihp-2015-survey-release-12-3-15-330pm.pdf]. Accessed 17 Sept 2017.
47. Groves RM. Nonresponse rates and nonresponse bias in household surveys. Public Opin Q. 2006;70:646–75.

13

Cost-effectiveness of nurse-delivered cognitive behavioural therapy (CBT) compared to supportive listening (SL) for adjustment to multiple sclerosis

I. Mosweu[1*], R. Moss-Morris[2], L. Dennison[3], T. Chalder[4] and P. McCrone[1]

Abstract

Background: Cognitive Behavioural Therapy (CBT) reduces distress in multiple sclerosis, and helps manage adjustment, but cost-effectiveness evidence is lacking.

Methods: An economic evaluation was conducted within a multi-centre trial. 94 patients were randomised to either eight sessions of nurse-led CBT or supportive listening (SL). Costs were calculated from the health, social and indirect care perspectives, and combined with additional quality-adjusted life years (QALY) or improvement on the GHQ-12 score, to explore cost-effectiveness at 12 months.

Results: CBT had higher mean health costs (£1610, 95% CI, −£187 to 3771) and slightly better QALYs (0.0053, 95% CI, −0.059 to 0.103) compared to SL but these differences were not statistically significant. This yielded £301,509 per QALY improvement, indicating that CBT is not cost-effective according to established UK NHS thresholds. The extra cost per patient improvement on the GHQ-12 scale was £821 from the same perspective. Using a £20,000, threshold, CBT in this format has a 9% probability of being cost effective. Although subgroup analysis of patients with clinical levels of distress at baseline showed an improvement in the position of CBT compared to SL, CBT was still not cost-effective.

Conclusion: Nurse delivered CBT is more effective in reducing distress among MS patients compared to SL, but is highly unlikely to be cost-effective using a preference-based measure of health (EQ-5D). Results from a disease-specific measure (GHQ-12) produced comparatively lower Incremental Cost-Effectiveness Ratios, but there is currently no acceptable willingness-to-pay threshold for this measure to guide decision-making.

Keywords: Multiple sclerosis, Cost-effectiveness, Costs, Cognitive behavioural therapy, Distress, Anxiety

Background

The clinical effects of multiple sclerosis (MS) and subsequent ambulatory complications associated with managing the condition may have psychological effects, which may not necessarily be treated with drugs. MS patients report very high levels of emotional distress and levels of major depression as high as 20% annually and 50% over a lifetime [1–3]. Depression in MS patients has been linked to disability, negative effects on quality of life, self-harming tendencies, as well as low adherence, which may eventually result in the discontinuation of disease modifying therapies (DMTs) [4, 5]. However, elevated levels of distress or comorbid psychological disorders in MS are often overlooked in treatment [6]. There are particularly stressful moments in the trajectory of the illness (such as MS diagnosis, relapse, disease progression) and other critical life changing events when elevated levels of distress are to be expected [7].

Treating depression appears to improve adherence to Interferon beta-1B [8], and cognitive behavioural therapy (CBT) is increasingly being used to manage symptoms

* Correspondence: iris.mosweu@kcl.ac.uk
[1]King's Health Economics, Institute of Psychiatry, Psychology & Neuroscience, King's College London, Box 024, The David Goldberg Centre, De Crespigny Park, Denmark Hill, London SE5 8AF, UK

and enhance psychosocial outcomes for people with chronic conditions [7, 9, 10]. In MS, there is evidence that CBT may be helpful in reducing depression, anxiety, fatigue, disability, problems in dealing with cognition in addition to improving quality of life [7, 10–14]. A recent meta-analysis suggested psychological interventions (most of which were CBT-based) were at least moderately effective in treating depression in MS [14]. To date only one trial [15] has reported on the cost-effectiveness of a psychological adjustment group therapy for MS, and due to the significant amount of missing data in the quality of life data, quality-adjusted-life-years (QALYs) were not estimated, and the Beck Depression Inventory-II was used to report a cost per point reduction on the scale of £118. Two pilot studies showed that web based CBT and SKYPE delivered mindfulness groups [16] may have the potential to be cost-effective in reducing fatigue and distress in MS respectively. However, these studies had no long-term follow up and data are preliminary.

A randomised controlled trial (RCT) of a nurse-led cognitive behavioural therapy for adjusting in the early stages of multiple-sclerosis reported that CBT is more effective in reducing distress for MS patients compared to supportive listening (SL) [17] up to one year follow up. The gains for CBT were also significantly greater for those who had clinically significant levels of distress at baseline. This paper reports on a cost-effectiveness study nested within this trial. We explored both cost-effectiveness and cost utility in the whole cohort. We also conducted a subgroup analysis of patients who entered the trial with clinically significant levels of distress.

Methods
Design and setting
The study was a two-arm, randomised, multicentre parallel-group controlled trial. Patients were recruited from MS centres in Hampshire and South London, and randomly assigned to receive either CBT or SL. Full details of the trial methods, intervention components and findings have been reported previously [10, 18].

Interventions
Both interventions were delivered by general nurses specifically trained to provide eight one-on-one sessions, over a 10-week period. The sessions were delivered as a combination of two face-to-face meetings and six telephone calls.

Self-reported outcomes
Patients completed detailed measures at baseline, 15 weeks (end of treatment), 6 and 12 months post-randomisation with 12 months being the primary outcome point. The primary outcome was adjustment (defined as psychological well-being) measured using the

General Health Questionnaire (GHQ-12) [19]. The GHQ-12 uses a Likert scoring method, where high scores indicate higher distress, and to allow for a meaningful cost-effectiveness analysis, the GHQ 12 score was reported as a change score, multiplied by –1 to get an inverted score in which higher figures denote better outcomes.

Quality of life was assessed using (EQ-5D-3L) [20]. EQ-5D-3L is a brief self-reported preference-based measure which considers five dimensions of health (mobility, self-care, usual activities, pain/discomfort and anxiety/depression) each consisting of three levels of functioning (e.g. the levels for the pain dimension are no pain, moderate pain and extreme pain). This measure produces a possible 243 distinct health states ranging from 11111 (full health) to 33333 (worst) [21]. Value sets estimated from general population based studies were applied to the health states to produce preference-based scores between 0 (worse health) and 1 (full health). The measure also has a visual analogue scale ranging from 0 (the worst health you can imagine) to 100 (the best health you can imagine). Quality-adjusted-life-years (QALYS) were derived from transformed EQ-5D-3L scores, using the area-under-the-curve method [22].

Service use and costs
Contacts with the CBT and SL interventions were centrally recorded. Self-reported six-month retrospective health and social services data were collected at baseline, six- and 12-month follow-up, using an adapted version of the Client Service Receipt Inventory (CSRI) [23]. To ensure we captured relevant services the CSRI was adapted based on available literature and expert guidance. Patients provided details of their retrospective use of medication, inpatient, out-patient appointments, laboratory tests and scans, emergency department, contact with community professionals (GPs, neurologists, etc.) and informal care including access to social welfare benefits.

Service use was combined with nationally applicable unit costs [24–26] to derive total costs. Costs were measured in UK prices (£) for 2008/09, and given the one-year time horizon, there was no need to discount either costs or effects. Interventions costs were estimated by multiplying the unit cost of nurses providing the intervention by the number of sessions attended. Informal carers are not paid for their support to patients but there is still a value to this time. Informal care cost was estimated using the unit cost of a local authority home care worker as a proxy value [24]. Productivity costs were estimated through the human capital approach, which involves applying national wage rates to days off work due to illness.

Statistical analysis

Data were analysed using Stata 11 and patients were assessed using an intention-to-treat analysis. Missing costs and QALY data were imputed using a regression-based method adjusting for baseline variables costs, EQ-5D-3L scores, GHQ-12 score, and the type of MS. Non-parametric bootstrapping methods were used to account for non-normality in the distribution of cost data [27]. Outcomes and costs were presented as mean values with standard deviations, and compared between groups at baseline and 12-months follow-up.

The economic evaluation was conducted from both a health and social care, and societal perspectives. If one intervention had lower costs and better outcomes than the comparator, then it would be considered 'dominant'. In the event of the intervention having higher costs and better outcomes, cost-effectiveness would be assessed using incremental cost-effectiveness ratios (ICERs).

Cost-effectiveness planes (CEP) and cost-effectiveness acceptability curves (CEAC) were created to address the uncertainty around points estimates of the ICERs. For the CEP plane, non-parametric bootstrapping was used to create a joint distribution of incremental costs and outcomes, and plotting these differences on a scatter plot (one axis represents incremental costs and the other incremental outcome), to show the probability of the intervention being (i) cost-saving and more effective, (ii) cost-saving and less effective, (iii) cost-increasing and more effective and (iv) cost-increasing and less effective. The probability of the intervention being cost-effective was explored through the use of cost-effectiveness acceptability curve (CEAC), which were created by calculating a series of net benefits for a range (£0–£60,000) of plausible values defined as a decision maker's willingness to pay for an additional unit improvement of health outcomes (e.g. QALYs) [28].

Sub-group analysis

The concurrent trial found that patients who had clinically significant distress at baseline showed meaningfully greater benefits from CBT over SL than those who were not distressed [7]. We conducted a sub-group analysis exploring cost-effectiveness for the distressed only, i.e. patients who scored three and above on GHQ-12 using the GHQ 0011 scoring method [29].

Results

Descriptive and clinical characteristics of participants

48 participants were randomised to CBT and 48 to SL. Patient characteristics at baseline were broadly similar across groups (Table 1), except that the SL group had a slightly higher mean age (43.1 vs. 40.3); were more distressed (GHQ-12), disabled (EDSS scores), with slightly lower quality of life scores (EQ-5D-3L). The proportion (23%) reporting use of antidepressants was higher for the CBT group (25 vs. 22), and more than half (60.6%) had clinically significant distress levels.

Service use and costs

There were minimal differences in service use between the two groups. Participants accessed a wide range of health and social care services (Table 2), but the most intensively used were the GP (84% at baseline) and MS nurse (82% at baseline), followed by neurologists (66%). The proportion with GP contacts had decreased by 12-month follow-up for both groups. The percentage in contact with neurologists and MS nurses was reduced over the follow-up period, with more reductions evident in the SL group for neurologists. Most participants reported the use of at least one medication (particularly disease modifying therapies) in both groups at baseline. Physiotherapists and alternative therapists had consistently low use over the entire study period for both groups.

Despite low admissions (10%), the CBT group had substantially more inpatient days at 12 months. More than

Table 1 Baseline characteristics of participants

	CBT (n = 48) Mean(S.D.)	SL (n = 46) Mean(S.D.)
Mean age in years (SD)	40.3 (8.6)	43.1 (10.1)
Number of female participants (%)	35 (72.9)	30 (65.2)
Number of Married/cohabiting participants (%)	30 (62.5)	24 (52.2)
Number of White British participants (%)	38 (79.2)	33 (71.7)
Number of participants with A level or higher (%)	35 (72.9)	30 (65.2)
Mean EDSS score (SD)	4.9 (1.4)	5.1 (1.0)
Mean GHQ score (SD)	14.0 (5. 5)	16.4 (6.8)
Mean EQ-5D score (SD)	0.66 (0.22)	0.60 (0.26)
Number treated for depression in the past year (SD)	12 (25)	10 (22)
Number diagnosed with relapsing remitting MS (SD)	37 (77)	36 (78)

Table 2 Patient's use of services at baseline, six and twelve months of the evaluation period

Service	Baseline				6 months				12 months			
	CBT (n = 48)		SL (n = 46)		CBT (n = 45)		SL (n = 38)		CBT (n = 41)		SL (n = 43)	
	Users	Contacts	Users	Contacts	Users	Contacts	Users	Contacts	Users	Contacts	Users	Contacts
	N (%)	Mean (S.D.)	N (%)	Mean (S.D.)	N (%)	Mean(S.D.)	N (%)	Mean(S.D.)	N (%)	Mean (S.D.)	N (%)	Mean (S.D.)
General practitioner	41 (85)	2.9 (2.6)	38 (83)	2.0 (1.1)	41 (85)	2.8 (2.1)	29 (62)	2.8 (3.8)	32 (67)	2.4 (1.8)	31 (67)	1.7 (0.8)
Neurologist	33 (69)	1.6 (1.2)	29 (63)	1.1 (0.4)	22 (46)	1.2 (0.4)	16 (35)	1.1 (0.5)	22 (46)	1.2 (0.7)	15 (33)	1.0 (0)
Other doctors (including dentist)	26 (54)	4.3 (11.7)	18 (39)	1.7 (1.1)	16 (33)	4.9 (8.1)	18 (39)	2.9 (3.3)	20 (42)	2.0 (1.8)	20 43	1.8 (1.3)
MS nurse	39 (81)	2.3 (4.1)	38 (83)	1.5 (1.0)	28 (58)	1.4 (0.6)	22 (48)	1.7 (1.2)	23 (48)	1.6 (1.2)	24 (52)	1.4 (0.8)
Pharmacist	9 (19)	1.8 (1.1)	8 (17)	1.8 (1.2)	7 (15)	1.9 (1.1)	4 (9)	2.0 (0.8)	3 (6)	1.0 (0)	9 (20)	3.3 (6.3)
Therapist	2 (67)	5.5 (3.5)	1 (2)	3.0 (.)	5 (10)	5.0 (2.2)	3 (7)	3.7 (4.6)	1 (2)	6.0 (.)	4 (9)	6.0(3.6)
Physiotherapist	12 (46)	5.4 (8.1)	14 (30)	4.2 (3.2)	5. [10]	9.2 (11.7)	8 (17)	4.0 (2.7)	8 (17)	8.1 (5.1)	10 (22)	8.6 (9.9)
Alternative therapy	9 (41)	5.3 (4.5)	13 (28)	3.0 (2.2)	7 (15)	5.4 (4.3)	10 (22	4.5 (5.1)	11 (23)	6.5 (5.6)	13(28)	9.9 (8.8)
Other community-based professionals	1 (2)	20.0 (.)	0	—	9 (19)	228.6 (340.7)	10 (22)	50.8 (39.1)	11 (23)	7.4 (7.5)	7 (15)	3.7 (3.4)
Medicine	43 (90)		33 (72)		39 (81)		33 (72)		37 (77)		37 (80)	
Hospital-based services												
In-patient (length of stay)	4 (8)	1.3 (0.5)	5 (11)	1.0 (0)	2 (4)	14.0 (15.6)	3 (7)	1.0 (0)	2 (4)	12.5 (16.3)	1 (2)	14.0 (.)
Accident and emergency	4 (8)	1.5 (0.7)	3 (7)	1.0 (0)	3 (6)	1.0 (0)	2 (4)	1 (0)	2 (4)	1.5 (0.7)	3 (7)	1.0 (0)
Investigations (blood test, MRI, x-ray, CT/CAT scan, EEG)	34 (71)	2.5 (1.6)	33 (72)	2.4(1.3)	27 (56)	2.0 (1.2)	18 (39)	2.3 (1.6)	23 (48)	2.5 (2.2)	25 (54)	1.6(0.8)
Time off work (days)	7 (15)	11 (16)	7 (11)	7 (11)	9 (19)	11 (30)	7 (15)	6 (8)	9 (19)	19 (34)	7 (15)	23 (44)
Informal care (hours per/week)	48 (100)	9 (15)	45 (98)	6 (10)	42 (88)	8 (16)	38 (83)	5 (11)	40 (83)	9 (14)	42 (91)	9 (13)

two thirds (71%) reported investigations (e.g. blood tests, MRI, x-rays, CT/CAT and EEGs) at baseline, but at follow-up the proportions had decreased for both groups. The mean number of tests remained the same (2.5) for the CBT group, but had decreased (1.6) for the SL group. Almost all (99%) patients reported informal care at baseline, and while this had decreased at follow-up, the mean hours/week were not so different. The mean cost of CBT was £307 compared to £306 for SL over 12 weeks. At baseline, mean service costs were fairly similar between the groups (Table 3), but higher informal care costs for the CBT group (£4378 vs. £2903), contributed to much more societal costs at baseline compared to the SL group. Over the whole follow-up period, mean costs were higher in the CBT group. Drug costs contributed the highest share to health and social care costs while informal care added the greatest proportion to societal costs. Although the number receiving informal care were similar, the CBT group had greater intensity of use hence higher costs. From the health and social care (NHS) perspective CBT had higher mean costs at follow-up compared to SL (£7331 vs. £5026), but this difference, adjusted for baseline costs (£1610) was not statistically significant (bootstrapped 95% CI, –£187 to 3771). The difference in mean costs from the societal perspective (£2871), was also not statistically significant (bootstrapped 95% CI, –£2028 to £7793).

Cost-effectiveness analysis and cost-utility-analyses

At baseline GHQ-12 scores were lower for the CBT group (13.98 vs. 16.40), and at 12 months both groups showed reductions in distress but the improvement in mean scores was better for the CBT group (2.69 vs. 1.97) and the difference(1.9572) statistically significant (bootstrapped 95% CI, –5.41 to –1.05) [17]. Based on the change score, CBT produced an ICER of £821/GHQ-12 score compared to SL from the health and social care perspective, indicating that for a one-point improvement on the GHQ-12 the NHS should pay £821. The ICER from the societal perspective is £1242/GHQ-12.

QALY results were also better for the intervention group at 12 months (0.6627 vs. 0.6197) but the difference (0.0053) was not statistically significant (bootstrapped 95% CI, –0.059 to 0.103). CBT was therefore more effective at improving quality of life, but expensive, yielding an ICER of £303,774 from the health and social care perspective and £541,698 from the societal perspective.

Subgroup analysis of those with clinical levels of distress at baseline

Results from the subgroup analysis revealed a mean cost difference of £1362 (bootstrapped 95% CI, –781 to 3612) from the NHS perspective and £3506 (bootstrapped 95% CI, –2704 to 9611) from the wider societal perspective. A statistically significant difference in the GHQ12 score (4.257 bootstrapped at 95% CI, 1.109 to 7.521) produced a corresponding ICER of £320 from the NHS perspective and £825 from the societal perspective.

For the same analysis, a mean difference in QALYs of 0.0108 (bootstrapped 95% CI, –0.051 to 0.068) indicates that the NHS would have to pay £126,111 for an additional QALY, while the society pays £324,630. Both these figures are higher than the UK cost-effectiveness threshold, but are substantially lower than the ICER in the base-case analysis.

The Cost-Effectiveness Plane (CEP) (Fig. 1) illustrates uncertainty around the estimated ICERs and it shows

Table 3 Summary of service costs and outcomes at baseline, six and twelve months

Cost category	Treatment A (CBT) n = 48			Treatment B (Supportive listening) n = 46		
	baseline Mean (S.D)	6 months Mean (S.D)	12 months Mean (S.D)	baseline Mean (S.D)	6 months Mean (S.D)	12 months Mean (S.D)
Intervention	0	307 (170)	0	0	306 (148)	0
Medication (drugs)	2079 (1938)	2724 (3427)	2531 (4656)	1928 (2373)	1476 (2094)	1882 (2644)
Community services (contacts with professionals)	657 (1130)	422 (430)	483 (715)	466 (402)	305 (331)	395 (482)
Hospital services	185 (559)	133 (692)	204 (956)	96 (340)	91 (393)	119 (466)
Investigations	79 (148)	35 (77)	33 (78)	78 (123)	20 (60)	15 (43)
Total hospital and social care costs	3000 (2098)	3621 (3751)	3251 (5134)	2568 (2295)	2198 (2507)	2412 (2654)
Informal care	4378 (6970)	3807 (7463)	4162 (6352)	2903 (4550)	2192 (4993)	4064 (6242)
Productivity loss	1096 (2726)	704 (3151)	388 (1742)	719 (2471)	147 (428)	385 (1987)
Total societal costs	8473 (8212)	8132 (9036)	7802 (8819)	6190 (6183)	4538 (5605)	6862 (6922)
Social benefits	1210 (1282)	1430 (1320)	1229 (1349)	1325 (1259)	1360 (1448)	1640 (1562)
EQ-5D score	0.659 (0.215)	0.661 (0.216)	0.644 (0.267)	0.595 (0.262)	0.641 (0.198)	0.622 (0.274)
GHQ-12	13.977 (5.449)		11.289 (4.63)	16.391 (6.771)		14.422 (7.316)

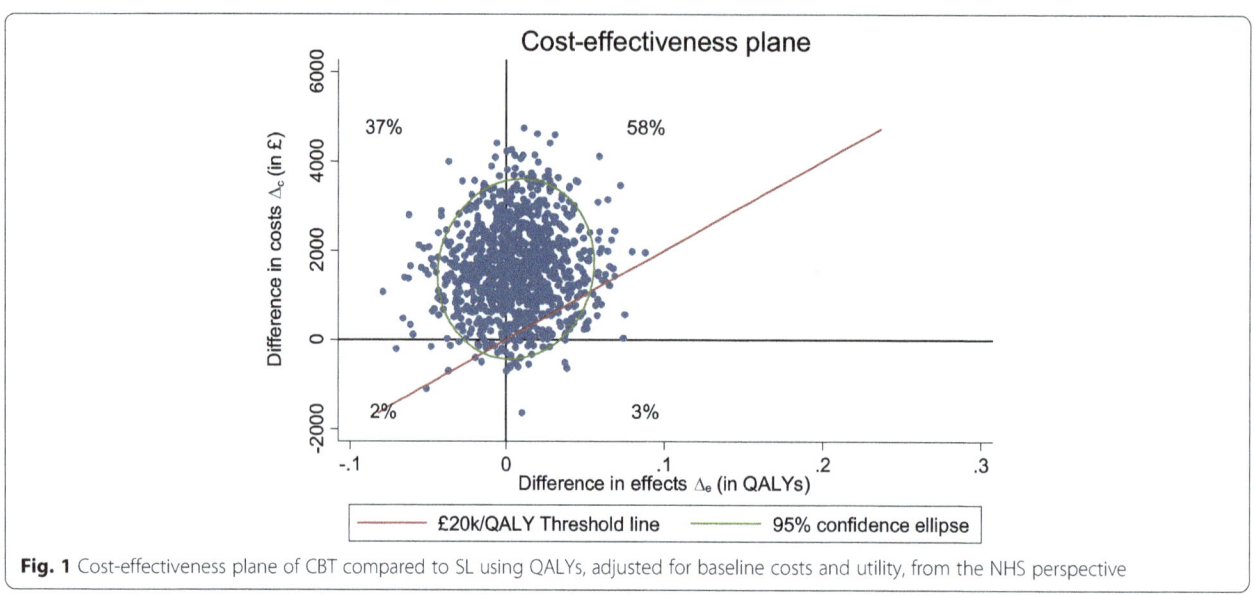

Fig. 1 Cost-effectiveness plane of CBT compared to SL using QALYs, adjusted for baseline costs and utility, from the NHS perspective

most (58%) of the scatter points fall on the north-east quadrant which implies that CBT produces higher costs and better QALYs. The £20,000 threshold line has very few points below it, indicating that the probability of cost-effectiveness is likely to be very low at that willingness-to-pay threshold. The CEAC (Fig. 2) demonstrates the probability of the intervention being cost-effective at varying willingness-to-pay thresholds per improvement in QALYs. Adjusted for baseline costs and utility scores, the CEAC indicates a 9% probability of CBT being cost-effective at £20,000/QALY from the health and social care perspective, which confirms the CEP findings. The second CEP (Fig. 3) produced using the GHQ-12 score and cost from a similar perspective, however show 91% of the bootstrapped ICERs falling on the north-east quadrant, indicating that CBT is better at

reducing psychological distress, albeit at higher costs, compared to SL.

Discussion

We have established that nurse-led CBT produces slightly better QALYs and is more effective in reducing psychological distress for MS, compared to SL. However, when the small effects are combined with incremental costs, CBT is not considered cost-effective compared to SL, according NICE guidelines. This conclusion was drawn from results of the ICER based on the EQ-5D-3L which show a cost per QALY of £303,774 from the health and social care perspective and £541,698 from the societal perspective. Sub-group analysis of patients meeting thresholds for clinical distress at baseline indicates a large improvement in the ICER (£126,111) from the NHS and societal (£324,629) perspectives, but still substantially higher than the recommended threshold in the UK. Results of the CEAC are also consistent with the ICER, showing only a 9% probability for CBT being cost-effective at the £20, 000 threshold when compared with SL. Comparatively, the GHQ-12 results produced much lower ICERs from both the health and social care (£821), and the societal perspective (£1242). These figures are even lower when only the distressed group is analysed; £320/GHQ-12 from the NHS perspective and £825 from the societal perspective.

The difference in the ICERs is mainly driven by incremental differences in the outcome measures, whereupon the GHQ-12 detected sizeable differences and the EQ-5D-3L produced very minimal differences. This could point to the insensitiveness of the EQ-5D-3L in patients with MS for all the five domains as illustrated in other previous work [30–32]. It is also possible that the EQ-

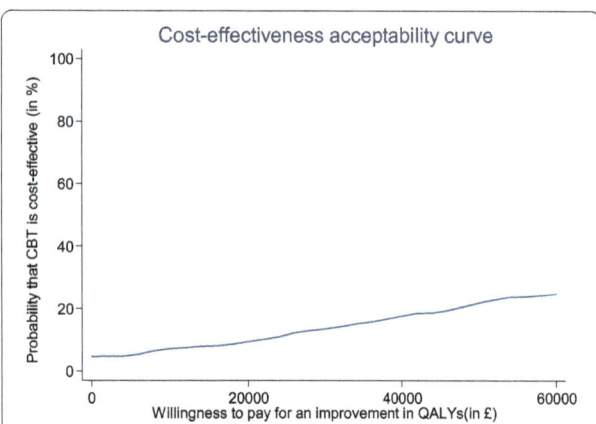

Fig. 2 Cost-effectiveness acceptability curve of CBT compared to SL, adjusted for baseline costs and utility, from the NHS perspective

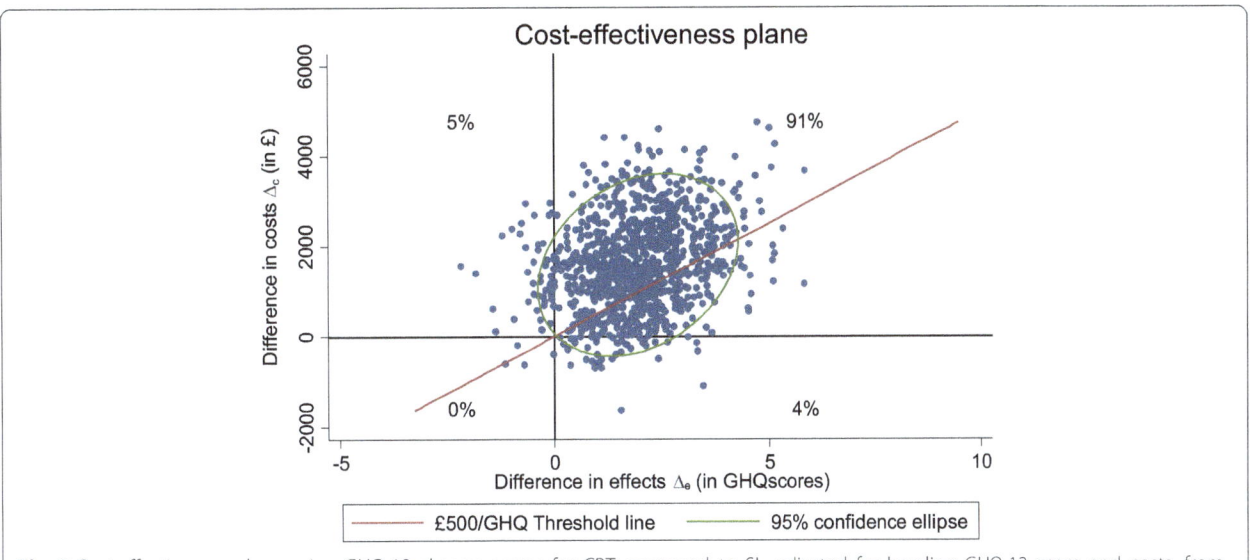

Fig. 3 Cost-effectiveness plane using GHQ-12 change scores for CBT compared to SL, adjusted for baseline GHQ-12 score and costs, from the NHS perspective

5D-3L is unable to detect the treatment effects of psychological interventions in MS patients. This is substantiated by previous work [15], in which the EQ-5D-3L failed to detect an effect in mood for MS patients. The sample size was estimated based on the primary clinical outcome, and it is possible that it was underpowered to demonstrate a significant difference in cost-effectiveness.

These results can assist in guiding researchers and policy-makers on areas to prioritise when considering interventions for MS patients.

As far as we know, this is the first economic evaluation of CBT for adjusting to multiple sclerosis. Whilst CBT has been found to be cost-effective in other disease areas such as depression [33], our results indicate that investing in nurse-led CBT may not proffer value for money compared to the same number of sessions of nurse-led SL for MS patients.

More work needs to be done to explore the potential cost-effectiveness of CBT in MS. Providing booster sessions at follow up may improve quality of life gains as the treatment effect for CBT at the end of treatment was greater than at follow-up [17]. It is also possible that there are subgroups within MS patients that could be targeted for future trials. It may be that future clinical trials target the therapy to those who need it most, like people with less social support or those screened and found to be distressed. Although our subgroup analysis did not produce cost-effective results, other studies [15] reported clinical and cost-effectiveness of group psychological therapy for MS patients with low mood. The control group in Humphreys et al. [15], unlike ours, received usual care (without psychological interventions), which is a closer reflection of the current reality. Most patients with MS do not receive

formal therapy for their distress so it may be that compared to treatment as usual, SL or CBT could be cost effective options. More work is needed to test this hypothesis.

Limitations

Limitations of the trial are outlined in our clinical paper [17], but the economic study had its own specific challenges. As is common in economic evaluations, there is a possibility of recall bias as participants reported on six months' retrospective service use. There is ongoing debate relating to the appropriateness of collecting resource use data, and for this trial the most pragmatic method was self-report and the recall period was determined by the trial design. There is currently no societal value linked to a unit improvement on the GHQ-12 score, making it hard to advice on the cost-effectiveness of CBT using this measure.

We used data from a clinical trial for our economic analysis. Sample size calculations in trials are generally based on the primary clinical outcome and not costs. However, most economic evaluations (including this one) focus on probabilities rather than testing for statistical significance in cost-effectiveness. Having said that, small samples do mean that we need to be cautious in our interpretation of findings and this small sample size is a limitation. We have referred to this in the discussion.

Conclusion

Nurse-led CBT compared to SL is not cost-effective for adjustment to MS using EQ-5D-3L but produces reasonable ICERs using GHQ-12. However, there is currently no acceptable willingness-to-pay threshold for this measure to guide in decision-making.

Implications for health care provision and use, health policies, and future research

Further research in this area could be directed at designing CBT trials targeted to those who need it most, such as people with distress, as well as using alternative utility measures validated for psychological interventions in MS patients. We also know little about the cost-effectiveness of different levels of clinical expertise. In this study, senior nurses who received a two-month training course provided the CBT. It is possible that experienced clinical psychologists, although costlier, may facilitate larger treatment effects and cost savings. Finally, recent evidence [34] suggests online therapy for depression may be an effective treatment in MS. Providing minimal therapy support alongside online therapy may be a cost-effective solution.

Abbreviations

CBT: Cognitive Behavioural Therapy; CEAC: Cost-Effectiveness Acceptability Curve; CEP: Cost-Effectiveness Plane; CSRI: Client Service Receipt Inventory; CT: Computerised Tomography; DMT: Disease Modifying Therapy; EDSS: Expanded Disability Status Scale; EEG: Electroencephalogram; EQ-5D: EuroQol Five Dimensions; GHQ-12: General Health Questionnaire; GP: General Practitioner; ICER: Incremental Cost-Effectiveness Ratio; MRI: Magnetic Resonance Imaging; MS: Multiple sclerosis; NHS: National Health Service; NICE: National Institute for Health and Care Excellence; QALY: Quality-Adjusted-Life-Year; RCT: Randomised Controlled Trial; SL: Supportive Listening

Acknowledgements
Open access for this article was funded by King's College London.

Funding
This paper summarises independent research funded by the MS Society in the UK (award number 872/07). The views expressed in this publication are those of the author(s) and not necessarily those of the NHS, the National Institute for Health Research or the Department of Health. Trial registration: Current Controlled Trials ISRCTN91377356.

Authors' contributions
All authors meet the criteria for authorship in accordance with HER having made: a) substantial contributions to the conception or design of the study; or the data acquisition, analysis, or interpretation of data; b) drafting the manuscript or revising it critically for important intellectual content; c) final approval of the version to be published; and d) agree to be accountable for all aspects of the work in ensuring that questions related to the accuracy or integrity of any part of the work are appropriately investigated and resolved. IM is guarantor for the manuscript and data contained within. IM affirms that the manuscript is an honest, accurate, and transparent account of the study being reported; that no important aspects of the study have been omitted.

Competing interests
The authors declare that they have no competing interests.

Author details
[1]King's Health Economics, Institute of Psychiatry, Psychology & Neuroscience, King's College London, Box 024, The David Goldberg Centre, De Crespigny Park, Denmark Hill, London SE5 8AF, UK. [2]Department of Psychology, Institute of Psychiatry Psychology & Neuroscience, King's College London, London, UK. [3]School of Psychology, University of Southampton, Southampton, UK. [4]Department of Psychological Medicine, King's College London, Cutcombe Road, London SE5 9RJ, UK.

References
1. Patten SB, Beck CA, Williams JV, Barbui C, Metz LM. Major depression in multiple sclerosis: a population-based perspective. Neurology. 2003;61(11): 1524–7.
2. Siegert R, Abernethy D. Depression in multiple sclerosis: a review. J Neurol Neurosurg Psychiatry. 2005;76(4):469–75.
3. Kern S, Schrempf W, Schneider H, Schultheiss T, Reichmann H, Ziemssen T. Neurological disability, psychological distress, and health-related quality of life in MS patients within the first three years after diagnosis. Mult Scler. 2009;15(6):752–8.
4. Patti F, Amato M, Trojano M, Bastianello S, Tola M, Picconi O, et al. Quality of life, depression and fatigue in mildly disabled patients with relapsing-remitting multiple sclerosis receiving subcutaneous interferon beta-1a: 3-year results from the COGIMUS (COGnitive Impairment in MUltiple Sclerosis) study. Mult Scler J. 2011;17(8):991–1001.
5. Feinstein A. Multiple sclerosis, depression, and suicide. British medical Journal. 1997;BMJ. 315:691(0959–8138 (Print)).
6. Simpson R, McLean G, Guthrie B, Mair F, Mercer S. Physical and mental health comorbidity is common in people with multiple sclerosis: nationally representative cross-sectional population database analysis. BMC Neurol. 2014;14(1):128.
7. Dennison L, Moss-Morris R. Cognitive-behavioral therapy: what benefits can it offer people with multiple sclerosis? Expert Rev Neurother. 2010;10(9): 1383–90.
8. Mohr DC, Goodkin DE, Likosky W, Gatto N, Baumann KA, Rudick RA. Treatment of depression improves adherence to interferon beta-1b therapy for multiple sclerosis. Arch Neurol. 1997;54(5):531–3.
9. Skokou M, Soubasi E, Gourzis P. Depression in Multiple Sclerosis: A Review of Assessment and Treatment Approaches in Adult and Pediatric Populations. ISRN Neurology. 2012;2012:6.
10. Moss-Morris R, Dennison L, Landau S, Yardley L, Silber E, Chalder T. A randomized controlled trial of cognitive behavioral therapy (CBT) for adjusting to multiple sclerosis (the saMS trial): does CBT work and for whom does it work? J Consult Clin Psychol. 2013;81(2):251–62.
11. Mohr DC, Hart S, Vella L. Reduction in disability in a randomized controlled trial of telephone-administered cognitive-behavioral therapy. Health Psychol. 2007;26(5):554–63.
12. van Kessel K, Moss-Morris R, Willoughby E, Chalder T, Johnson MH, Robinson E. A randomized controlled trial of cognitive behavior therapy for multiple sclerosis fatigue. Psychosom Med. 2008;70(2):205–13.
13. Cosio D, Jin L, Siddique J, Mohr DC. The effect of telephone-administered cognitive-behavioral therapy on quality of life among patients with multiple sclerosis. Ann Behav Med. 2011;41(2):227–34.
14. Fiest KM, Walker JR, Bernstein CN, Graff LA, Zarychanski R, Abou-Setta AM, et al. Systematic review and meta-analysis of interventions for depression and anxiety in persons with multiple sclerosis. Multiple Sclerosis and Related Disorders. 2016;5:12–26.
15. Humphreys I, Drummond Ae Fau - Phillips C, Phillips C Fau - Lincoln NB, Lincoln NB. Cost-effectiveness of an adjustment group for people with multiple sclerosis and low mood: a randomized trial. Clinical rehabilitation. 2013;0(1477–0873 (Electronic)).
16. Bogosian A, Chadwick P, Windgassen S, Norton S, McCrone P, Mosweu I, et al. Distress improves after mindfulness training for progressive MS: A pilot randomised trial. Multiple Sclerosis Journal.
17. Moss-Morris R, Dennison L, Landau S, Yardley L, Silber E, Chalder T. A Randomized Controlled Trial of Cognitive Behavioral Therapy (CBT) for Adjusting to Multiple Sclerosis (the saMS Trial): Does CBT Work and for Whom Does It Work? J Consult Clin Psychol. 2012;81(2):251–62.

18. Moss-Morris R, Dennison L, Yardley L, Landau S, Roche S, McCrone P, et al. Protocol for the saMS trial (supportive adjustment for multiple sclerosis): a randomized controlled trial comparing cognitive behavioral therapy to supportive listening for adjustment to multiple sclerosis. BMC Neurol. 2009;9:45.

19. Goldberg D. General health questionnaire (GHQ-12). Nfer-Nelson: Windsor, UK; 1992.

20. Williams A. The role of the EuroQol instrument in QALY calculations: Centre for Health. Economics Discussion Paper [Internet]. 1995; 130. .

21. Rabin R, de Charro F. EQ-5D: a measure of health status from the EuroQol Group. Ann Med. 2001;33(5):337–43.

22. Brazier J, Ratcliffe J, Salomon J, Tsuchiya A. Measuring and Valuing Health Benefits for Economic Evaluation. Oxford: Oxford University Press; 2007.

23. Beecham J, Knapp M, editors. Costing psychiatric interventions, in Measuring Mental Health Needs. Gaskell: London; 2001.

24. Curtis L, editor. Unit Costs of Health and Social Care. : Personal Social Services Research Unit, University of Kent, 2008; 2008.

25. Department of Health. National Health Service Schedule of Reference Costs 2007/08 London2009 [Available from: http://webarchive.nationalarchives. gov.uk/+/http://www.dh.gov.uk/en/Publicationsandstatistics/Publications/ PublicationsPolicyAndGuidance/DH_095859.

26. British Medical Association RPS. British National Formulary, 49. London, 2008: RMJ Publishing,; 2008.

27. Barber JA, Thompson SG. Analysis of cost data in randomized trials: an application of the non-parametric bootstrap. Stat Med. 2000;19(23):3219–36.

28. Fenwick E, Byford S. A guide to cost-effectiveness acceptability curves. The British journal of psychiatry : the journal of mental science. 2005;187:106–8.

29. Nicholl CR, Lincoln NB, Francis VM, Stephan TF. Assessment of emotional problems in people with multiple sclerosis. Clin Rehabil. 2001;15(6):657–68.

30. Jones KH FD, Jones PA, et al. How People with Multiple Sclerosis Rate Their Quality of Life: An EQ-5D Survey via the UK MS Register. Reindl M, ed. PLoS ONE. 2013;8(6):e65640. doi:https://doi.org/10.1371/journal.pone.0065640. PLoS ONE. 2013;8(6).

31. Svensson M, Fajutrao L. Costs of Formal and Informal Home Care and Quality of Life for Patients with Multiple Sclerosis in Sweden. Mult Scler Int. 2014;2014:7.

32. Kuspinar A, Mayo NE. Do generic utility measures capture what is important to the quality of life of people with multiple sclerosis? Health Qual Life Outcomes. 2013;11(1):71.

33. Hollinghurst S, Carroll FE, Abel A, Campbell J, Garland A, Jerrom B, et al. Cost-effectiveness of cognitive-behavioural therapy as an adjunct to pharmacotherapy for treatment-resistant depression in primary care: economic evaluation of the CoBalT Trial. Br J Psychiatry. 2014;204(1):69–76.

34. Fischer A, Schröder J, Vettorazzi E, Wolf OT, Pöttgen J, Lau S, et al. An online programme to reduce depression in patients with multiple sclerosis: a randomised controlled trial. The Lancet Psychiatry. 2015;2(3):217–23.

14

The net effects of medical malpractice tort reform on health insurance losses: the Texas experience

Patricia H. Born[2], J. Bradley Karl[3] and W. Kip Viscusi[1*]

Abstract

In this paper, we examine the influence of medical malpractice tort reform on the level of private health insurance company losses incurred. We employ a natural experiment framework centered on a series of tort reform measures enacted in Texas in 2003 that drastically altered the medical malpractice environment in the state. The results of a difference-in-differences analysis using a variety of comparison states, as well as a difference-in-difference-in-differences analysis, indicate that ameliorating medical malpractice risk has little effect on health insurance losses incurred by private health insurers.

Keywords: Medical malpractice, Health insurance, Tort reform, Liability

JEL codes: K13, I10, G22

Introduction

The motivations for reforming the medical malpractice tort environment, beginning in some states several decades ago, include assertions that limitations on liability would reduce expenditures on unnecessary health care services, specifically those services provided solely in defense of potential liability claims. In reducing defensive medicine practices, these reforms would thereby reduce overall health care costs. This assertion relies on health care providers' responses to a reduction in perceived malpractice risk. Physicians may reduce services provided, but unless they are otherwise penalized for providing unnecessary services (e.g., through managed care plans' profiling activities), they may be reluctant to reduce the income associated with these services. In fact, reducing providers' expected liability could also lead to potentially *more* health care services provided, that is, a wider range of procedures supplied or more intensive treatments. If more health care services are provided, insurers will experience an increase in claims, rather than a reduction.

The markets for medical malpractice insurance and health insurance are linked via the provision of health care services. A comprehensive evaluation of reform activity in either market consequently should recognize the potential spillover effects of the reform in one market to the other. Several prior studies have addressed the relationship between a change in medical malpractice liability exposure and healthcare costs (for example, [1, 2]). A subset of these studies find evidence of provider responses to a reduction in liability within samples of patients with certain diagnoses, or among a sample of the population (for example, Medicare patients). There is little evidence of how private health insurers generally fare following reform activity. Studies that specifically consider health insurance markets examine the extent to which changes in the medical malpractice environment affect insurance premiums and coverage rates (for example, [3, 4]). However, little evidence exists regarding the extent to which a change in the medical malpractice environment, such as the implementation of a cap on noneconomic damage levels, might influence losses in the private health insurance market.

In this paper, we use the experience in Texas to evaluate the effect of medical malpractice tort reform on losses in the private health insurance market. In 2003,

* Correspondence: kip.viscusi@vanderbilt.edu
[1]Vanderbilt University Law School, 131 21st Avenue South, Nashville, TN 37203, USA
Full list of author information is available at the end of the article

Texas passed a series of sweeping medical malpractice reform measures aimed at reducing the medical professional liability exposure of health care providers in the state. The enactment of these reforms provides an opportunity to examine the influence of the malpractice environment on insured health losses using a natural experiment design. Using insurance company financial data from the National Association of Insurance Commissioners (NAIC), we perform a series of Difference-in-Differences (DD) and Difference-in-Difference-in-Differences (DDD) analyses to provide evidence that tort reform in Texas had little effect on the levels of losses incurred by private health insurers on behalf of insured patients (in other words, claims for healthcare services).

More specifically, our analysis yields no support for the hypothesis that the Texas medical malpractice reforms had and substantial, persistent influence on levels of health insurance losses. We do find some evidence that suggests health insurance losses incurred by Texas insurers *increased* in the initial two years following the reform and our estimates indicate that this increase was between $400 and $500 per enrollee. However, we find no other evidence that Texas health insurer losses were affected by the reform during any other post-reform year, suggesting that the spillover effects of the reforms were, at best, short-lived. Taken in its entirety, our analysis leads us to conclude that medical malpractice reforms had little influence on reducing the cost of medical care paid for by private health insurers.

The paper proceeds as follows. In Section II we discuss the existing literature that addresses the effects of medical malpractice tort reform. We note that there are numerous studies that measure the effects of reform on the target market (that is, the influence of medical malpractice legal reforms on the profitability of medical malpractice insurers), but only a few studies evaluate the spillover to the health care environment. In Section III we derive our hypothesis, and in Section IV we describe our data. Section V presents our empirical methodology, which includes several approaches to estimate the influence of the reform using DD and DDD analyses. Section V also details our results and Section VI provides a discussion of the policy implications and a conclusion.

Background

Numerous studies have evaluated medical malpractice liability exposure from varying perspectives. Some of the earliest research examines the extent to which demographic, medical, and legal factors influence the frequency and severity of medical malpractice insurance claims (for example, [5, 6]). Subsequent studies specifically consider the influence of tort reform on medical malpractice payments and provide evidence that tort reform measures have a non-trivial influence on medical malpractice

damage awards (for example, [7]). Similarly, many studies find that the tort reform is associated with lower levels of incurred losses and lower loss ratios for medical malpractice insurance companies (for example, [8–10, 11, 12, 13, 14]). The thrust of the empirical evidence is that medical malpractice reform generates a cost-restraining effect on medical malpractice costs. Of particular relevance to our analysis is that these studies suggest that caps on non-economic damages have the greatest influence on loss levels incurred by medical malpractice insurers.

There is no consensus in the empirical literature regarding how the malpractice environment influences the actions of healthcare providers and physicians.[1] The consequences of a state reducing malpractice liability could have a number of effects, theoretically. Providers could discontinue providing services that were solely defensive in nature. Alternatively, providers could be willing bear risky exposures that they had previously avoided. This response would be evident not only in providers offering riskier procedures, but deciding to practice in riskier specialty areas (for example, obstetrics). More far-reaching consequences include attracting of physicians from other states, thereby increasing the supply of services.

Some studies find no evidence of a relation between malpractice risk and physician behavior. For example, Sloan and Shadle [2], using survey data as well as Medicare data, conclude that medical decisions are not significantly affected by tort reform measures. Other studies provide evidence that physicians respond to higher levels of malpractice risk by practicing "positive" defensive medicine and supply additional services which are of no marginal value to the patient. For example, Kessler and McClellan [1] find that liability-reducing tort reform measures reduce the rates of defensive medicine in a sample of Medicare beneficiaries and their finding of the existence of defensive medicine practices is echoed by other studies in the literature.[2] Still other studies provide evidence that physicians react to higher levels of malpractice risk by practicing "negative" defensive medicine whereby physicians distance themselves from certain patient interactions or, in the extreme case, withdraw from a particular healthcare market.[3] For example, Currie and MacLeod [15] find that the implementation of caps on non-economic damages increased the frequency of C-sections among a large sample of individual births from 1989 to 2001.

The literature also provides evidence that, via its effect on physician behavior, tort reform influences private health insurance market operations.[4] An example is Avraham and Schanzenbach [3], who use individual-level survey data from 1982 through 2007 to test the hypotheses that either 1) tort reform may reduce damage awards and defensive medicine costs or 2) tort reform may increase providers' costs by reducing physicians' caretaking incentives. In support for their first hypothesis, Avraham and Schanzenbach [3] find that tort reform increases insurance coverage rates. In a more recent paper, Avraham and Schanzenbach [16] find that treatment intensity for heart attack victims declines following a cap on noneconomic damages. Similarly, Avraham, Dafny, and Schanzenbach [17] find that the enactments of various tort reform measures reduce group self-insured health insurance premiums by 1 to 2%. Karl, Born, and Viscusi [18] also find that the professional liability climate has a non-trivial influence on the dollar amount of state-level health insurance losses per capita, though their results suggest that lower levels of professional liability exposure are associated with higher levels of health insurance losses.

A number of studies also specifically examine the Texas market following the state's comprehensive medical malpractice reform in 2003.[5] While the inefficiency of the tort system was one motivating factor for reform, the effort also recognized problems in the availability and affordability of medical malpractice coverage. It was suggested by some that "crisis" was evident in the preceding years: Texas reportedly had the lowest number of physicians per capita in the nation, and one in every four physicians had a malpractice claim filed against them each year [19].[6] The Texas reform measures, shown in Table 1, addressed several dimensions of liability and the most striking of the reform was the measure to cap non-economic damages. The 2003 reforms drastically changed the medical malpractice environment in the state and evidence suggests that the reform resulted in a 60% reduction in medical malpractice claims rates and a 30% reduction in payouts per claim [20, 21].

Of the studies that specifically consider the consequences of the Texas tort reform measures enacted in 2003, the most pertinent to our study is Paik et al. [22]

Table 1 Texas Reform Measures, 2003

Limits noneconomic damages to $250,000

Defendants can appeal class certification directly to the Texas Supreme Court to decide up front, not after years of costly litigation, if the plaintiff has a class action.

Law ensures that lawyers are paid in coupons if clients in a class-action suit get paid in coupons.

A new standard to ensure sued parties pay only their proportionate responsibility.

Reformed product liability laws so retailers are not liable for a manufacturer's mistake.

Enacted liability limits for good Samaritans, volunteer firefighters, charity volunteers and teachers.

Closed loopholes that allowed trial lawyers to venue shop.

Notes: This table provides summary information regarding the tort reform measures enacted in Texas in 2003

who examine how Medicare spending changed after the enactment of the Texas reform measures.[7] Using both a county-level and state-level analysis, they find no evidence that Medicare spending declined after the enactment of the reform and provide a degree of evidence that spending increased following the 2003 reforms. The analysis of Paik et al. [22] is insightful because it suggests that physicians in Texas did not alter defensive medicine practices in a way that led to lower health insurance cost. In fact, the reform in Texas may have altered provider behavior in ways that *increase* healthcare costs, which is the opposite effect that many proponents of the Texas tort liability reform had predicted.

In summary, there exists considerable evidence that medical malpractice reform measures reduce medical malpractice awards and also the losses incurred by medical malpractice insurance companies. There is also disagreement in the literature regarding the extent to which medical malpractice reforms have any meaningful influence on the provider-patient interaction. However, some studies provide evidence that tort reform's influence on provider behavior ultimately leads to consequences for health insurance markets but, again, there is no general consensus in the literature as to if and how tort reforms influence insured loss levels in health insurance markets.

Methods
Hypothesis development

Theory and empirical evidence to date suggest that the indirect effects of tort reform on health insurance costs are ambiguous. We develop our main hypothesis under the assumption that risk of a medical malpractice lawsuit influences the nature of the medical care given by health care providers and, more broadly, the provider marketplace. Prior to reform, a state's medical malpractice insurance regulation and unique demographic characteristics are associated with a level of medical malpractice insurance claims which reflects, among other things, the litigiousness of the population and expertise of health care providers. We hypothesize that providers perceive their risk of being sued for medical malpractice in a rational manner, guided by their prior experience, information about malpractice claims being brought against other providers, or the cost of medical malpractice insurance.[8] Assuming that the medical malpractice environment affects the expected liability costs, there will be an incentive for medical malpractice providers to take actions to reduce exposure to risk. For example, a provider who perceives an increase in liability exposure could order more tests for insured patients, see fewer patients with specific health issues, or even exit the geographic market altogether. These behavioral changes will generate a change in levels of health insurance claims, and we might expect to find a significant relationship between changes in the legal environment for medical malpractice and losses incurred by health insurers. However, since providers may respond in ways that either increase health care costs or reduce health care costs, the direction of this relationship, when evaluated in the aggregate, is ambiguous. To the extent that changes in behavior might, in effect, all cancel each other out in the aggregate, we provide the following null hypothesis:

H_o: *Liability-reducing reform in the medical malpractice market has no effect on the level of health insurance losses.*

If we are able to reject the null hypothesis, then we find in favor of an alternative hypothesis that medical malpractice reform leads to changes in provider behavior that significantly increases or decreases health insurance losses. To the extent that providers do not instantaneously comprehend the consequences of the reforms at the time of enactment, the effect on the health insurance market may be potentially delayed. However, efforts to over-treat for defensive reasons will result in an increase in health insurance losses while efforts to avoid certain patients will result in a reduction in health insurance losses. We note that rejection of the null hypotheses could also result from changes in provider behavior outside of simply interacting with the patient. Reforms could lead to an expansion in the number of physicians in the state and the supply of medical care. Medical malpractice market reforms also could influence the nature of rents demanded by physicians from health insurance companies, thereby potentially influencing health insurance losses without changing the nature of provider-patient interactions. As such, evidence on the validity of our hypothesis will not evaluate the specific nature of a medical professionals' behavior changes surrounding medical malpractice reforms, but rather the ultimate effect of the changes on health insurance losses.

Examining the experience of the private health insurers in Texas before and after the malpractice reform effort would provide evidence on whether malpractice reforms have implications for health insurance markets as well as the direction of these effects. Specifically, if the reforms passed in Texas had no effect on provider behavior, then we would expect the levels of health insurance losses incurred by Texas health insurers to be equal before and after the reform. Such a result would provide support for our null hypothesis. Alternatively, if the Texas reforms altered physician behavior in a way that resulted in either higher or lower levels of health insurance losses, then we would expect levels of health insurance losses incurred by health insurers in Texas before the reforms to differ from the levels after the

implementation of the reforms. Such a result would support our alternative hypothesis that the ramifications of medical malpractice reforms for health insurance are consequential.

Data

We identify several sources of data to test our hypothesis. Data on state tort reform measures comes from the American Tort Reform Association (ATRA) and the Database of State Tort Law Reforms [23]. State demographic data, added to the analysis for a further robustness check, is obtained from the Centers for Disease Control (CDC) and the U.S. Census Bureau. "Health Status" is a variable provided by the CDC that indicates the overall health status of a given state in a given year and is increasing in good health. "Dependents" is the number of persons under the age of 18 per capita in a given state in a given year. "Females" is the proportion of a state's population that is female in a particular year. "Median Income" is the median income level for residents of a given state during a given year. "Unemployment Rate" is the proportion of a particular state's available workforce that is not employed in a given year.

Testing of our hypothesis also requires state-specific data pertaining to health insurance losses. We use insurer financial data from the state pages of the National Association of Insurance Commissioners (NAIC) statutory filings for the years 2001 through 2010.[9] This dataset provides the most complete and comprehensive database of private health insurance losses.[10] We then apply several filters to this raw dataset in order to screen out insurers that do not have a significant level of business in a given state.[11] Since we are interested in examining the extent to which loss levels incurred by health insurers changed following the Texas reform, it would be inappropriate to include firms that enter a state market after the reform. As such, if insurer i does not operate in state j from 2001 to 2003, we remove that insurer-state observation for all future years.[12]

To test our hypothesis relating to the influence of tort reform on health insurance losses, we use the NAIC data to calculate health insurance losses per enrollee (LPE). This variable is defined as total health insurance losses incurred for insurer i in state j during year t scaled by total health enrollees for insurer i in state j during year t and is ideal for our analysis because it provides a standardized metric of health insurance losses which facilitates comparison across all firms.[13] In all tables and figures presented in this analysis, LPE is always expressed as scaled by \$1000 for ease of formatting.

Our analysis focuses on insurers operating in Texas, New Jersey, Colorado, and three additional subsamples of states that did not enact significant medical malpractice reforms during our sample period. Table 2 provides

Table 2 Health Insurance Losses per Enrollee for Different Samples

Health Insurance Losses per Enrollee

Panel A

	Texas			New Jersey			Colorado		
Year	Mean	St. Dev.	Insurers	Mean	St. Dev.	Insurers	Mean	St. Dev.	Insurers
2001	1.56	1.85	45	1.78	1.08	18	1.78	1.21	18
2002	1.53	1.49	41	1.45	1.48	34	1.99	1.36	20
2003	1.88	1.79	43	1.41	1.53	34	1.96	1.40	18
2004	1.99	2.09	39	1.51	1.75	34	2.02	1.47	18
2005	2.04	2.22	38	1.71	2.38	34	2.22	1.60	18
2006	1.99	2.23	38	1.39	1.56	31	2.33	1.71	18
2007	2.25	2.52	38	1.47	1.74	30	2.45	1.85	18
2008	2.22	2.62	37	1.50	1.82	30	2.30	1.97	16
2009	2.52	3.00	34	1.71	2.07	29	2.57	2.30	16
2010	2.10	2.67	32	1.72	2.29	28	2.53	2.38	15

Panel B

	41 State Subsample			18 State Subsample			9 State Subsample		
Year	Mean	St. Dev.	Insurers	Mean	St. Dev.	Insurers	Mean	St. Dev.	Insurers
2001	1.95	3.99	545	1.90	1.27	223	1.94	1.26	96
2002	1.87	1.70	588	2.02	1.72	241	2.07	1.70	108
2003	1.96	1.72	587	2.16	2.01	248	1.98	1.69	110
2004	2.14	1.89	554	2.38	2.17	234	2.14	1.79	103
2005	2.13	1.79	533	2.31	1.89	222	2.21	1.93	96
2006	2.30	1.99	520	2.57	2.26	218	2.53	2.34	95
2007	2.46	2.09	491	2.71	2.30	207	2.64	2.40	92
2008	2.56	2.27	483	2.92	2.57	205	2.67	2.45	89
2009	2.73	2.46	463	3.15	2.83	196	2.90	2.80	88
2010	2.76	2.55	440	3.19	2.88	191	2.97	2.88	86

Notes: This table provides summary information regarding health insurance firms' Losses per Enrollee (LPE) for each of the subsample of firms used in our analysis, during each year of our sample period. LPE is defined as the dollar amount of health insurance losses incurred by a given insurer, in a given state, during a given year, scaled by the number of plan enrollees for a given insurer, in a given state, during a given year. LPE is also scaled by 1000. Panel A provides information pertaining to LPE for a subsample of insurers operating in Texas, New Jersey, or Colorado. Panel B provides information pertaining to LPE for three subsamples of insures operating in states identified by Paik et al. [24]. "Mean" refers to the mean value of LPE, "St. Dev." refers to the standard deviation of LPE, and "Insurers" refers to the number of insurers (observations)

summary statistics of health insurance LPE, scaled by $1000, for the insurers operating in these states from 2001 to 2010 in terms of 2010 dollars.[14] The table indicates that LPE generally increased over our sample period in all state samples and suggests that healthcare costs are rising, in general. Summary inspection of the Texas data, in particular, indicates that insurers' mean LPE increased by roughly about $1000 from the beginning to the end of our sample period. However, there is no obvious break in this trend surrounding the enactment of the Texas reforms, which is consistent with our null hypothesis.

Figure 1a – 1f show the mean LPE, and the 95% confidence interval around the mean for the different samples of insurers in our analysis across our sample period. The figures reinforce our observations in the summary

data. The gradual upward trend in Texas LPE is easily observable and, with the exception of New Jersey, largely mirrors the trends observed in the other non-reforming states. However, the figure does highlight a relatively sudden increase in LPE in Texas in 2003 – the year the reforms were enacted – relative to 2002. The magnitude of this increase in mean LPE is approximately $300 and may suggest that reforms had the initial effect of increasing health insurance losses incurred by Texas insurers. We investigate this possibility in more detail in the ensuing sections.

Difference-in-differences analysis

The dramatic overhaul of Texas' medical professional liability climate in 2003 resulting from the enactment of medical malpractice reforms presents an ideal setting

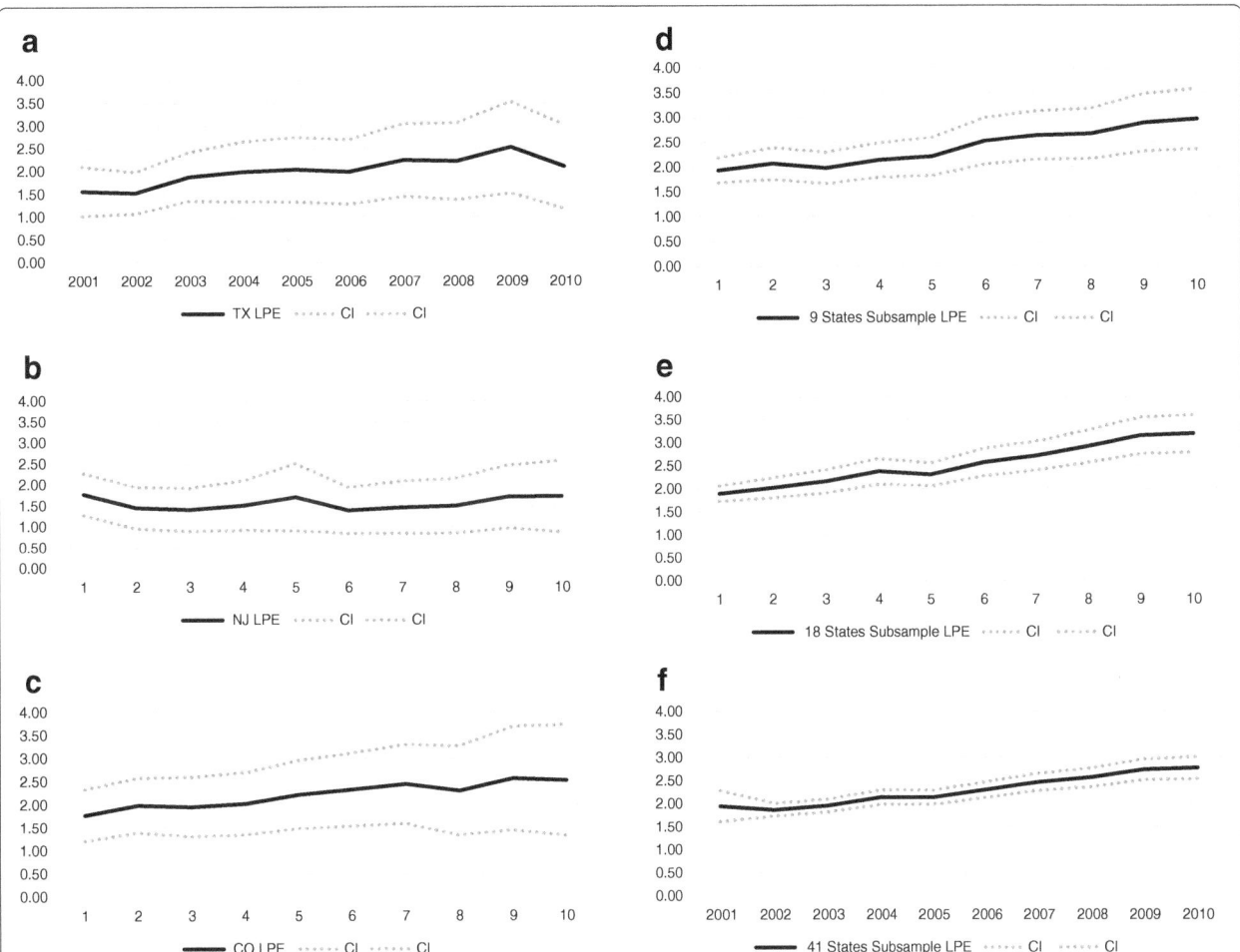

Fig. 1 a Trends in health insurance losses per enrollee (LPE) – Texas. **b** Trends in health insurance losses per enrollee (LPE) – New Jersey.**c** Trends in health insurance losses per enrollee (LPE) – Colorado. **d** Trends in health insurance losses per enrollee (LPE) – 9 State Subsample. **e** Trends in health insurance losses per enrollee (LPE) – 18 State Subsample. **f** Trends in health insurance losses per enrollee (LPE) - – 41 State Subsample.Notes: These figures display trends in health insurance firms' Losses per Enrollee (LPE), for each of the subsample of firms used in our analysis during our sample period. LPE is defined as the dollar amount of health insurance losses incurred by a given insurer, in a given state, during a given year, scaled by the number of plan enrollees for a given insurer, in a given state, during a given year. LPE is also scaled by 1000

for testing our hypothesis using a natural experiment design.[15] If, as our alternative hypothesis predicts, the change in the medical malpractice environment led to changes in the way medical providers behave in the healthcare market, which ultimately led to changes in health insurance losses, then we would not expect health insurance loss levels before the reform to equal loss levels after the reform. Further, since the reform measures only apply to the legal environment in Texas after the implementation of the new law, we would not expect the law passed in Texas to have an influence on the insurance markets of other states pre- or post- Texas reform. Therefore, comparing the difference in Texas health insurance losses levels pre- and post- Texas reform to the difference in the health insurance losses levels pre- and post- the Texas reform of a state

unaffected by the losses allows us to isolate the direct influence of the tort reform measures on the health insurance market in Texas.

For robustness in the DD, we first identify insurers operating in two different non-treated states – New Jersey and Colorado, and perform two separate DD analyses. Neither state had major upheaval in the health insurance marketplace (such as health insurance reforms) in the time closely preceding and following the implementation of the Texas tort reforms. Further, neither state enacted any major medical malpractice insurance reforms during the time of the Texas tort reforms. Of note is that Colorado had several tort reform measures in place prior to 2003, including caps on non-economic damages (enacted in 1987), while New Jersey had relatively few tort reform measures in place and no caps on non-economic damages.

Following Paik et al. [22], we also identify three additional non-treated subsamples, comprised of insurers operating in states unaffected by tort reforms during our sample period. The first subsample consists of insurers operating in the 41 states that did not enact a major tort reform from 2001 to 2010.[16] The second subsample consists of insurers operating in the 18 states that never enacted a cap on non-economic damages or total damages during the sample period.[17] The third subsample consists of insurers operating in nine states that did not enact a cap on damages and, as suggested by Paik et al. [22], are similar to Texas both geographically and culturally.[18] Using the same non-treated states as Paik et al. [22] adds another element of robustness to our individual state comparisons and allows us to consider their conclusions in the context of private health insurance markets.[19]

In theory, implementation of the DD analysis involves comparing the difference in mean health insurance LPE between insurers operating in Texas and insurers in the non-treated samples before the enactment of the Texas reform. This difference is then compared to the difference in mean health insurance LPE between insurers operating in Texas and insurers in the non-treated samples after the Texas reform. While the Texas reforms went into effect in the latter part of 2003, their first full year of implementation was 2004. As a result, our DD analysis considers how losses changed in 2004 and onward relative to 2003 and before.

In practice, the DD analysis is implemented using a regression framework.[20] We estimate several unique model specification that take the general form of the following OLS model:

$$LPE_{it} = a + \beta_1 Treat_{it} + \beta_2 Reform_t + \beta_3 Treat_{it}$$
$$* Reform_t + \varepsilon_{it} \qquad (1)$$

where.

Treat = a dummy variable indicating insurer i is a member of the treatment group in year t and captures differences between the treatment and control group. In our analysis, *Treat* is equal to one for insurers operating in Texas and zero for insurers operating in the other non-treated states described previously;

Reform = a dummy variable equal to one if the year is greater than or equal to 2004 and 0 if the year is less than 2004; and.

*Treat*Reform* = a dummy variable equal to one for insurers that are members of the treatment group in the years after the enactment of the tort reforms.

The coefficient on *Treat*Reform*, β_3, is the DD estimator. Formally,

$$\beta_3 = \left(\overline{LPE}_{Treat=1, Reform=1} - \overline{LPE}_{Treat=1, Reform=0} \right)$$
$$- \left(\overline{LPE}_{Treat=0, Reform=1} - \overline{LPE}_{Treat=0, Reform=0} \right).$$

The numerical value of this coefficient is the difference in the differences of mean health insurance LPE in Texas and the control state before and after the implementation of the reforms. The t-test of the coefficient indicates if the difference-in-difference estimate is statistically significant. A statistically insignificant β_3 would prevent us from rejecting the null hypothesis that the Texas reforms influenced physician behavior in a way that spilled over into the health insurance marketplace. A statistically significant and positive (negative) β_3 would provide support for our alternative hypothesis that the enactment of the Texas tort reforms influenced physician behavior in a way that, in the aggregate, increased (decreased) health insurance losses.

Difference-in-difference-in-differences analysis

In an effort to provide further evidence on the validity of our hypothesis, we employ a difference-in-difference-in-differences (DDD) analysis where we include, as an additional control group, a sub-sample insurers operating in lines of business not related to health insurance or medical malpractice markets. The identification assumptions of the DDD are more robust than that of a DD analysis and helps to confirm the findings of the previous section. In particular, a DDD strategy controls for the potentially confounding trend of changes in health insurance losses over time that are not related to medical malpractice reform[21] and also controls for the confounding effects of state-specific factors that affect insurance losses, generally. As such, the DDD framework improves on the shortcomings of the DD analysis by controlling for a broad set of other influences. If our results are robust to a DDD analysis, this would suggest that our results are not due to spurious developments in the state's health insurance environment.

To implement the DDD, we select as the additional control group a subsample of insurers operating in private passenger automobile physical damage insurance in Texas, New Jersey, Colorado, and the three multi-state subsamples identified by Paik et al. [22].[22] We quantify the losses incurred by these insurers in the given states as losses per automobile (LPA), calculated as the amount of private passenger automobile physical damage losses incurred by insurer i in state j during year t scaled by a weighted measure of the number of automobiles insured by insurer i in state j during year t.[23] We then compare the difference-in-differences between LPE and LPA in Texas pre and post Texas tort reform with the difference-in-differences between LPE and LPA in the control state(s) pre and post Texas tort reform.

In practice, the DDD analysis is implemented using a regression framework. We estimate several unique model specifications that take the general form of the following OLS model:

$$Losses_{it} = a_i + \beta_1 Treat + \beta_2 Control + \beta_3 Treat \\ * Control + \beta_4 Reform + \beta_5 Treat \\ * Reform + \beta_6 Control * Reform \\ + \beta_7 Treat + Control * Reform + \varepsilon_{it} \quad (2)$$

where.

Losses = insurer *i*'s LPE if the insurer is a health insurer or insurer *i*'s LPA if the insurer is an auto insurer in a given state in a given year;

Treat = a dummy variable indicating insurer *i* is a member of the treatment group in year *t* and captures differences between the treatment and control group. In our analysis, *Treat* is equal to one for insurers operating in Texas and zero for insurers operating in the other states described previously;

Control = a dummy variable indicating insurer *i* is a health insurer in year *t* and captures the effects that the insurance market, in general, may have on health insurance losses levels. In our analysis, *Control* is equal to one if the insurer is operating in health insurance lines and equal to zero if the insurer is operating in automobile insurance lines in a given state in a given year;

Reform = a dummy variable equal to one if the year is greater than or equal to 2004 and 0 if the year is less than 2004; and.

*Treat*Control*Reform* = a dummy variable equal to one if insurer *i* is a health insurer operating in a non-treated state in year 2004 or later.

The coefficient on *Treat*Control*Reform*, β_7, is the difference-in-differences-in-differences estimator. The numerical value of this coefficient is the difference-in-differences-in-differences of mean LPE and LPA in Texas and the control state before and after the implementation of the reforms. The t-test of the coefficient indicates if the DDD is statistically significant. A statistically insignificant β_7 would prevent us from rejecting the null hypothesis that the Texas reforms influenced physician behavior in a way that spilled over into the health insurance marketplace. A statistically significant and positive (negative) β_7 would provide support for our alternative hypothesis that the enactment of the Texas tort reforms influenced physician behavior in a way that, in the aggregate, increased (decreased) health insurance losses.

Results and discussion

Table 3 displays the results of estimating eq. 1 for five distinct model specifications, where each specification differs only by the sample of insurers designated as non-treated. For all specifications, we cluster standard errors at the firm level. As shown in the table, none of the coefficients on the DD estimator are statistically significant at conventional levels. This result suggests that the mean change in Texas health insurers' LPE was not statistically different from the mean change in non-reform state

Table 3 Basic Difference-in-Differences Regression Analyses of Texas Reforms

	New Jersey	Colorado	41 State Subsample	18 State Subsample	9 State Subsample
DD Estimator	0.4276	0.0687	−0.0039	−0.1983	−0.0706
	[0.268]	[0.304]	[0.243]	[0.251]	[0.269]
Treatment Dummy	0.1557	−0.2526	−0.2653	−0.3743	−0.3398
	[0.319]	[0.342]	[0.233]	[0.243]	[0.262]
Reform Dummy	0.0689	0.4278**	0.5004***	0.6948***	0.5671***
	[0.138]	[0.209]	[0.091]	[0.114]	[0.150]
Constant	1.5024***	1.9107***	1.9234***	2.0323***	1.9979***
	[0.232]	[0.282]	[0.113]	[0.144]	[0.175]
Observations	687	560	5589	2570	1348
R-squared	0.0182	0.0137	0.0110	0.0260	0.0202

Notes: This table presents the results of several difference-in-differences analyses obtained using the regressions described generally in eq. 1. The dependent variable, Losses per Enrollee (LPE), is defined as the dollar amount of health insurance losses incurred by a given insurer, in a given state, during a given year, scaled by the number of plan enrollees for a given insurer, in a given state, during a given year. LPE is also scaled by 1000. In the table, "DD estimator" is the difference-in-differences estimator, "Treatment dummy" indicates firms operating in Texas, and "Reform Dummy" indicates years following the enactment of the Texas reform measures. Each column of output represents a separate analysis that differs only by the subsample of firms used as non-treated groups. Clustered standard errors are presented in parentheses and ***indicates $p < 0.01$, and **indicates $p < 0.05$

health insurers' LPE from in the years 2004–2010 relative to 2001–2003. This evidence is consistent with our null hypothesis that the Texas tort reform efforts had no spillover effects that substantially influenced the losses incurred by health insurers.

The results presented in Table 4 confirm that, with one exception, the results displayed in Table 3 are not sensitive to the inclusion of state-level demographic control variables. The exception is that we find that mean changes in LPE were *larger* in for Texas insurers in the years following the reform relative to their New Jersey counterparts. The magnitude of this coefficient, which is significant at the 10% level, indicates that, relative to New Jersey, insurers operating in Texas experience an increase in LPE of approximately $519, on average, in the years following the reforms. This result is consistent with our alternative hypothesis and other findings in the literature (e.g., [22]) that the reforms in Texas actually bent the healthcare cost curve upward. However, in light of the fact that the DD estimator is not statistically significant in the other model specifications, the results of

the New Jersey specification do not provide compelling support for the rejection of our null hypothesis.

As a robustness exercise, we compare differences in losses levels in 2002 to differences in losses levels in 2004, 2005, 2006, 2007, 2008, 2009, and 2010. These estimates help to illustrate the significance and magnitude of the difference in LPE in the year immediately preceding the enactment of the reforms, to each individual year following the reform. The results of this year-by-year DD analysis for the insurers operating in the subsample of 9 states as the control group are given in Table 5.[24] For the sake of brevity, we discuss the results of the other subsamples, where relevant, instead of reporting the full year-by-year analysis for all subsamples.[25] As shown in the table, the DD estimator is statistically significant at the 10% level only in the 2002–2004 period. This result indicates that, relative to the year 2002, mean LPE increased at a greater rate for Texas insurers than the non-Texas insurers in the 9 state subsample for the year 2004 through 2010. The magnitude of the coefficient suggest the change in LPE experienced by Texas

Table 4 Difference-in-Differences Regression Analyses of Texas Reforms Including Full Variable Set

	New Jersey	Colorado	41 State Subsample	18 State Subsample	9 State Subsample
DD Estimator	0.5193*	0.1734	0.0566	−0.1421	−0.1018
	[0.292]	[0.291]	[0.249]	[0.262]	[0.276]
Treatment Dummy	−0.5373	−0.1091	0.2461	0.1101	−0.3308
	[0.748]	[0.578]	[0.331]	[0.545]	[0.755]
Reform Dummy	0.1043	0.2086	0.3786***	0.5063**	0.6322**
	[0.163]	[0.139]	[0.130]	[0.199]	[0.247]
Health Status	−0.0056	0.0253	−0.0285	−0.0319	−0.0535
	[0.037]	[0.043]	[0.027]	[0.042]	[0.038]
Dependents	0.2297	−0.0202	−0.1281***	−0.0814	0.0458
	[0.215]	[0.200]	[0.048]	[0.121]	[0.198]
Females	−0.0646	−0.0173	−0.0125	0.0355	0.0006
	[0.063]	[0.118]	[0.073]	[0.085]	[0.109]
Median Income	0.0000	0.0000	−0.0000	0.0000	−0.0000
	[0.000]	[0.000]	[0.000]	[0.000]	[0.000]
Unemployment Rate	0.0774***	0.0347	0.0607***	0.0714**	0.0600*
	[0.023]	[0.031]	[0.021]	[0.029]	[0.033]
Constant	−1.9597	1.2360	6.0315	1.6430	1.6183
	[5.237]	[7.573]	[4.276]	[5.848]	[9.012]
Observations	687	560	5589	2570	1348
R-squared	0.0202	0.0161	0.0197	0.0370	0.0276

Notes: This table presents the results of several difference-in-differences analyses obtained using the regressions described generally in eq. 1. The dependent variable, Losses per Enrollee (LPE), is defined as the dollar amount of health insurance losses incurred by a given insurer, in a given state, during a given year, scaled by the number of plan enrollees for a given insurer, in a given state, during a given year. LPE is also scaled by 1000. "DD estimator" is the difference-in-differences estimator, "Treatment dummy" indicates firms operating in Texas, and "Reform Dummy" indicates years following the enactment of the Texas reform measures. "Health status", "Dependents", "Females", "Median income" and "Unemployment rate" are all state-level demographic control variables previously described. Each column of output represents a separate analysis that differs only by the subsample of firms used as non-treated groups. Clustered standard errors are presented in parentheses and ***indicates $p < 0.01$, **indicates $p < 0.05$, and *indicates $p < 0.1$

Table 5 Difference-in-Differences Regression Analyses of Texas Reforms for Nine State Sample and Multiple Time Periods

	2002–2004	2002–2005	2002–2006	2002–2007	2002–2008	2002–2009	2002–2010
DD Estimator	0.3914*	0.3710	0.0004	0.1473	0.0909	0.1681	−0.3316
	[0.235]	[0.255]	[0.260]	[0.323]	[0.342]	[0.426]	[0.381]
Treatment Dummy	−0.5408*	−0.5408*	−0.5408*	−0.5408*	−0.5408*	−0.5408*	−0.5408*
	[0.293]	[0.293]	[0.293]	[0.293]	[0.293]	[0.293]	[0.293]
Reform Dummy	0.0739	0.1404	0.4590***	0.5727***	0.6043***	0.8266***	0.9023***
	[0.117]	[0.131]	[0.169]	[0.190]	[0.189]	[0.233]	[0.255]
Constant	2.0696***	2.0696***	2.0696***	2.0696***	2.0696***	2.0696***	2.0696***
	[0.201]	[0.201]	[0.201]	[0.201]	[0.201]	[0.201]	[0.201]
Observations	291	283	282	279	275	271	267
R-squared	0.0130	0.0143	0.0276	0.0321	0.0333	0.0438	0.0502

Notes: This table presents the results of several difference-in-differences analyses obtained using the regressions described generally in eq. 1 and only using the subsample of firms operating in 9 states as the non-treated group. The dependent variable, Losses per Enrollee (LPE), is defined as the dollar amount of health insurance losses incurred by a given insurer, in a given state, during a given year, scaled by the number of plan enrollees for a given insurer, in a given state, during a given year. LPE is also scaled by 1000. In the table, "DD estimator" is the difference-in-differences estimator, "Treatment dummy" indicates firms operating in Texas, and "Reform Dummy" indicates years following the enactment of the Texas reform measures. Each column of output represents a separate analysis that compares LPEs in the year 2002 to a given, single year in the future. Clustered standard errors are presented in parentheses and ***indicates $p < 0.01$, and *indicates $p < 0.1$

health insurers was approximately $390 greater than their counterparts in the 9 state subsample.

In unreported analysis, we also find changes in Texas LPE in 2004, relative to 2002, were greater than the changes experienced by health insurers operating in New Jersey and Colorado over the same period. However, regardless of the sample examined, we find no other evidence that changes in Texas LPE in any ensuing year (i.e. 2005 to 2010) were significantly greater than those experienced by insurers operating in other states. Taken together, this year-by-year DD analysis suggests that the spillover effects of the Texas reforms into the health insurance market were, at best, short-lived and influenced Texas health insurers only during 2004. While this result does favor our alternative hypothesis, the evidence is weak and does not provide compelling evidence that the Texas reforms had a long-lasting and substantial effect on the health insurance market.

Considered in their entirety, the results presented in Tables 3 through 5 provide little support for the hypothesis that the Texas reforms had a significant influence on the health insurance market – the vast majority of our model specifications fail to find a significant change in Texas LPE after the enactment of tort liability reforms. In the few instances we do find a statistically significant spillover effect, our estimates suggest the reforms had the effect of *increasing* LPE. However, in these cases, the results are not robust across all subsample analyses and/or the effect is short-lived and we therefore are unable to reject null hypotheses based on the evidence in the DD analysis. In the ensuing subsection, we explore the robustness of our findings by extending our DD analysis to control for other potential confounding factors.

Table 6 displays the results of estimating eq. 2, our DDD model, for five distinct model specifications, where each specification differs only by the sample of insurers designated as non-treated.[26] The DDD estimator is statistically insignificant in all but one of the five model specifications which provides little support for the hypothesis that the Texas liability reforms had any meaningful impact on losses incurred by health insurers operating in Texas. However, the DDD estimator is statistically significant at the 5 % level when the New Jersey insurer subsample is used and the magnitude of the coefficient indicates the net increase in LPE incurred by Texas insurers in the post-reform time period was approximately $620. The results in Table 7 further suggest that our DDD analysis is robust to the addition of several state-level demographic control variables.[27] The DDD analysis, therefore, provides little evidence in favor of our alternative hypothesis.

In Table 8, we provide the results of a DDD analysis where LPE in 2002 is compared to the years 2004 through 2010 in an effort to illustrate the significance and magnitude of difference in LPE in the year immediately preceding the enactment of the reforms, to each individual year following the reform.[28] The table indicates that, relative to the non-treated group of insurers operating in the nine-state subsample, mean LPE in Texas were higher and statistically different from zero in the first two years following the reform. In particular, the magnitude of the DDD estimator coefficient suggests that the net increase in mean LPE for Texas insurers in 2004, relative to 2002, was approximately $490 and this same increase was approximately $435 in 2005 relative to 2002. Again, this evidence suggests that, at best, the spillover effect of the Texas reforms on the health insurance market was short-lived. In unreported analysis using the New Jersey insurers, Colorado insurers, and the 41 state subsample of insurers, we find further evidence of

Table 6 Basic Differences-in-Differences-in-Differences Regression Analyses of Texas Reforms

	New Jersey	Colorado	41 State Subsample	18 State Subsample	9 State Subsample
DDD Estimator	0.6191**	0.2000	0.1505	−0.0424	0.0821
	[0.270]	[0.305]	[0.245]	[0.253]	[0.271]
Treatment Dummy	0.3992***	0.2950***	0.3064***	0.3221***	0.2984***
	[0.038]	[0.039]	[0.037]	[0.037]	[0.038]
Control Dummy	1.2416***	1.5457***	1.5698***	1.6944***	1.6363***
	[0.231]	[0.280]	[0.113]	[0.143]	[0.174]
Control*Treatment	−0.2435	−0.5476	−0.5717**	−0.6964***	−0.6382**
	[0.320]	[0.342]	[0.236]	[0.246]	[0.264]
Reform Dummy	−0.0138	−0.0741***	−0.0509***	−0.0494***	−0.0527***
	[0.016]	[0.012]	[0.005]	[0.006]	[0.008]
Treatment*Reform	−0.1916***	−0.1312***	−0.1544***	−0.1560***	−0.1527***
	[0.041]	[0.039]	[0.037]	[0.037]	[0.037]
Control*Reform	0.0827	0.5019**	0.5513***	0.7442***	0.6198***
	[0.138]	[0.208]	[0.091]	[0.114]	[0.150]
Constant	0.2608***	0.3650***	0.3536***	0.3379***	0.3616***
	[0.011]	[0.011]	[0.005]	[0.006]	[0.008]
Observations	2447	2873	42,436	21,281	11,603
R-squared	0.2338	0.3113	0.3469	0.4252	0.3794

Notes: This table presents the results of several difference-in-differences-in-differences analyses obtained using the regressions described generally in eq. 2. The dependent variable, Losses per Enrollee (LPE), is defined as the dollar amount of health insurance losses incurred by a given insurer, in a given state, during a given year, scaled by the number of plan enrollees for a given insurer, in a given state, during a given year. LPE is also scaled by 1000. "DDD estimator" is the difference-in-differences-in-differences estimator, "Treatment dummy" indicates firms operating in Texas, "Reform Dummy" indicates years following the enactment of the Texas reform measures, "Control dummy" indicates health insurers, "Control*Treatment" is the interaction of Control dummy and Treatment dummy, "Treatment*Reform" is the interaction of Treatment dummy and Reform dummy, and "Control*Reform" is the interaction of Control dummy and Reform dummy. Each column of output represents a separate analysis that differs only by the subsample of firms used as non-treated groups. Clustered standard errors are presented in parentheses and ***indicates p < 0.01, **indicates p < 0.05, and *indicates $p < 0.1$

statistically significant increases in mean LPE in the initial year or two following the reform that do not persist to future years.

As a whole, the results of the DDD analysis provide additional support for the conclusion drawn in the DD analysis. There is very little evidence to suggest that the Texas tort liability reforms had a substantial prolonged spillover effect on health insurers operating in Texas in the years following the reforms. We do find some evidence that mean LPE in Texas increased at a greater rate than that of New Jersey, but this result does not hold for any of the four other subsamples of insurers used as controls. In addition, we find some evidence that LPE in Texas increased to a greater degree than non-Texas insurers in the year immediately following the reform but this effect does not persist to other future years. As a result, we are unable to definitively reject the null hypothesis, as there does not appear to be sufficient evidence in favor of the alternative.

Conclusion

Using a difference-in-differences (DD) analysis, we find evidence that the Texas tort reform measures enacted in 2003 had little influence on the levels of health

insurance losses per enrollee incurred by Texas health insurers. We utilize several non-treated groups and find that this result is not sensitive to the selection of the non-treated group. In an effort to control for state-specific insurance climates in general, we also consider automobile physical damage losses incurred by insurers in our sample and employ a difference-in-difference-in-differences (DDD) analysis, the results of which are largely consistent with the DD analysis. Our results provide support for our null hypothesis that reform measures in the medical malpractice market did not have a significant, persistent effect on health insurance losses.

Interestingly, our analysis does provide some evidence that the reforms had an immediate, but short-term spillover effect on health insurance markets. In particular, we find that the LPE for Texas insurers increased to a greater degree than non-Texas insurers in the first two years following the enactment of the reform. This evidence is consistent with the work of Paik et al. [22], who present evidence that Texas' tort reform did not bend the healthcare cost curve downward as was suggested by many proponents of tort liability reform. However, since we find no other evidence that the reforms influenced the levels of health insurance losses incurred by Texas

Table 7 Difference-in-Differences-in-Differences Regression Analyses of Texas Reforms Including Full Variable Set

	New Jersey	Colorado	41 State Subsample	18 State Subsample	9 State Subsample
DDD Estimator	0.6221**	0.2013	0.1516	−0.0432	0.0817
	[0.269]	[0.305]	[0.245]	[0.253]	[0.271]
Treatment Dummy	0.1862	0.0750	0.3041***	0.2471***	0.0820
	[0.215]	[0.118]	[0.044]	[0.061]	[0.077]
Control Dummy	1.2415***	1.5460***	1.5711***	1.6950***	1.6355***
	[0.232]	[0.280]	[0.114]	[0.143]	[0.174]
Control*Treatment	−0.2435	−0.5480	−0.5730**	−0.6969***	−0.6375**
	[0.321]	[0.342]	[0.236]	[0.246]	[0.263]
Reform Dummy	−0.0218	−0.0665***	−0.0412***	−0.0263	0.0145
	[0.052]	[0.023]	[0.013]	[0.017]	[0.023]
Treatment*Reform	−0.1455***	−0.1113***	−0.1523***	−0.1608***	−0.1607***
	[0.052]	[0.040]	[0.037]	[0.038]	[0.038]
Control*Reform	0.0805	0.5010**	0.5507***	0.7452***	0.6208***
	[0.136]	[0.208]	[0.091]	[0.114]	[0.150]
Health Status	0.0124	0.0149	−0.0033	−0.0060	−0.0051
	[0.012]	[0.010]	[0.003]	[0.005]	[0.004]
Dependents	0.0529	0.0553	0.0003	0.0226*	0.0641***
	[0.071]	[0.040]	[0.005]	[0.013]	[0.021]
Females	−0.0160	0.0069	0.0009	−0.0017	−0.0223*
	[0.025]	[0.024]	[0.010]	[0.011]	[0.012]
Median Income	0.0000	0.0000	−0.0000	−0.0000	−0.0000
	[0.000]	[0.000]	[0.000]	[0.000]	[0.000]
Unemployment Rate	0.0215***	0.0178***	0.0101***	0.0095**	0.0077*
	[0.008]	[0.007]	[0.003]	[0.004]	[0.004]
Constant	−0.7595	−1.9630	0.4092	−0.0350	0.0713
	[1.976]	[1.368]	[0.571]	[0.674]	[0.954]
Observations	2447	2873	42,436	21,281	11,603
R-squared	0.2342	0.3118	0.3472	0.4260	0.3831

Notes: This table presents the results of several difference-in-differences-in-differences analyses obtained using the regressions described generally in eq. 2. The dependent variable, Losses per Enrollee (LPE), is defined as the dollar amount of health insurance losses incurred by a given insurer, in a given state, during a given year, scaled by the number of plan enrollees for a given insurer, in a given state, during a given year. LPE is also scaled by 1000. In the table, "DDD estimator" is the difference-in-differences-in-differences estimator, "Treatment dummy" indicates firms operating in Texas, "Reform Dummy" indicates years following the enactment of the Texas reform measures, "Control dummy" indicates firms operating as health insurers, "Control*Treatment" is the interaction of Control dummy and Treatment dummy, "Treatment*Reform" is the interaction of Treatment dummy and Reform dummy, and "Control*Reform" is the interaction of Control dummy and Reform dummy. "Health status", "Dependents", "Females", "Median income" and "Unemployment rate" are all state-level demographic control variables previously described. Each column of output represents a separate analysis that differs only by the subsample of firms used as non-treated groups. Clustered standard errors are presented in parentheses and ***indicates $p < 0.01$, **indicates $p < 0.05$, and *indicates $p < 0.1$

insures after 2005, our conclusion is that reforming the malpractice environment has largely insignificant economic implications for health insurance markets.

Our analysis provides novel and valuable insight into the consequences of tort reform. Proponents of tort liability reforms often suggest that reforms reduce defensive medicine practices, thereby reducing healthcare costs. Our analysis suggests that, if there are any persistent effects of tort reforms on provider-patient interactions, they do not spillover into health insurance markets. If anything, our analysis suggests these reforms may lead to initial, short-term increases in costs borne by health insurers. As

such, our analysis should suggest to policy makers that, while there are potentially many economic benefits to tort liability reforms, reforms do not appear to be useful for influencing outcomes in health insurance markets.

An important consideration when interpreting our results is that our analysis provides evidence that the Texas reform had little influence on levels of health insurance losses, *in the aggregate*, across a variety of patient groups and provider specialties. That is, because health insurance companies reporting to the NAIC engage in a variety of health insurance lines, such as individual and group comprehensive healthcare, dental

Table 8 Differences-in-Differences-in-Differences Regression Analyses of Texas Reforms for Nine State Sample and Multiple Time Periods

	2002–2004	2002–2005	2002–2006	2002–2007	2002–2008	2002–2009	2002–2010
DDD Estimator	0.4919**	0.4347*	0.0733	0.2393	0.0666	0.2097	−0.1943
	[0.235]	[0.255]	[0.260]	[0.322]	[0.343]	[0.424]	[0.379]
Treatment Dummy	0.2154***	0.2154***	0.2154***	0.2154***	0.2154***	0.2154***	0.2154***
	[0.023]	[0.023]	[0.023]	[0.023]	[0.023]	[0.023]	[0.023]
Control Dummy	1.7160***	1.7160***	1.7160***	1.7160***	1.7160***	1.7160***	1.7160***
	[0.199]	[0.199]	[0.199]	[0.199]	[0.199]	[0.200]	[0.200]
Control*Treatment	−0.7563***	−0.7563***	−0.7563***	−0.7563***	−0.7563***	−0.7563***	−0.7563***
	[0.292]	[0.292]	[0.292]	[0.292]	[0.292]	[0.292]	[0.292]
Reform Dummy	−0.0404***	−0.0584***	−0.0429***	−0.0415***	−0.0299**	−0.0555***	−0.0442***
	[0.008]	[0.007]	[0.007]	[0.007]	[0.014]	[0.008]	[0.007]
Treatment*Reform	−0.1005***	−0.0637**	−0.0730**	−0.0920***	0.0243	−0.0416	−0.1374***
	[0.025]	[0.029]	[0.029]	[0.026]	[0.041]	[0.026]	[0.025]
Control*Reform	0.1144	0.1988	0.5020***	0.6142***	0.6341***	0.8821***	0.9465***
	[0.117]	[0.131]	[0.168]	[0.189]	[0.189]	[0.232]	[0.253]
Constant	0.3537***	0.3537***	0.3537***	0.3537***	0.3537***	0.3537***	0.3537***
	[0.006]	[0.006]	[0.006]	[0.006]	[0.006]	[0.006]	[0.006]
Observations	2682	2563	2520	2461	2433	2374	2335
R-squared	0.4285	0.4238	0.4177	0.4220	0.4073	0.4083	0.4079

Notes: This table presents the results of several difference-in-differences-in differences analyses obtained using the regressions described generally in eq. 2 and only using the subsample of firms operating in 9 states as the non-treated group. The dependent variable, Losses per Enrollee (LPE), is defined as the dollar amount of health insurance losses incurred by a given insurer, in a given state, during a given year, scaled by the number of plan enrollees for a given insurer, in a given state, during a given year. LPE is also scaled by 1000. In the table, "DDD estimator" is the difference-in-differences-in-differences estimator, "Treatment dummy" indicates firms operating in Texas, and "Reform Dummy" indicates years following the enactment of the Texas reform measures. Each column of output represents a separate analysis that compares LPEs in the year 2002 to a given, single year in the future. Clustered standard errors are presented in parentheses and ***indicates $p < 0.01$, **indicates $p < 0.05$, and *indicates $p < 0$

and vision, Medicaid, Medicare, and Federal Employee Health Benefits, our analysis captures the net result of changes in medical professionals' behavior among a heterogeneous group of provider and patient types. This degree of heterogeneity is often not present in studies of malpractice liability's influence on physician behavior and healthcare costs (for example [1, 2, 22]). As a result, if tort reform's effects on provider behavior differ by the provider's specialty type or the type of patient, then different analyses presented in the literature, utilizing different but relatively homogenous samples of provider or insured types, may yield conflicting results regarding the influence of malpractice exposure on healthcare cost and health insurance markets. Further research may consider how specific provider specialties and patient groups are influenced by changes in medical malpractice liability exposure.

Endnotes

[1]Reasons for the disagreement in the literature could arise from a number of sources including differences in sample characteristics, time periods, or econometric methods. As such, the additional evidence on the influence of malpractice exposure on the frequency/cost of services rendered by medical providers, presented in our

analysis, is a valuable contribution to the ongoing debate in the literature.

[2]For example, using data from the Physician Insurance Association of America (PIAA), Kessler and McClellan [24] find evidence that direct malpractice reforms reduce defensive medicine practices but do not influence health outcomes. Baicker, Fisher, and Chandra [25] find a positive relation between Medicare spending, especially on imaging services, and malpractice awards which provides support for the hypothesis that malpractice awards drive defensive medicine rates.

[3]For example, Mello et al. [26] provide evidence that suggests physicians reduce or eliminated "high risk" aspects of their practice. Kessler, Sage, and Becker [27] provide evidence that tort reforms increase the supply of physicians.

[4]This is not a universal sentiment in the literature. For example, Morrisey, Kligore, and Nelson [4] do not find any evidence that damage caps reduce the cost of employer sponsored health insurance. Given somewhat conflicting results in prior literature, our analysis is valuable in that it provides insight into the ongoing debate regarding how the medical professional liability climate ultimately influences the health insurance market.

[5]In 2008 ten plaintiffs filed a federal lawsuit claiming the state's non-economic cap violates the U.S. Constitution. The suit, similar to those filed in other states with such caps, argued that the cap has a direct impact on an injured patient's potential jury award and, consequently, influences the value of filing the suit in the first place. A federal judge ruled that the cap was constitutional in 2012.

[6]Interestingly, Hyman et al. [28] evaluate physician supply in Texas before and after the 2003 reforms. They find that physician supply in Texas was not deteriorating before 2003 and "did not measurably improve after the reform" (p.203).

[7]Other Texas-specific studies include Friedson and Kniesner [29], who examine how the reform – specifically the non-economic damages cap – has affected pre-trial settlement speed and settlement amounts. They find that even though injured plaintiffs are compensated more quickly after reform, they receive a lower settlement. In addition, Paik, Black, Hyman, Sage, and Silver [20] evaluate the influence of the Texas reform on elderly patients. They find that tort reform strongly affected claim rates and payouts for all patients, but elderly claimants receive disproportionately lower payouts after reform. Further, a recent review of the Texas market indicates, among other things, that "the reform bill's most significant achievements have been increased access to health care and an unanticipated positive economic impact on the Texas economy. By the end of 2013, 10 years and three months after the effective date of HB4, the number of licensed physicians in the state will almost have doubled" [19].

[8]Paik et al. [22] posit a similar hypothesis regarding physicians' perception of malpractice risk.

[9]While much of our analysis relies on the NAIC's health insurance database, we also utilize the property-casualty database for private passenger automobile loss data. Both databases also contain information relating to overall company financial information (for example, assets, liabilities, organizational form). However, the analysis presented here relies strictly on data from the state pages.

[10]The dataset includes financial data filed with state insurance departments for all insurers classified as health insurers and much of the data, including premiums, claims, and enrollment, are reported separately for each state in which an insurer operates

[11]Specifically, we restrict our sample to firms with at least $100,000 in direct premiums written, $100,000 in direct losses incurred, and 1000 enrollees. The inclusion of these filters does not substantially reduce our sample size and helps to reduce the effects of outliers in our analysis. These filters ensure that the insurers included in our analysis are non-trivial market participants in a given state that are likely to be influenced by the operational and regulatory climate of a given state.

[12]This filter effectively ensures that we analyze firms that were operating before and after the Texas reform took effect.

[13]Previous studies similar in nature to ours (for example, [22]) evaluate relative spending levels scaled by enrollees. In addition, because the size of health insurance markets, in terms of premium levels and insurers vary widely across states, it would be inappropriate to evaluate raw, unscaled loss levels across states. Further, a loss measure scaled by premiums is more indicative of financial/operational performance of the health insurer while losses scaled by plan participants (enrollees) better quantifies the amount of claims that insurance companies incur due to patients' interactions with medical providers. We therefore believe that scaling by enrollees is the most appropriate method for our analysis.

[14]The NAIC Health Insurance database, due to changes in reporting requirements, does not provide consistent and reliable data that can be used in our study before 2001. As such, we are forced to limit the start of our sample to 2001.

[15]Such DD analyses are frequently used in the economics, finance, and insurance literature (for example, [22, 30, 31]). The method involves computing the difference between the pre- and post-, within-subjects differences of the treatment and control groups. As it applies to our analysis, the subjects are a sample of health insurance companies, the treatment group is a sub-sample of health insurers operating in Texas, and the non-treated group is a sub-sample of health insurers operating in other states.

[16]Health insurers operating in Florida, Georgia, Illinois, Mississippi, Nevada, Ohio, Oklahoma, Oregon, and South Carolina are not included in this subsample.

[17]These 18 states are Alabama, Arizona, Arkansas, Connecticut, Delaware, Iowa, Kentucky, Maine, Minnesota, New Hampshire, New York, North Carolina, Pennsylvania, Rhode Island, Tennessee, Vermont, Washington, and Wyoming. Paik et al. [22] also include the District of Columbia but, due to the unavailability of certain demographic data, we are forced to omit insurers operating there in our analysis.

[18]These 9 states are Alabama, Arizona, Arkansas, Iowa, Kentucky, Minnesota, Tennessee, Washington, and Wyoming.

[19]We recognize that some of the states in these subsamples enacted other reforms relating to medical malpractice during our sample period but, following Paik et al. [22], we believe these other reforms are not likely to cause major changes in losses per enrollee and are confident in the validity of these samples.

[20]Studies such as Bertrand, Duflo, and Mallainthan [32] and Donald and Lang [33] suggest that, in certain cases, econometric issues lead researchers to incorrectly reject the null hypothesis of the statistical significance of

a difference-in-differences coefficient. These studies provide evidence that clustering standard errors helps reduce the likelihood of a false rejection of the null. All results reported throughout the paper are from models with standard errors clustered at the firm level. In unreported results, we also implement another procedure found by Bertrand et al. [32] to reduce the likelihood of an inaccurate rejection of the null, the block bootstrap procedure. Our main results remain unchanged when the block bootstrap procedure is implemented. Further, our main results remain unchanged when we cluster standard errors by state and also when we include state and year effects (instead of the *Treat* and *Reform* dummies in the main specification). Therefore, we do not believe that the common econometric pitfalls of DD analysis described in the literature bias our results.

[21]For example, changes in the number of people with health insurance.

[22]We select private passenger automobile physical damage insurers because this line of business strictly relates to property losses. As such, factors associated directly with medical malpractice tort reform (for example, liability lawsuits, physician behavior, and the like) do not influence loss levels in this line of business. Similarly, factors associated directly with health insurance (doctors, healthcare costs, and so on) also do not influence loss levels in this line of business. Thus loss levels in private passenger automobile physical damage insurance are an appropriate control.

[23]More specifically, we assign each insurer a number of automobiles based on proportion of premiums insurer *i* writes relative to all other insurers in a given state in a given year. For example, assume total premiums written in Texas for all insurers in 2010 was $1 billion and Insurer A wrote $100 million in premiums in 2010. If there are 1 million automobiles in the state of Texas in 2010, then Insurer A would be assigned (100 million/1 billion) X 1 million automobiles. Therefore, LPA for Insurer A would be incurred automobile physical damage losses divided by 100,000.

[24]Note the "DD Estimator" coefficients and statistical significances reported are the regression coefficients of *Treat*Reform* from equation 1. However, in this output, *Reform* takes the value of 0 if the year is 2002 and 1 if the year is either 2004, 2005, 2006, 2007, 2008, 2009, or 2010, depending on the specification.

[25]These results are available from the authors upon request.

[26]For the same reasons described in a previous footnote, all reported results are from models with standard errors clustered at the firm level. In addition, all reported results are robust to different clustering strategies described in a previous footnote as well as various combinations of state-level control variables.

[27]These are the same control variables included in the DD analysis which are defined in a previous footnote. In addition, unreported analysis indicates that our main result is robust to the inclusion of additional/alternative demographic controls, such as uninsured rates and educational attainment.

[28]Note the "DDD" estimates and statistical significances reported in the table are the regression coefficients of *Treat*Control*Reform* from equation 2. However, in this output, *Reform* takes the value of 0 if the year is 2002 and 1 if the year is either 2004, 2005, 2006, 2007, 2008, 2009, or 2010, depending on the specification.

Acknowledgements
none.

Authors' contributions
All authors contributed equally. All authors read and approved the final manuscript.

Funding
not applicable.

Competing interests
The authors declare that they have no competing interests.

Author details
[1]Vanderbilt University Law School, 131 21st Avenue South, Nashville, TN 37203, USA. [2]Florida State University, College of Business, Tallahassee, FL, USA. [3]East Carolina University, College of Business, Greenville, NC, USA.

References
1. Kessler D, McClellan M. Do doctors practice defensive medicine? Q J Econ. 1996;111(2):353–90.
2. Sloan FA, Shadle JHl. There empirical evidence for "defensive medicine"? A reassessment. J Health Econ. 2009;28(2):481–91.
3. Avraham R, Schanzenbach M. The impact of tort reform on private health insurance coverage. Am law. Econ Rev. 2010;12(2):319–55.
4. Morrisey MA, Kilgore ML, Nelson L. Medical malpractice reform and employer-sponsored health insurance premiums. Health Serv Res. 2008; 43(6):2124–42.
5. Danzon P. The frequency and severity of medical malpractice claims. J Law Econ. 1984;27(1):115–48.
6. Danzon P. The frequency and severity of medical malpractice claims: new evidence. Law Contemp Probl. 1986;49(2):57–84.
7. Avraham R. An empirical study of the impact of tort reforms on medical malpractice settlement payments. J Leg Stud. 2007;36(S2):S183–229.
8. Born PH, Karl JB. The effect of tort reform on medical malpractice insurance market trends. J Emp Legal Studies. 2016;13(4):718–55.
9. Born PH, Viscusi WK. The distribution of the insurance market effects of tort liability reforms. Brookings Pap Econ Ac: Microecon. 1998:55–105.

10. Born PH, Viscusi WK, Baker T. The effect of tort reform on malpractice insurers' ultimate losses. J Risk Insur. 2009;76(1):197–219.

11. Grace MF, Leverty JT. How tort reforms affect insurance markets. J Law Econ Org. 2013;29(6):1253–78.

12. Viscusi WK, Zeckhauser R, Born PH, Blackmon G. The effects of the 1980s tort reform legislation on general liability and medical malpractice insurance. J Risk Uncertainty. 1993;6(2):165–86.

13. Viscusi WK. Born PH. Medical malpractice insurance in the wake of liability reform. J Leg Stud. 1995;24(2):463–90.

14. Viscusi WK. Born PH. Damage caps, insurability, and the performance of medical malpractice insurance. J Risk Insur. 2005;72(1):23–43.

15. Currie J, MacLeod WB. First do no harm? Tort reform and birth outcomes. Q J Econ. 2008;123(2):795–830.

16. Avraham R, Schanzenbach M. The impact of tort reform on intensity of treatment: evidence from heart patients. J Health Econ. 2015;39:273–88.

17. Avraham R, Dafny L, Schanzenbach M. The impact of tort reform on employer sponsored health insurance premiums. J Law Econ Org. 2013;28(4):657–86.

18. Karl JB, Born PH, Viscusi WK. The relationship between the markets for health insurance and medical malpractice insurance. App Econ. 2016;48(55):5348–63.

19. Nixon J. Ten years of tort reform in Texas: A review," Backgrounder #2830, The Heritage Foundation, 2013. Available from: http://www.heritage.org/research/reports/2013/07/ten-years-of-tort-reform-in-texas-a-review.

20. Paik M, Black B, Hyman D, Sage W, Silver C. How do the elderly fare in medical malpractice litigation, before and after tort reform? Evidence from Texas. Am law. Econ Rev. 2012;14(2):561–600.

21. Sage WM, Harding MC, Thomas EJ. Resolving malpractice claims after tort reform: experience in a self-insured Texas public academic health system. Health Serv Res 2016; 51. S3:2615–33.

22. Paik M, Black B, Hyman D, Silver C. Will tort reform bend the cost curve? Evidence from Texas. J Empirical Legal Stud. 2012;9(2):173–216.

23. Avraham R. Database of state tort law reforms. 5th ed; 2014.

24. Kessler D, McClellan M. Malpractice law and healthcare reform: optimal liability policy in an era of managed care. J Pub Econ. 2002;84(2):175–97.

25. Baicker K, Fisher ES, Chandra A. Malpractice liability costs and the practice of medicine in the Medicare program. Health Aff. 2007;23(3):841–52.

26. Mello MM, Studdert DM, DesRoches CM, Peugh J, Zapert K, Brennan TA, Sage WM. Effects of a malpractice crisis on specialist supply and patient access to care. Ann Surg. 2005;242(5):621–8.

27. Kessler DP, Sage WM, Becker DJ. Impact of malpractice reforms on the supply of physician services. J Am Med Assn. 2005;293(21):2618–25.

28. Hyman DA, Silver C, Black B, Paik M. Does tort reform affect physician supply? Evidence from Texas. Int Rev Law Econ. 2015;42:203–18.

29. Friedson AI, Kniesner TJ. Losers and losers: some demographics of medical malpractice tort reforms. J Risk Uncertainty. 2012;45(2):115–33.

30. Meyer B, Viscusi WK, Durbin D. Workers compensation and injury duration: evidence from a natural experiment. Am Econ Rev. 1995;85(3):322–40.

31. Viscusi WK, Born PH. The performance of the liability reform experiments: New York and Colorado. J Prod Toxics Liability. 1994;16(1):1–18.

32. Bertrand M, Duflo E, Mullainathan S. How much should we trust differences-in-differences estimates? Q J Econ. 2004;119(1):249–75.

33. Donald S, Lang K. Inference with difference-in-differences and other panel data. Rev Econ Stat. 2007;89(2):221–33.

15

National health insurance subscription and maternal healthcare utilisation across mothers' wealth status in Ghana

Edward Kwabena Ameyaw[1*], Raymond Elikplim Kofinti[2] and Francis Appiah[1]

Abstract

Introduction: This study is against the backdrop that despite the forty-nine percent decline in Maternal Mortality Rate in Ghana, the situation still remains high averaging 319 per 100,000 live births between 2011 and 2015.

Objective: To examine the relationship between National Health Insurance and maternal healthcare utilisation across three main wealth quintiles (Poor, Middle and Rich).

Methods: The study employed data from the 2014 Ghana Demographic and Health Survey. Both descriptive analysis and binary logistic regression were conducted.

Results: Descriptively, rich women had high antenatal attendance and health facility deliveries represented by 96.5% and 95.6% respectively. However, the binary logistic regression results revealed that poor women owning NHIS are 7% (CI = 1.76–2.87) more likely to make at least four antenatal care visits compared to women in the middle wealth quintile (5%, CI = 2.12–4.76) and rich women (2%, CI = 1.14–4.14). Similarly, poor women who owned the NHIS are 14% (CI = 1.42–2.13) likely to deliver in health facility than women in the middle and rich wealth quintile.

Conclusion: The study has vindicated the claim that NHIS Scheme is pro-poor in Ghana. The Ministry of Health should target women in the rural area to be enrolled on the NHIS to improve maternal healthcare utilisation since poverty is principally a rural phenomenon in Ghana.

Keywords: Antenatal care, Maternal healthcare utilisation, Wealth status, Women, Health insurance

Background

Maternal related complications constitute the major source of disabilities and mortality among women within reproductive age globally [1]. Despite the tremendous progress made by the global community in combating maternal related complications and mortality, 289,000 women still die yearly owing to pregnancy with low and middle income countries bearing the highest brunt [1]. The disparity between these countries and the developed countries presupposes that income disparities have consequences on maternal health status. The crucial nature of maternal and child health instigated the global community to devote the third Sustainable Development Goal (SDG) to reduction in maternal mortality, neonatal, infant and under five mortality rates [2].

Whilst studies indicate decline in maternal mortality rates since 1990s, the decline is not universal and still remains high in southern Asia and Africa [1, 3, 4]. For instance, it has been realised that risk of maternal mortality for a woman in Sub-Saharan Africa is forty-seven times higher as compared to someone in the United States, meanwhile most of these deaths are avoidable [5]. In the case of Ghana, despite the forty-nine percent decline in Maternal Mortality Rate (MMR), the situation still remains high because as noted by the World Bank, it averaged 319 per 100,000 live births between 2011 and 2015 [6].

The high rate of maternal complications emerge from the numerous threats confronting the health sector of most African countries and cost associated with healthcare

* Correspondence: edmeyaw19@gmail.com
[1]Department of Population and Health, Faculty of Social Sciences, University of Cape Coast, Cape Coast, Ghana

utilisation. Arguably, economic standing of women is critical to the extent to which maternal healthcare can be utilised and as indicated by Marmot [7], income relates to health in three principal ways: countries' gross national product; individual's income; and variation in income. In light of this, the poor are the most vulnerable in terms of maternal healthcare access [8, 9]. Since investment in maternal health constitutes not only social and political imperatives but also cost effective investment, a number of initiatives have been instituted manifesting in interventions such as health insurance scheme.

Health insurance exists as an essential pro-poor initiative and despite its enormous benefits, evidence suggests that maternal healthcare utilisation especially Antenatal Care (ANC) attendance and supervised delivery are still induced by maternal wealth status in some countries [10]. Through rise in health insurance subscription, a growing body of studies have investigated the essence of health insurance to utilisation of healthcare [11–14], meanwhile, the impact of health insurance on maternal healthcare utilisation across wealth status in Ghana has not gained recognition in literature.

The National Health Insurance Scheme (NHIS) commenced in 2005 as a demand side initiative to overcome financial obstacles to healthcare utilisation. As far as the link between NHIS ownership and maternal healthcare utilisation is concerned, some questions remain unanswered in the literature: (1) is NHIS a prerogative of the rich, the poor or both?; (2) which of these groups should be the primary target of the NHIS?; and (3) which of these groups are currently benefitting from NHIS ownership via maternal health utilisation? Whilst some evidence point out that women with higher socio-economic standing least utilise NHIS due to their access to multiple options to enhance their health status in terms of accessing quality and or private healthcare and good nutrition during pregnancy [15, 16], counter evidence have also been reported [17]. Considering the fact that divergent results have been reported in Ghana about NHIS and maternal healthcare utilisation [18, 19], this study intends to unearth the current direction as far as the relationship between health insurance and maternal healthcare utilisation across wealth status is concerned. There is therefore the need for this investigation with the 2014 Ghana Demographic Health Surveys (GHDS) to know the current status of how well the NHIS has impacted maternal healthcare utilisation (antenatal visits and place of delivery) across wealth status in Ghana.

Theoretical framework

Several and complex drivers influencing healthcare utilisation revolve around social, cultural, economic and religious factors [20, 21]. In order for the concept of healthcare utilisation and its drivers which are at the core of this paper to be well-understood and for conceptual clarity, it demands theoretical guidance. Anderson's Behavioural Model (BM) of healthcare utilisation [22, 23] shall guide this paper since the primary focus of the paper is to investigate the relationship between insurance subscription and maternal healthcare utilisation (measured by ANC attendance and place of delivery) across wealth status of women (poor, middle, rich).

The BM postulates that healthcare utilisation rest on predisposing, enabling and need factors operating at both individual and contextual domains [23, 24]. Within the predisposing factors, individual predisposing factors constitute the aggregate of demographic, biological and social while the contextual predisposing factors also encompass demographic, social composition of communities and cultural norms that interact to influence healthcare utilisation [23, 24]. The enabling factors include but not limited to one's income and wealth status that enables individuals to pay for healthcare services and the effective price of healthcare influenced by one's health insurance status. However, due to inherent weaknesses, the model was revised and as such healthcare systems, service availability, population-based factors and consumer satisfaction in the initial model are considered as drivers of healthcare utilisation.

Methods

Data from the 2014 GDHS was used for this study. Specifically, the women and child files were used for the study. GDHS is carried out by the Ghana Statistical Service and Macro International under the auspices of DHS programs. The survey captures data on various aspects of maternal health conditions within the country and as such was deemed suitable for this study. The dataset was requested online from Measure DHS website on the 16th October, 2015. In all, 9,396 women (aged 15–49) from 11,835 households nationwide were interviewed [25]. However, 4,294 women had birth history within the last 5 years preceding the survey and as such they constituted the sample size for this study.

The 2014 GDHS was conducted with an updated frame from the 2010 Population and Housing Census (PHC) prepared by the Ghana Statistical Service (GSS). The frame exempted institutional and nomadic groups including hotel occupants and prisoners. The survey constituted a two-stage sample design for the purpose of allowing estimates of core indicators at the national level. The initial phase constituted selection of sample points (clusters) involving enumeration areas (EAs) outlined for the 2010 PHC in which 427 clusters were designated in all constituting 216 from urban and 211 from rural areas. The next stage utilised systematic sampling of households in which household inventory operation was carried out in all the identified EAs between January and March 2014. Afterwards, the households to be considered for the survey were selected from the list randomly [25].

Econometric model

To investigate the effect of National Health Insurance Subscription (NHIS) on maternal healthcare utilisation across the three main wealth quintiles (Poor, Middle and Rich) in Ghana we relied on theorising maternal healthcare utilisation specified by Anderson [22, 23]. The study assumes that the mother derives utility from (1) making at least four antenatal care visits during pregnancy and, (2) delivering in a health facility/hospital, and that there is disutility to the mother and the husband in the form of complications during pregnancy and time of delivery when the mother fails to either make at least four antenatal care (ANC) visits or delivers at a health facility. It can be elaborated that the mother makes a conscious effort to improve her own survival and that of the child during pregnancy through investment in health care which can take the form of either curative or preventive health care. Therefore, it can be argued that the decision of the mother to utilise maternal health is the responsibility of the mother as Anderson [22] later considered individuals as the unit of analysis which goes beyond health care utilisation only.

The probability that the mother utilises maternal health care is a function of a key enabling factor of National Health Insurance Subscription NHIS (N) and the level of education of the mother (E_m), the level of education of the partner/husband (E_f). Some of the predisposing factors considered for the study are religious affiliation (R_A), household purchasing decision (HP) and household health care decision making (HC). The maternal health care probability production function of the mother is thus specified as:

$$MH_i = \pi\left(N, E_m, E_f, R_A, HP, HC, X\right) \qquad (1)$$

Where MH_i is the probability that the mother utilises the two maternal health care services: (1) probability that the mother makes at least four antenatal care visits; and (2) the probability that the woman delivers in a health facility, and X is a vector of other exogenous variables such as ecological zone and the urban dummy.

$$MH_i = \varphi_i\beta + \delta_i \text{ with } MH_i = \begin{cases} 1 \text{ if } MH_i > 0 \\ 0 \text{ otherwise} \end{cases} \qquad (2)$$

Where MH_i is the probability of maternal health care utilisation by the mother, which is broken up into two in this study: (1) the probability that the mother makes at least four antenatal care visits; and (2) the probability that the mother delivers in a health facility. Equation two is therefore estimated for the three wealth quintiles,

viz., poor, middle and rich. φ_i is a vector of exogenous factors influencing maternal health care utilisation; β is a vector of unknown parameters; and δ_i is an error term with zero mean and a constant variance, which also captures the unobserved factors in the model. In order to estimate equation (2), the maximum likely estimation (MLE) technique in logistic regression is employed. This is against the background that the logistic regression satisfies the main assumption underlying MLE, viz., the dependent variable, maternal health care utilisation, is dichotomous.

Dependent variables

Utilisation of maternal healthcare services, comprising ANC attendance and place of delivery, was the outcome variable. The first dependent variable, ANC visits was recoded into a binary outcome variable with zero '0' denoting less than four and one '1' at least four. Similarly, the second dependent variable, place of delivery, was recoded into a binary outcome variable with zero '0' denoting delivery at home and one '1' denoting delivery in a health facility.

Independent variables of interest

The main independent variable of the study was health insurance ownership which is a dummy variable where one '1' represents women who have subscribed to NHIS, and zero '0' otherwise. The effect of NHIS ownership on maternal healthcare utilisation was analysed across the wealth status of women. Wealth status is a categorical variable with zero '0' denoting women in the poor wealth quintile, one '1' denoting women in the middle wealth quintile and two '2' denoting women in the rich wealth quintile. As with any good model specification and taking into cognizance the theoretical literature review, other socio-demographic variables were controlled for in the estimation. These are residential status, religion, marital status, frequency of watching television and listening to radio, frequency of reading newspaper, ecological zone (made up of the ten administrative regions), occupation, partner's occupation and education, contraceptive usage and birth order.

Results

Descriptive statistics for the independent variables

Table 1 presents the descriptive statistics of the independent variables. The analysis indicated that across wealth status, the highest NHIS subscription occurred among the poor (42.9%) whilst the least subscription occurred among those in the middle wealth status (19.4%). Specifically, 67.1% of the poor had subscribed to the scheme, whereas 68.7% of those in the middle wealth category had subscribed. However, among the rich women, NHIS subscription stood at 72.9%. It was

Table 1 Descriptive Statistics for the Independent Variables

Variable	Poor Row (Col.)	Middle Row (Col.)	Rich Row (Col.)	N = 4,294
NHIS				
Owned	42.9 (67.1)	19.4 (68.7)	37.7 (72.9)	100
	45.0 (32.9)	21.8 (31.3)	33.2 (27.1)	100
Not Owned	(100)	(100)	(100)	
Residence				
Rural	77.1 (86.3)	16.7 (51.9)	6.2 (12.6)	100
Urban	17.2 (13.7)	21.8 (48.1)	61.0 (87.4)	100
	(100)	(100)	(100)	
Religion				
Others	65.6 (35.6)	16.0 (24.0)	18.4 (18.0)	100
Christianity	46.9 (64.4)	20.0 (76.0)	33.1 (82.0)	100
	(100)	(100)	(100)	
Marital Status				
Not Married	48.6 (32.1)	26.2 (48)	25.2 (30.1)	100
Married	54.1 (67.9)	15.0 (52)	30.9 (69.9)	100
	(100)	(100)	(100)	
Occupation				
Not working	45.4 (15.0)	24.1 (22.2)	30.5 (18.2)	100
Working	53.7 (85.0)	17.7 (77.8)	28.6 (81.8)	100
	(100)	(100)	(100)	
Partner's occupation				
Primary	87.5 (9.6)	9.6 (20.9)	2.9 (45.9)	100
Secondary	23.9 (76.3)	30.7 (25.0)	45.4 (4.6)	100
Tertiary	23.1 (14.1)	16.9 (54.1)	60.0 (49.5)	100
	(100)	(100)	(100)	
Education				
No education	80.6 (51.4)	12.0 (21.2)	7.4 (8.5)	100
Primary	61.6 (23.9)	20.3 (21.8)	18.1 (12.7)	100
At least secondary	27.8 (24.7)	23.1 (56.9)	49.1 (78.9)	100
	(100)	(100)	(100)	
Partner's education				
No education	85.9 (48.4)	8.5 (14.2)	5.5 (5.6)	100
Primary	38.8 (50.3)	21.7 (83.0)	39.5 (93.1)	100
At least secondary	44.1 (1.3)	32.2 (2.8)	23.7 (1.3)	100
	(100)	(100)	(100)	
Ecological zone				
Coastal	27.1 (14.7)	23.7 (35.6)	49.2 (48.1)	100
Savannah	81.2 (33.6)	8.3 (49.9)	10.5 (39.8)	100
Forest	45.6 (51.7)	24.4 (14.5)	30.0 (12.1)	100
	(100)	(100)	(100)	
Frequency of listening to radio				
Not at all	69.8 (25.7)	14.9 (15.2)	15.3 (10.1)	100

Table 1 Descriptive Statistics for the Independent Variables *(Continued)*

Less than once a Week	50.1 (29.4)	21.8 (35.5)	28.1 (29.8)	100
At least once a week	46.7 (44.9)	18.6 (49.4)	34.7 (60.1)	100
	(100)	(100)	(100)	
Water source				
Pipe	5.3 (1.0)	13.3 (5.1)	81.4 (20.2)	100
Others	48.0 (99.0)	21.0 (94.9)	31.0 (79.8)	100
	(100)	(100)	(100)	
Contraceptive usage				
No modern contraceptive	43.3 (75.5)	19.8 (71.7)	36.9 (73.9)	100
Uses modern	44.6 (24.5)	22.1 (28.3)	33.3 (26.1)	100
Contraceptive	(100)	(100)	(100)	
Healthcare decision making				
Alone	46.3 (19.0)	20.3 (25.3)	33.4 (24.4)	100
Not alone	54.7 (81.0)	16.7 (74.7)	28.6 (75.6)	100
	(100)	(100)	(100)	
Household purchase decision making				
Alone	50.7 (17.9)	19.6 (20.9)	29.7 (18.7)	100
Not alone	53.4 (82.1)	16.9 (79.1)	29.7 (81.3)	100
	(100)	(100)	(100)	
Decision making on visits				
Alone	48.9 (20.2)	18.9 (23.7)	32.0 (23.5)	100
Not alone	53.9 (79.8)	17.0 (76.3)	29.0 (76.5)	100
	(100)	(100)	(100)	
Shared toilet facility				
No	1.7 (0.6)	8.4 (5.9)	90.0 (58.3)	100
With other household only	53.2 (99.4)	22.9 (94.1)	23.9 (41.7)	100
	(100)	(100)	(100)	

Computed from GHDS 2014 Data

found that most poor women reside in rural settings (77.1%) as compared to women in other wealth categories. Within the poor, rural residents accounted for 86.3%. This observation implies that most poor women in Ghana reside in rural settings. This residential status might have potential implications on their access to maternal health services. Poor women affiliated to non-Christian religious bodies (65.6%) exceeded their non-Christian counterparts in middle (16.0%) and rich (18.4%) wealth categories. The proportion of poor women who were Christians (46.9%) was the highest.

It was found that across wealth status, marriage was high among poor women (54.1%). Similarly, marriage stood at 69.9% among the rich women. With regard to occupation across wealth status, it was realised that the greatest proportion of working women were poor (53.7%) with the least being women in the middle wealth status (17.7%). As depicted in Table 1, most women whose partners were engaging in primary occupation

were poor (87.5%) when considered across wealth status. On education, most uneducated women were poor (80.6%) whereas the highest proportion of those with at least secondary education was recorded among rich women (49.1%). Specifically, 51.4% of the poor were uneducated with 24.7% having at least secondary education. Also, majority of the rich women had at least secondary education (78.9%) whilst only 8.5% had no formal education. This finding imply that at least two out of ten Ghanaian women in the reproductive age group have had some formal education.

Upon analyzing partners' education, it was noted that partners of most poor women were uneducated (85.9%). Investigation among the poor indicated that half of their partners had attained primary education (50.3%) as indicated in Table 1. Similarly, majority of the rich women's partners had attained primary education (93.1%). Although educational attainment is generally high among the women, it is obvious that women from wealthier homes have dominated. It was evident from the study that a significant share of the rich women were within the Coastal zone (49.2%) with major of the poor residing in the Savanna zone (81.2%). Further analysis indicated half of the poor women were within the Forest zone (51.7%).

Most poor women were found not to listen to radio at all (69.8%) as compared with women in other wealth categories. Among the poor, 44.6% were listening to radio at least once a week with 25.7% not listening at all. With respect to the rich, 60.1% were listening to radio at least once a week whilst 10.1% were not listening to radio. Upon exploring among women in these wealth categories, it was noted that almost all poor women obtained water from sources other than pipe (99.0%). Among those in the middle wealth status, 94.9% were obtaining water from other sources. Hence, a greater proportion of Ghanaian women obtain water from sources other than pipe. As such, it is more probable that sources such as bole holes, wells and streams are much utilised, meanwhile, the health implications of these sources are sometimes adverse.

Investigation into contraceptive use revealed that as compared to women in other wealth categories, non-use was high among poor women (43.3%). Specifically, 75.5% of the poor were not using contraceptives, meanwhile the proportion of the rich who were not using contraceptives stood at 73.9%. Analysis of decision making on healthcare unraveled that women who were not taking the decision alone were predominantly poor (54.7%) as compared with middle and rich women. Among the poor, 81.0% were not taking the decision alone, whereas 74.7% of those in the middle wealth status were also not taking the decision alone. Almost all poor women were sharing (99.4%) and this was not so different from the observation made among those in the middle wealth status as 94.1% were sharing toilet facility with other households.

Maternal healthcare utilisation by wealth status

Assessment of delivery in health facility across wealth status revealed that generally the rich tend to deliver in health facilities more than their poor counterparts. This is because 95.6% of rich women delivered in health facilities compared to 57.2% health facility deliveries among poor women as illustrated in Fig. 1. Similarly, attendance of antenatal care was relatively high among rich women (96.5%) than their poor counterparts (80.6%). The Figure has indicated a trend whereby the rich appears to make more use of maternal healthcare services (place of delivery and antenatal visits). The low utilisation among the poor do not necessarily indicate that they are not interested in accessing the services but might be disadvantaged by their low economic status. This is because the rich are more likely to have multiple avenues of accessing these services which the poor might not be able to utilise. From the Figure, more than half of poor mothers deliver at home (43%) compared to the mothers in the middle wealth quintile (22%) and rich mothers (4%). Similarly, majority of mothers who fail to make the recommended WHO healthy antenatal visits of four are poor, thus 19.9% compared to mothers in the middle and rich wealth quintile of 12.5 and 3.5% respectively.

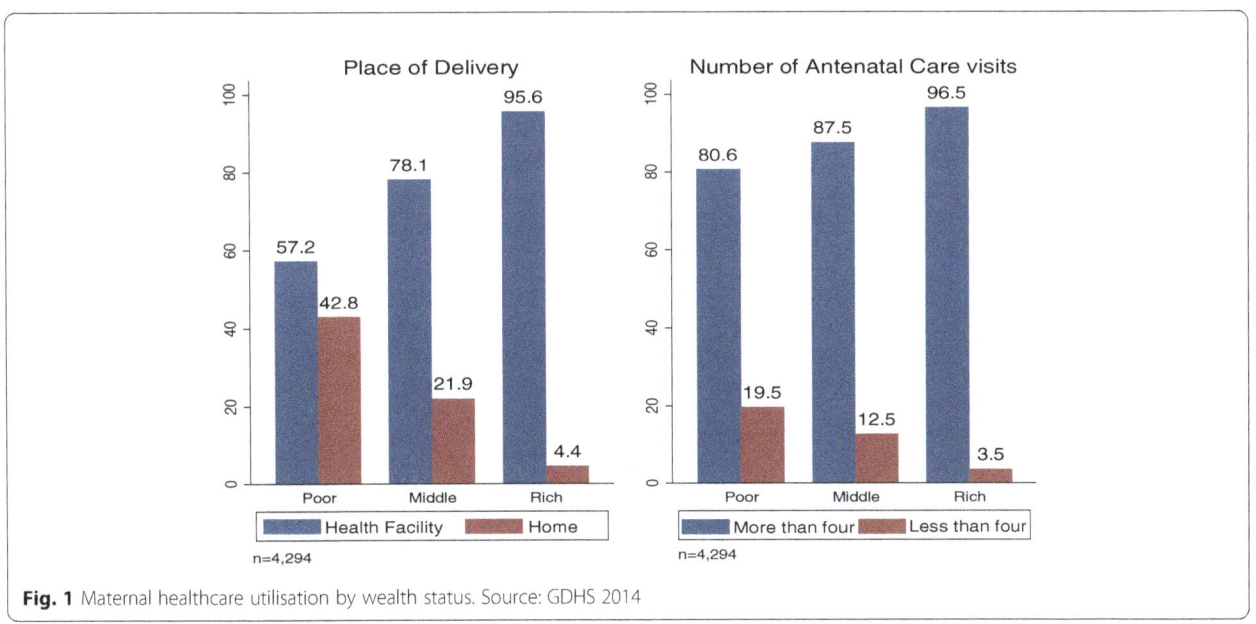

Fig. 1 Maternal healthcare utilisation by wealth status. Source: GDHS 2014

Maternal healthcare utilisation by wealth and zonal distribution

It was observed that home deliveries dominated among poor women in all the three zones of the country namely Coastal Poor (43.6%), Forest Poor (38.9%) and Savannah Poor (45.1%). At the same time, poor women in rural settings were noted to have the highest prevalence of home deliveries (45.2%) as depicted in Table 2. It is not surprising that rural poor women have high prevalence of home deliveries considering the poor road networks linking these rural areas to health facilities coupled with refusal of healthcare providers to accept postings to rural settings. When ANC visit was viewed across Rural–urban dimension, it was clear that having at least four visits was prevalent among both Rural Rich (97.4%) and Urban Rich (96.4%) as projected in Table 2.

Results of econometric models (logistic regression)
Logistic regression results on ANC visit

In all, six logistic regression models were constructed in explaining the effect of health insurance ownership on maternal healthcare utilisation across wealth status. Table 3 presents the results of antenatal care visit whilst Table 4 presents the results of place of delivery. With regard to antenatal care (ANC) visits, the logistic regression analysis indicated that poor women who were subscribed to the NHIS were about 7% (CI = 1.76–2.87) likely to have more ANC visits than poor women who have not subscribed to the scheme. Whilst urban poor residents were about 3% (CI = 1.66–3.21) more probable to attend ANC than rural

residents, poor Christians were about 5% less likely to attend ANC (–4.5%, CI = 0.67–1.34) as compared to poor women affiliated to other religions. Married women in the poor category were noted to have about 7% (CI = 1.41–2.44) likelihood of accessing ANC than the un-married. Meanwhile, poor women who were working were 10% (CI = 1.11–2.26) more likely to access ANC than their non-working counterparts (reference category). Common knowledge would argue that non-working women might have had enough time to attend ANC as compared to working women but that is not the case in the Ghanaian context. This, however, points to the notion that attendance or non-attendance of ANC is not only a function of availability of time but perception about the need to access such service.

Poor women with primary education (–1.0%, CI = 0.86–1.69) and those with at least secondary education were all less probable to utilise ANC as compared to those without formal education, meanwhile, contrary observation was made among those whose partners had at least secondary education (2.3%, CI = 0.98–1.96). It was also evident that ANC visits among poor women listening to radio at least once a week was 10% (CI = 1.83–3.28) higher than those who did not listen to radio at all. Less possibility of ANC attendance was associated with poor women who could not decide on their healthcare alone (–5%, CI = 1.21–3.43) as compared to those taking such decision on their own. However, poor women who were unable to decide household purchases (8%, CI = 2.32–4.51) and visits (2%, CI = 1.32–4.12) alone were more probable to utilise ANC as compared to those taking such decisions alone.

Among those in the middle wealth status, higher likelihood of ANC visits was observed among those subscribed to the NHIS as compared to those who had not subscribed (5%, CI = 2.12–4.76). This is expected, considering the fact that maternal health services are absorbed by the NHIS. Consequently, women who are subscribed to the scheme will be highly exposedto access the service as compared to their counterparts who are not subscribed to the scheme. Unlike the observation made among the poor, urban residents were less probable to utilise ANC as compared to rural women (–3%, CI = 0.98–1.64), however, married women in this category were more likely to utilise ANC than the unmarried (8%, CI = 0.74–2.86). Those residing in the Savannah zone were more probable to utilise ANC (2%, CI = 0.49–1.52) unlike their Forest zone counterparts (–3%, CI = 0.64–1.73) when compared with those in the Coastal zone (reference category).

Women in the middle wealth quintile who were obtaining water from sources other than pipe were relatively less probable to utilise ANC (–9%, CI = 0.65–2.71), however, those using modern contraceptives were more likely to utilise ANC (7%, CI = 0.95–2.63) as compared to those

Table 2 Maternal Healthcare Utilisation by Wealth and Zonal Distribution

	Place of delivery			ANC visit		
	Home	Health facility	Total	<4	≥4	Total
Coastal Poor	43.6	56.4	100	17.9	82.1	100
Coastal Middle	29.0	70.9	100	11.9	88.1	100
Coastal Rich	5.7	94.3	100	3.2	96.8	100
Forest Poor	38.9	61.0	100	21.2	78.8	100
Forest Middle	18.4	81.6	100	13.6	86.4	100
Forest Rich	3.1	96.9	100	4.1	95.9	100
Savannah Poor	45.1	54.9	100	18.8	81.2	100
Savannah Middle	16.2	83.8	100	10.3	89.7	100
Savannah Rich	3.3	96.7	100	2.7	97.4	100
Rural Poor	45.2	54.8	100	20.4	79.6	100
Rural Middle	28.3	71.7	100	10.8	89.2	100
Rural Rich	9.1	90.9	100	2.6	97.4	100
Urban Poor	27.9	72.1	100	13.7	86.3	100
Urban Middle	14.8	85.2	100	14.4	85.6	100
Urban Rich	3.7	96.3	100	3.6	96.4	100

Computed from GHDS 2014 Data

Table 3 Logistic regression results on ANC visit

Variable	Poor	95% CI	ANC Middle	95% CI	Rich	95% CI
Health Insurance						
Not-subscribed		1,1		1,1		1,1
Subscribed	0.067**(0.028)	1.76–2.87	0.045 (0.031)	2.12–4.76	0.017 (0.013)	1.14–4.14
Residence						
Rural		1,1		1,1		1,1
Urban	0.026 (0.039)	1.10–2.68	−0.034 (0.026)	0.98–1.64	−0.012 (0.015)	0.28–2.73
Religion						
Others		1,1		1,1		1,1
Christianity	−0.045 (0.028)	0.67–1.34	0.034 (0.034)	0.46–2.51	0.005 (0.022)	0.59–4.21
Marital Status						
Not Married		1,1		1,1		1,1
Married	0.067*(0.031)	1.41–2.44	0.080**(0.031)	0.74–2.86	0.021 (0.016)	0.75–3.16
Occupation						
Not working		1,1		1,1		
Working	0.104**(0.044)	1.11–2.26	0.095**(0.036)	1.75–4.31	0.049**(0.018)	
Partner's occupation						
Primary		1,1		1,1		1,1
Secondary	0.048 (0.032)	1.15–2.65	−0.002 (0.031)	2.31–3.99	0.010 (0.027)	0.23–2.30
Tertiary	0.129***(0.029)	1.27–3.87	0.027 (0.036)	1.54–2.56	0.019 (0.025)	0.65–5.42
Education						
No education		1,1		1,1		1,1
Primary	−0.009 (0.035)	0.86–1.69	0.012 (0.043)	0.77–1.75	−0.030 (0.025)	0.63–2.71
At least secondary	−0.001 (0.037)	0.91–3.01	0.049 (0.040)	0.94–1.88	0.005 (0.017)	0.97–1.72
Partner's education						
No education		1,1		1,1		1,1
Primary	−0.019 (0.040)	0.80–1.64	−0.029 (0.049)	0.82–1.66	0.040 (0.035)	1.21–3.22
At least secondary	0.023 (0.036)	0.98–1.96	−0.007 (0.039)	0.78–1.84	0.041 (0.033)	2.12–4.21
Ecological zone						
Coastal		1,1		1,1		1,1
Savannah	0.015 (0.039)	0.58–1.37	0.015 (0.039)	0.49–1.52	0.001 (0.022)	0.82–2.45
Forest	−0.033 (0.030)	0.46–1.02	−0.033 (0.030)	0.64–1.73	−0.005 (0.012)	0.94–1.63
Frequency of listening to radio						
Not at all		1,1		1,1		1,1
Less than once a Week	0.042 (0.041)	1.00–1.84	0.042 (0.041)	2.02–4.89	−0.013 (0.017)	2.42–5.21
At least once a week	0.106***(0.036)	1.83–3.28	0.106**(0.036)	1.86–3.72	0.009 (0.012)	2.01–4.21
Water source						
Pipe		1,1		1,1		1,1
Others	0.281 (0.154)	0.45–2.14	0.089**(0.033)	0.65–2.71	0.009 (0.015)	0.72–2.71
Contraceptive usage						
No modern contraceptive		1,1		1,1		1,1
Uses modern Contraceptive	0.064**(0.025)	1.43–2.70	0.065**(0.024)	0.95–2.63	0.000**(0.012)	0.52–2.61
Birth order	−0.004*(0.032)	0.33–2.01	0.001 (0.154)	1.22–3.28	0.024 (0.031)	0.74–3.82

Table 3 Logistic regression results on ANC visit *(Continued)*

Healthcare decision making						
Alone		1,1		1,1		1,1
Not alone	−0.050 (0.028)	1.21–3.43	−0.052 (0.030)	1.63–3.21	−0.015 (0.011)	1.82–2.73
Household purchase decision making						
Alone		1,1		1,1		1,1
Not alone	0.080 (0.042)	2.32–4.51	0.070 (0.041)	2.41–4.22	−0.016 (−0.013)	0.54–2.82
Decision making on visits						
Alone		1,1		1,1		1,1
Not alone	0.021 (0.036)	1.32–4.12	0.075*(0.038)	0.56–2.61	0.004 (0.016)	0.82–2.64
Shared toilet facility						
No		1,1		1,1		1,1
With other household only	−0.026 (0.036)	2.11–4.24	−0.066 (0.053)	2.31–4.46	−0.026*(0.012)	2.14–4.62
Public	−0.004 (0.032)	0.97–2.54	−0.051 (0.049)	1.11–3.01	−0.013 (0.012)	1.85–3.22
Hosmer and Lemeshow's Gof	9		12.7		9.7	

Co-efficient; standard error in bracket; 95% confidence interval *$p < 0.10$; **$p < 0.05$; ***$p < 0.001$

who were not. This has indicated that Ghanaian women using contraceptive also usually utilise ANC. As such, it can be inferred that women who are conscious about timing of their pregnancies are also much concerned about their pregnancies and unborn children. Those sharing toilet facility with other households (7.5%, CI = 0.56–2.61) together with those using public toilets (−5%, CI = 1.11–3.01) were less likely to access ANC as compared to women who were not sharing.

Urban rich women were relatively less probable to utilise ANC than rural rich women (−1%, CI = 0.28–2.73). This raises a number of concerns because it was expected that the rich who have wherewithal would make active use of all available health services. However, the emerging trend of wealthier women especially in the urban areas having the means of accessing other health care services they deem as 'quality' coupled with the general perception in the country that the NHIS is pro-poor could be adduced to the disinclination in usage stemming from the urban rich women. As compared to unmarried women, married women were more probable to access ANC (2%, CI = 0.75–3.16). Whilst low tendency of ANC utilisation was noted among those with primary education as compared with those without formal education (−3%, CI = 0.63–2.71), a contrary observation was made among women with at least secondary education (1%, CI = 0.63–2.71).

Logistic regression on place of delivery
Upon analysing the poor and place of delivery, poor women subscribed to the NHIS were 14% (CI = 1.42–2.13) more probable to deliver in health facilities than poor women who had not subscribed whilst poor urban residents also had a little higher propensity of delivering

in health facilities (3%, CI = 1.66–3.21) over their rural counterparts (reference category) as indicated in Table 4. As compared to poor women who are affiliated to other religions, Christians were 9% (CI = 1.16–1.78) more likely to deliver in health facilities and a similar observation was made among married women as compared to unmarried ones (4%, CI = 1.08–1.71). Those listening to radio at least once a week had 10% (CI = 1.40–2.26) higher likelihood of delivering in health facilities than those who were not listening to radio at all.

Poor women resident in Savannah (9%, CI = 0.85–1.65) and Forest zones (5%, CI = 0.73–1.39) were more likely to deliver in health facilities just as working women when compared with non-working ones (5%, CI = 0.90–1.60). As shown in Table 4, poor women whose partners were engaging in secondary and tertiary occupation were more probable to deliver in health facilities (5%, CI = 0.86–1.60 and 7%, CI = 1.42–3.09 respectively). At the same time, poor women sharing toilet facilities with other households (1%, CI = 0.77–1.01) and those using public toilets (5%, CI = 0.98–1.23) were also more inclined towards health facility delivery than those who were not sharing toilet facilities (reference category).

Among women in the middle wealth status, those subscribed to the NHIS were 7% (CI = 1.00–2.10) more likely to deliver in health facilities over those who were not subscribed. Urban residents in the middle wealth status were 17% (CI = 1.63–3.44) more likely to deliver in health facilities than their rural counterparts whilst Christians were similarly more probable to deliver in health facilities than those affiliated to other religions (8%, CI = 0.75–1.80). With regard to educational status, women with primary (2%, CI = 0.98–1.15) and at least secondary education (9%, CI = 1.01–2.75) were more

Table 4 Logistic regression on place of delivery

Variable	Poor	95% CI	Middle	95% CI	Rich	95% CI
Health Insurance						
Not-subscribed		1,1		1,1		1,1
Subscribed	0.139***(0.037)	1.42–2.13	0.074*(0.039)	1.00–2.10	0.048*(0.017)	1.02–3.18
Residence						
Rural		1,1		1,1		1,1
Urban	0.033 (0.053)	1.66–3.21	0.168***(0.035)	1.63–3.44	0.041 (0.022)	1.60–5.92
Religion						
Others		1,1		1,1		1,1
Christianity	0.087*(0.042)	1.16–1.78	0.076 (0.047)	0.75–1.80	0.029 (0.021)	0.71–2.97
Marital Status						
Not Married		1,1		1,1		1,1
Married	0.043 (0.040)	1.08–1.71	0.044 (0.038)	0.70–1.44	−0.001 (0.015)	0.70–2.96
Highest Education						
No education		1,1		1,1		1,1
Primary	0.075 (0.469)	1.09–1.84	0.024 (0.058)	0.98–1.15	−0.041 (0.024)	0.82–3.01
At least Secondary Education	0.171***(0.477)	1.53–2.80	0.094 (0.056)	1.01–2.75	0.011 (0.019)	1.12–2.84
Partner's Education						
No education		1,1		1,1		1,1
Primary	−0.067 (0.051)	1.06–1.87	0.108 (0.078)	2.13–3.08	0.043 (0.039)	1.88–2.76
At least secondary Education	−0.018 (0.045)	0.93–1.60	0.094 (0.068)	1.75–2.37	0.053 (0.034)	2.71–3.98
Frequency of listening to radio						
Not at all		1,1		1,1		1,1
Less than once a week	−0.019 (0.050)	0.98–1.66	−0.065 (0.054)	2.07–3.55	−0.007 (0.021)	0.63–2.75
At least once a week	0.102**(0.045)	1.40–2.26	−0.041 (0.052)	1.89–2.33	0.020 (0.018)	2.71–4.87
Ecological Zone						
Coastal		1,1		1,1		1,1
Savannah	0.086 (0.053)	0.85–1.65	−0.015 (0.071)	0.82–1.99	0.026 (0.023)	1.53–3.44
Forest	0.049 (0.043)	0.73–1.39	0.017 (0.040)	2.14–3.11	0.027*(0.013)	2.31–5.44
Occupation						
Not working		1,1		1,1		1,1
Working	0.047 (0.049)	0.90–1.60	0.070 (0.049)	1.78–2.56	0.021 (0.018)	2.55–4.21
Partner's occupation						
Primary		1,1		1,1		1,1
Secondary	0.048 (0.048)	0.86–1.60	−0.034 (0.043)	2.76–3.44	0.072 (0.040)	0.74–2.55
Tertiary	0.073 (0.056)	1.42–3.09	0.020 (0.057)	1.99–3.76	0.068 (0.041)	2.11–4.31
Water source						
Pipe		1,1		1,1		1,1
Others	−0.001 (0.119)	1.93–2.01	−0.081 (0.082)	2.12–3.71	−0.020 (0.014)	0.98–3.11
Contraceptive usage						
No modern contraceptive		1,1		1,1		1,1
Uses modern Contraceptive	0.022 (0.036)	1.18–1.87	0.009 (0.039)	1.53–2.76	−0.017 (0.015)	1.77–3.21
Birth order	0.018 (0.028)	0.78–1.98	0.025 (0.087)	2.33–3.81	0.038 (0.051)	0.84–3.22

Table 4 Logistic regression on place of delivery *(Continued)*

Healthcare decision making						
Alone		1,1		1,1		1,1
Not alone	0.025 (0.468)	2.54–2.98	−0.049 (0.047)	0.63–1.21	−0.016 (0.015)	2.01–4.72
Household purchase decision making						
Alone		1,1		1,1		1,1
Not alone	−0.023 (0.048)	1.53–2.07	0.087 (0.057)	0.74–1.52	0.015 (0.021)	0.82–2.60
Decision making on visits						
Alone		1,1		1,1		1,1
Not alone	0.004 (0.049)	1.32–1.96	−0.014 (0.053)	0.69–2.11	0.001 (0.015)	2.03–4.82
Shared toilet facility						
No		1,1		1,1		1,1
With other household only	0.010 (0.048)	0.77–1.01	0.038 (0.070)	0.52–1.74	−0.019 (0.015)	0.93–3.11
Public	0.045 (0.044)	0.98–1.23	0.013 (0.067)	1.55–3.02	−0.032 (0.016)	1.71–3.85
Hosmer and Lemeshow's Gof	9.9		13.5		7.3	

Co-efficient; standard error in bracket; 95% confidence interval *$p < 0.10$; **$p < 0.05$; ***$p < 0.001$

probable to deliver in health facilities than their counterparts without any formal education as indicated in Table 4. As compared with Coastal zone, women in the Savannah zone were less likely to deliver in health facilities (−2%, CI = 0.82–1.99) unlike Forest zone middle wealth status women (2%, CI = 2.14–3.11). Women who were working had 7% (CI = 1.78–2.56) higher likelihood of health facility delivery over non-working women.

Those who were not alone in terms of decision making about healthcare (−5%, CI = 0.63–1.21) and visits (−1%, CI = 0.69–2.11) were less probable to deliver in health facilities as compared to those taking those decisions alone (reference category). This points to the notion that in order for a woman be able to utilise health services, her decision making rights ought to be safe-guarded. However, women who were not deciding on household purchases alone were 9% more probable to deliver health facilities over those taking the decision alone. Again, as compared to those not sharing toilet facilities, women sharing with other households (4%, CI = 0.52–1.74) and those using public toilets (1%, CI = 1.55–3.02) were more inclined toward health facility delivery as shown in Table 4.

With regard to rich women, those subscribed to the NHIS were 5% (CI = 1.02–3.18) more likely to deliver in health facilities over those who were not subscribed and similar observation was made among rural residents (4%, CI = 1.60–5.92). At the same time, Christians were 3% (CI = 0.71–2.97) more probable to deliver in health facilities than other religious' affiliates. Whilst those with at least secondary education were likely to deliver in health facilities (1%, CI = 1.12–2.84), rich women with primary education were less probable to deliver in health facilities as compared to their counterparts without any formal education (−4%, CI = 0.82–3.01) as shown in Table 4. Rich women whose partners had

attained primary (4%, CI = 1.88–2.76) and at least secondary education (5%, CI = 2.71–3.98) were more likely to deliver in health facilities as compared to those whose partners had not been educated.

The study indicated that rich women who listened to radio at least once a week were 2% (CI = 2.71–4.87) more likely to deliver in health facilities over those who do not listen at all. Again, residents of Savannah (3%, CI = 1.53–3.44) and Forest zone (3%, CI = 2.31–5.44) more probable to deliver in health facilities than those in the Coastal zone. Working rich women were similarly more likely to deliver in health facilities than their non-working counterparts (2%, CI = 2.55–4.21) whilst those whose partners were engaged in secondary (7%, CI = 0.74–2.55) and tertiary occupation (7%, CI = 2.11–4.31) were more likely to deliver in health facilities over those whose partners were into primary occupation (reference category). Both rich women sharing toilet facility with other households (−2%, CI = 0.93–3.11) and using public toilet (−3%, CI = 1.71–3.85) were less likely to deliver in health facilities as compared with those who did not share as noted in Table 4. At 95% confidence interval, the three models fit reasonably well at probability values of 9.9%, 13.5% and 7.3% for the poor, middle and rich models respectively.

Discussion

This study was motivated by reported evidence of variation in maternal healthcare utilisation across wealth status driven by diverse factors [20, 21]. It is evident from the study that utilisation of health service is a function of NHIS subscription as also revealed by an earlier study in Ghana [26]. From the descriptive results, majority of the poor subscribed to insurance compared to the middle and the rich, perhaps the reason for this can be the observed group of the emerging "intervened poor" in Ghana where NGOs are aiding the poor especially in the savannah zone of the country. It was evident from the study that NHIS subscription was low among women in the middle wealth status. Though unexpected, it is not surprising because to subscribe or otherwise is purely a choice or decision to be made and it was evident that among poor, middle and the rich independence in decision making on healthcare, household purchase and visit was least among women in the middle wealth status. Consequently, this might account for the observed poor NHIS subscription among women with middle wealth status.

The study has revealed that rich women are more inclined toward both ANC visits and health facility delivery than poor women. Rich women might be more likely to have easy financial access of any health services of their choice and as such can easily utilise maternal health services unlike their poor counterparts. Although ANC is free in Ghana, cost of transportation can be a barrier to dissuade poor women from regularly attending ANC thereby possibly accounting for the relatively low maternal healthcare utilisation among them despite the fact that no much variation persisted with regard to NHIS subscription. The inclination of high wealth status toward maternal healthcare utilisation buttresses some earlier findings [4, 24] that enabling factors motivating healthcare utilisation constitutes one's wealth status just as also purported by the Behavioural Model [23].

The study has therefore pointed to the fact that in order for a woman to enjoy optimum access to maternal health services, she needs to be economically endowed. It is therefore not surprising for the high prevalence of maternal mortality to occur in developing countries where most women lack the economic capacity for accessing healthcare [1, 4]. Meanwhile obtaining better maternal healthcare assures desirable delivery outcomes which implies that as long as variation persist among the economically endowed and poor women, the latter will persistently fall prey to maternal induced complications.

Although poor women generally had lower utilisation of maternal health services, those subscribed to the NHIS were noted to have a relative higher access to ANC more than their unsubscribed counterparts. NHIS as cost cutting intervention has therefore proven be of extreme benefit in the quest to enhance maternal utilisation of healthcare especially among the poor. This indicates that NHIS serves as enabling factor irrespective of one's wealth status as posited by the Behavioural Model (BM) of healthcare utilisation.

Urban poor women were noted to have relatively high tendency of ANC attendance than their rural counterparts. This is not surprising considering the fact that most health facilities in Ghana are clustered in urban settings. Again this observation may fit into the contextual predisposing factors postulated by the BM as comprising demographic and social composition of communities having the capacity to induce healthcare utilisation [23, 24]. Considering pattern of distribution of health facilities in Ghana, urban women generally have a relative advantage over rural women and as such their geographical access to health facilities may be easier as compared to rural residents thereby contributing to this observation.

Poor married women were more probable to access ANC. Women in marital unions are more likely to enjoy social support manifesting in either accompaniment to ANC by one's partner or being reminded by the partner about ANC schedules. However, unmarried women will be lacking such social benefits and might thereby may be less motivated to access ANC especially when males who impregnated these women deny fathering the child. It has been similarly noted in Nepal that demographics such as being in a marital union is a source of social support that have higher inclination towards effective utilisation of health services [27].

Working poor women were having a higher tendency of utilising ANC as compared to non-working poor women. This finding may be as a result of relative higher exposure among working women arising from their frequent interaction with co-workers with whom they are more likely to discuss matter pertaining to their household arrangement and their health and wellbeing issues. As co-workers, they are likely to draw inspiration from each other; a social support that non-working women might lack. In this context, been employed or working will denote a motivating factor as inherent in the Behavioural Model.

Poor women whose partners had at least secondary education were noted to have higher ANC visits than those whose partners had no formal education. It is not surprising that such women have relatively high tendency to utilise ANC because education endows people to appreciate the essence of seeking healthcare at each stage of life and as such men with at least secondary education might urge their wives on the need to regularly access ANC without obstructing them. Juley-Anne [28] also found that educational attainment of both women and their partners is a major motivation for accessing health services and this was also earlier revealed [29].

Radio been one of the dominant mediums of mass media communication in Ghana was realised to have higher inclination toward ANC utilisation as poor women listening to radio at least once a week were 10% higher to utilise ANC than their counterparts who do not listen at all. This finding therefore highlights the instrumental role of mass media in shaping people's lives as posited earlier [30].

The study revealed that poor women who could not decide independently for their own healthcare were less likely to access ANC as compared to those who could decide on their own. However, those who could decide on matters pertaining to household purchases and visits had higher propensities of ANC utilisation. This indicates how women's autonomy feeds into critical spheres of their lives and therefore implies that autonomy of women is a prerequisite for enhancing their utilisation of healthcare services [31].

Among those in the middle wealth status category, on the contrary to what was found among poor women, urban residents were less probable to access ANC as compared with their rural counterparts. This might however originate from increasing job demands and overcrowding in urban settings as compared to rural areas. In one's quest to make ends meet within urban settings, women are more likely to postpone ANC in order to meet job schedules and deadlines. Meanwhile those who might desire to regularly seek the ANC service might be discouraged by the crowd they would have to compete with.

The study has revealed that utilisation of ANC is facilitated within the domains of poor and middle wealth status women's NHIS subscription, marriage, occupation as well as decision making autonomy with regard to owns' healthcare, household purchases and visits. Again, usage of modern contraceptives manifested in high inclination toward ANC utilisation among women in the middle wealth status stratum as also noted among poor folks.

Among rich women, although it was realised that those who had subscribed to the NHIS were highly inclined toward ANC, it was less as compared to subscribed poor women with high ANC utilisation. This indicates that interventions geared toward enhancement of maternal healthcare utilisation and combating adverse occurrences aligned with maternity must focus on poor women. This is because literature have continuously highlighted less utilisation of healthcare among poor women and even when they use, they usually access substandard care due to the element of cost [26, 32].

With regard to place of delivery, most factors that favoured ANC utilisation were noted to also favour health facility delivery across all wealth quintiles. This is an indication that motivating factors aligned with a specific maternal service utilisation might be a universal facilitator as far as maternal healthcare access is concerned. On the contrary, it implies that factors obstructing a specific maternal healthcare service use may obstruct utilisation of all maternal healthcare services.

Specifically, subscription to NHIS, marriage and educational attainment were all contributing factors towards health facility delivery among poor women. It can therefore be inferred that a woman's ability to deliver in

healthcare facility is hinged on numerous factors [33–35]. It was also noted that poor women residing in savannah and forest zones were more probable to deliver in health facilities. This might imply that enabling factors available to these women abound as purported by Anderson's Behavioural Model. Since women usually desire better health conditions for themselves and their children alike, they are more likely to utilise health facility for delivery purposes whenever an enabling environment avails itself [33] and as such manifesting in high utilisation of health facilities for delivery.

With rich women in context, they exhibited similar traits as their colleagues in the poor and middle wealth categories. This indicates that to a greater extent, obstructing and enabling factors surrounding maternal healthcare are near universal except few domains. However, the study has illustrated that as compared with rich women, cost saving interventions are much beneficial to the poor.

Limitations of the study

It is worthy to acknowledge that the study has some limitations. The study made use of cross sectional data and as such could not explore cause and effects of the findings observed. Also, the study was unable to investigate the motivation that urged women to attend ANC and also utilise health facilities for delivery due to the secondary data used. In spite of these, limitations the results present a credible reflection on the interaction between maternal healthcare utilisation and NHIS subscription and further offer practical measures that would aid to further improve maternal healthcare utilisation in the country.

Conclusions

With the aid of the Anderson's Behavioural Model (BM) of healthcare utilisation, this study has drawn attention to some key interventions worth instituting to accelerate maternal healthcare utilisation in the country. For instance, it has demonstrated the need for well-tailored maternal healthcare interventions such as offering motivation in terms of providing gifts to women who regularly attend ANC and those utilising health facilities for delivery. This is likely to boost maternal healthcare utilisation in the country and such interventions must target the poor and less privileged in society in order to further enhance maternal healthcare utilisation. It can be achieved through collaboration between the Ghana Health Service and other donor agencies committed to maternal and child health in the country such as Savanna Signatures and Care Net Ghana. There is also the need for the Reproductive and Child Health (RCH) unit of the Ghana Health Service to intensify mass media campaigns projecting the essence of ANC and delivery in health facilities since mass media (specifically radio and television) have proven to have higher inclination towards maternal healthcare utilisation. Again, female education must be targeted and promoted in order for them to ascend on the academic ladder since the study has revealed that highly educated women utilise maternal health services; that is having high tendency of attending ANC and utilising health facilities for delivery more than their uneducated counterparts.

Acknowledgement
The authors are most grateful to Measure DHS for making data accessible for the study.

Funding
No funding was obtained for the study.

Authors' contributions
EKA and REK conceived the study and carried out the analysis. FA prepared the background and theoretical framework. All authors substantially revised the manuscript for important intellectual content. All authors read and approved the final manuscript.

Competing interests
The authors declare that they have no competing interests.

Author details
[1]Department of Population and Health, Faculty of Social Sciences, University of Cape Coast, Cape Coast, Ghana. [2]Department of Economics, Faculty of Social Sciences, University of Cape Coast, Cape Coast, Ghana.

References
1. World Health Organization. Trends in maternal mortality: 1990 to 2010. WHO, UNICEF, UNFPA and The World Bank estimates. 2012. Available from http://www.unfpa.org/webdav/site/global/shared/documents/publications/2012/Trend_in_maternal_mortality_A4-1.pdf. Accessed on 18 Apr 2016
2. Leadership Council of the Sustainable Development Solutions Network. Indicators and a Monitoring Framework for the Sustainable Development Goals: Launching a data revolution for the SDGs. Geneva: United Nations; 2015.
3. Ir P, Horemans D, Souk N, Van DW. Using targeted vouchers and health equity funds to improve access to skilled birth attendants for poor women: a case study in three rural health districts in Cambodia. BMC Pregnancy Childbirth. 2010;10:1.
4. Chomat AM, Solomons NW, Montenegro G, Crowley C, Bermudez OI. Maternal health and health seeking behaviors among indigenous Mam mothers from Quetzaltenango, Guatemala. Rev Panam Salud Publica. 2014;35(2):113–20.
5. U.S. Agency for International Development (USAID). Ending Preventable Maternal Mortality. Washington: USAID Maternal Health Vision for Action; 2014.
6. World Bank. Maternal Mortality Ratio (modelled estimate, per 100,000 live births). 2016. Retrieved from http://data.worldbank.org/indicator/SH.STA.MMRT on 19th April, 2016.
7. Marmot M. The Influence of Income on Health: Views of an Epidemiologist. Health Aff. 2002;21(2):31–46.
8. Gonzalez R, Requejo JH, Nien JK, Merialdi M, Bustreo F, Betran AP. Tackling Health Inequities in Chile: Maternal, Newborn, Infant, and Child Mortality between 1990 and 2004. Am J Public Health. 2009;99:1220–6.
9. Arthur E. Wealth and antenatal care use: implications for maternal healthcare utilisation in Ghana. Heal Econ Rev. 2012;2:14.
10. WHO & UNICEF. Antenatal care in developing countries: promises achievements and missed opportunities. An analysis of trends, levels and differentials, 1990–2001. Geneva: Center for Communication Programs; 2003.
11. Mensah J, Oppong JR, Schmidt CM. Ghana's national health insurance scheme in the context of the health MDGs: An empirical evaluation using propensity score matching. Health Econ. 2010;19:95–106.
12. Hong R, Ayad M, Ngabo F. Being Insured Improves Safe Delivery Practices in Rwanda. J Community Health. 2011;36(5):779–84.
13. Dong H. Book Review: The Impact of Health Insurance in Low- and Middle-Income Countries, edited by C.C. Griffin, M.L. Escobar, and R.P. Shaw, Washington DC, USA: The Brookings Institution Press. J Int Dev. 2012;24(4):529–30.
14. Giedion U, Alfonso EA, Diaz BY. The Impact of Universal Coverage Schemes in the Developing Countries. Washington: The World Bank; 2013.
15. Owoo SN, Lambon-Quayefio PM. National Health Insurance, Social Influence and Antenatal Care use in Ghana. Heal Econ Rev. 2013;3:19.
16. Bosomprah S, Ragno PL, Gros C, Banskota H. Health Insurance and Maternal, Newborn services utilisation and under-five mortality. Archives of Public Health. 2015;73:51.
17. Agyare-Kwabi P. Policy Brief: Gender, Social Inclusion and Health in Ghana. Star Ghana: UKaid, USAID & DANIDA; 2013.
18. Kumi-Kyereme A, Amo-Adjei J. Effects of spatial location and household wealth on health insurance subscription among women in Ghana. BMC Health Serv Res. 2013;13:221.
19. Amu H, Dickson KS. Health insurance subscription among women in reproductive age in Ghana: do socio-demographics matter? Heal Econ Rev. 2016;6:24.
20. Lindelow M. The utilisation of curative healthcare in Mozambique: does income matter? J Afr Econ. 2016;14(3):435–82.
21. Amin R, Shah NM, Becker S. Socioeconomic factors differentiating maternal and child health-seeking behaviour in rural Bangladesh: A cross-sectional analysis. Int J Equity Health. 2010;9:9.
22. Andersen R, Newman JF. Societal and individual determinants of medical care utilization in the United States. Milbank Mem Fund Q Health Soc. 1973; 51(1):95–124.
23. Andersen RM. National health surveys and the behavioral model of health services use. Med Care. 2008;46(7):647–53.
24. Babitsch B, Gohl D, Von Lengerke T. Re-revisiting Andersen's Behavioral Model of Health Services Use: A systematic review of studies from 1998 to 2011. GMS Psycho-Social-Medicine. 2012;9:1–15.
25. Ghana Statistical Service (GSS), Ghana Health Service (GHS), and ICF International. Ghana Demographic and Health Survey 2014. Rockville: GSS, 395 GHS and ICF International; 2015.
26. Bonfrer I, Breebaart L, Van de Poel E. The Effects of Ghana's National Health Insurance Scheme on Maternal and Infant Health Care Utilization. PLoS ONE. 2016;11:11.
27. Sharma RS, Poudyal AK, Devkota BM, Singh S. Factors associated with place of delivery in rural Nepal. BMC Public Health. 2014;14:306.
28. Juley-Anne BM. Factors influencing delivery practices among pregnant women in Kenya: A Case of Wareng' District in Uasin Gishu County, Kenya. Int J Innov Sci Res. 2014;10(1):50–8.
29. Gabrysch S, Campbell O. Still too far to walk: literature review of the determinants of delivery service use. BMC Pregnancy Childbirth. 2009;9:34.
30. Navaneetham K, Dharmalingam A. Utilization of Maternal Healthcare Services in South India. Paper presented in faculty seminar at the Centre for Development Studies. Kerala: Thiruvananthapuram; 2000.
31. Dangal G, Bhandari TR. Women's autonomy: new paradigm in maternal healthcare utilization. GJMEDPH. 2014;3:5.
32. Dixon J, Tenkorang EY, Luginaah IN, Kuuire VZ, Boateng GO. National health insurance scheme enrolment and antenatal care among women in Ghana: Is there any relationship? Trop Med Int Health. 2014;19(1):98–106.
33. Adegoke A, Utz B, Msuya SE, et al. Skilled birth attendants: who is who? A descriptive study of definitions and roles from nine sub-Saharan African countries. PLoS ONE. 2012;7:e40220.
34. Sakeah E, Doctor H, McCloskey L, Bernstein J, Yeboah-Antwi K, Mills S. Using the community-based health planning and services program to promote skilled delivery in rural Ghana: socio-demographic factors that influence women utilization of skilled attendants at birth in Northern Ghana. BMC Public Health. 2014;14:344.
35. Amoakoh-Coleman M, Ansah EK, Agyepong IA, et al. Predictors of skilled attendance at delivery among antenatal clinic attendants in Ghana: a cross-sectional study of population data. BMJ Open. 2015;5: e007810.

16

Assessing the impact of state "opt-out" policy on access to and costs of surgeries and other procedures requiring anesthesia services

John E. Schneider[1], Robert Ohsfeldt[2], Pengxiang Li[3], Thomas R. Miller[4] and Cara Scheibling[5*]

Abstract

In 2001, the U.S. government released a rule that allowed states to "opt-out" of the federal requirement that a physician supervise the administration of anesthesia by a nurse anesthetist. To date, 17 states have opted out. The majority of the opt-out states cited increased access to anesthesia care as the primary rationale for their decision. In this study, we assess the impact of state opt-out policy on access to and costs of surgeries and other procedures requiring anesthesia services. Our null hypothesis is that opt-out rule adoption had little or no effect on surgery access or costs. We estimate an inpatient model of surgeries and costs and an outpatient model of surgeries. Each model uses data from multiple years of U.S. inpatient hospital discharges and outpatient surgeries. For inpatient cost models, the coefficient of the opt-out variable was consistently positive and also statistically significant in most model specifications. In terms of access to inpatient surgical care, the opt-out rules did not increase or decrease access in opt-out states. The results for the outpatient access models are less consistent, with some model specifications indicating a reduction in access associated with opt-out status, while other model specifications suggesting no discernable change in access. Given the sensitivity of model findings to changes in model specification, the results do not provide support for the belief that opt-out policy improves access to outpatient surgical care, and may even reduce access to outpatient surgical care (among freestanding facilities).

Background

In 2001, the U.S. federal government released a rule that allowed states to "opt-out" of the federal requirement that a physician supervise the administration of anesthesia by a nurse anesthetist. The "November 13" rule was effective upon publication in the November 13, 2001 *Federal Register*. [1] For a state to opt-out of the federal supervision requirement, the state's governor must send a letter of attestation to the Centers for Medicare and Medicaid Services [1]. The letter must attest that: 1) the state's governor has consulted with the state's boards of medicine and nursing about issues related to access to and the quality of anesthesia services in the state; 2) it is in the best interests of the state's citizens to opt-out of the current federal physician supervision requirement; and 3) the opt-out is consistent with state law.

To date, as shown in Appendix Table 6, 17 states have opted out. [2] The majority of the opt-out states cited increased access to anesthesia care as the primary rationale for their decision. [2] Collectively, in 2015 these states had about 73 million residents, or about 23% of the total resident population of the United States. [3] The majority of the opt-out states were sparsely populated states (e.g., Iowa, North Dakota, and Montana), with the notable exception of California, which nonetheless includes large rural areas interior to the heavily populated Pacific coast.

Following the implementation of the November 13 rule, the U.S. Agency for Healthcare Research and Quality (AHRQ) was charged with assessing whether anesthesia outcomes differed between opt-out states and other states.

* Correspondence: Cara.scheibling@avalonecon.com
[5]Avalon Health Economics, 26 Washington Street, 3rd Fl., 07960 Morristown, NJ, USA

The study analyzed Medicare data for 1999 through 2005, and found no evidence that opting out of the oversight requirement resulted in increased inpatient deaths or complications. [4] Similarly, a recent Cochrane review concluded there was insufficient evidence to conclude whether quality of anesthesia care differed across nurse and physician anesthesiologists [5]. However, among the stated goals of the opt-out rule was to improve access to anesthesia care and control growth in its costs. [6] At the time of the rule, there was a potential shortage of anesthesiologists, at least in some regions and states. [7] The presumption was that allowing nurse anesthetist to practice without physician supervision would alleviate these shortages and thus enhance access to anesthesia care. The lower professional service costs for nurse anesthetist practicing without physician supervision also was presumed to lower anesthesia care costs.

Despite the importance of the presumed cost and access benefits of the opt-out rule, to date few studies have attempted to quantify changes in access and costs attributable to the opt-out rules. Sun et al. [8] utilize data from the National Inpatient Sample (NIS) to assess whether opt-out was associated with an increase in the percentage of patients receiving a therapeutic procedure among patients admitted for appendicitis, bowel obstruction, choledocholithiasis, or hip fracture. In a similar vein, using claims data for Medicare fee-for-service enrollees, Sun et al. [9] examine differences in average anesthesia utilization rates three years before and after out-out for opt-out states grouped by year of opt-out, compared to differences in average anesthesia utilization rates over the same time period in non-opt-out states. Both studies conclude the adoption of the opt-out rule had no significant impact on access to anesthesia care.

In this study, we extend the literature on the impact of state opt-out policy by adding an assessment of its impact on costs of surgeries, and by assessing its impact on a wider variety of procedures requiring anesthesia services than in prior studies. Our hypothesis is that opt-out states exhibited changes in access to surgery and changes in surgery costs similar to non-opt-out states; that is, that the opt-out laws had little or no effect on surgery access or costs. We estimate models of inpatient surgery costs and surgery volume, as well as a model for volume of outpatient surgeries. Each model uses data from multiple years of U.S. inpatient hospital discharges and outpatient surgeries. Our results indicate that the opt-out policy is associated with higher inpatient surgery costs, with little or no impact on access for either inpatient or outpatient surgery.

Methods
We used two data sources that were appropriate for the study objectives. There has been continuous growth in outpatient surgery both in years before and years after passage of the opt-out law. [9] Thus, we believe that it is important to examine access and cost associated with inpatient *and* outpatient surgery. We used the Nationwide Inpatient Sample (NIS) for analysis of changes in inpatient surgery volume. The NIS is part of the Healthcare Cost and Utilization Project (HCUP), and is the largest publicly available all-payer inpatient health care database in the United States, yielding national estimates of hospital inpatient stays (https://www.hcup-us.ahrq.gov/nisoverview.jsp#data). Unweighted, the NIS contains data from more than 7 million hospital stays each year. Weighted, it estimates (or represents) more than 36 million hospitalizations nationally (around 20%). With more than 20 years of data, the NIS is ideal for longitudinal analyses.

However, the database has undergone changes over time, including the sampling and weighting strategy used. Beginning in 2012, sampling strategy for NIS was redesigned from formerly a random sample of hospitals and retaining all discharges from those sampled hospitals to a random sample of discharges from all hospitals participating in HCUP. To remove inconsistency due to change of sampling strategy, we did not include NIS data for hospitalizations after 2011. Thus, our NIS sample covers a 14-year time frame from 1998 to 2011 which allows for several years before and after the opt-out decisions by states. The unit of observation is "facility-year."

For outpatient surgery, we used the State Ambulatory Surgery and Services Databases (SASD). The SASD is also part of the HCUP system (https://www.hcup-us.ahrq.gov/sasdoverview.jsp). The SASD include encounter-level data for ambulatory surgeries and "may also include various types of outpatient services such as observation stays, lithotripsy, radiation therapy, imaging, chemotherapy, and labor and delivery." The specific types of ambulatory surgery and outpatient services included in the SASD vary by state and data year. SASD include data from hospital-owned ambulatory surgery facilities and nonhospital-owned facilities.

For the outpatient analysis, we included three opt-out states (California, Colorado, and Kentucky) and three non-opt-out states (Florida, Maryland, and New Jersey). These states were selected based on two criteria: [1] the state-level SASD contain all of the data we will need to estimate the models (e.g., procedure codes); and [2] the state SASD data contain the sufficient pre- and post-opt-out years. The unit of observation for the outpatient analysis is also the "facility-year."

Our outcomes include measures of access and cost. The access measures were the number of all inpatient and outpatient surgeries.[1] The cost measure was average cost per surgical inpatient stay, calculated by using hospital cost-to-charge ratios to deflate total charges per stay reported in the NIS. Nominal cost estimates were converted to constant 2011 dollars using the "Hospital and related services" component of the Consumer Price Index (http://www.bls.gov/cpi/). No cost-to-charge ratio estimates are available for the outpatient facilities in the SASD, and as a result, no average cost estimates are available for outpatient procedures.

A quasi-experimental study design was used to study the change in outcomes (access and costs) in "treatment" facilities (those located in opt-out states) before and after opt-out policy implementation, compared to facilities located in non-opt-out states over the same time period. The statistical analysis was based on panel data facility-level fixed-effect model which examined how the change of opt-out status affected changes in outcomes while removing facility-level time-invariant unmeasured confounders. We used robust standard error estimation adjusting for state level clustering. The null hypothesis is that opt-out states exhibited changes in access to surgery and changes in surgery costs similar to non-opt-out states; that is, that the opt-out laws had little or no effect on surgery access or costs.

The base statistical model of access is written as:

$$D_{it} = \alpha + \beta_1 OPT_{it} + \beta_n X_{it} + \beta_n T_t + U_i + \varepsilon_{it}$$

The unit of observation in the NIS is the discharge, and in the SASD is the procedure. In this equation, the dependent variable D_{it} refers to access (total number of surgeries) or cost (mean cost per surgery) for facility i in year t. The key right-hand side variable of interest is a dummy variable OPT_{it} indicating whether the facility is located in an opt-out state (OPT equal to 1 if the facility was located in an opt-out state and 0 otherwise) in year t (For example, CA adopted opt-out in 2009; thus $OPT_{it} = 0$ before 2009 and $OPT_{it} = 1$ since 2009 for CA). For a control state like FL, $OPT_{it} = 0$ during all the observed years [see Appendix Table 6]). X_{it} represents a vector of covariates likely to affect access or cost.

In the inpatient models, X_{it} includes facility characteristics (bed size[2] of hospital: [1] small, [2] medium, [3] large; control/ownership of hospital: (0) government or private, collapsed category, [1] government, nonfederal, public, [2] private, non-profit, voluntary, [3] private, invest-own, [4] private, collapsed category; rural or urban hospital; and teaching or non-teaching hospital).[3] The inpatient models also adjust for lagged (year t-1) facility-level patient summary measures, including the total number of hospitalizations, patient case mix (i.e. percentage of cases were female, mean length of stay, percentage of surgical cases, the mean of the Centers for

Medicare & Medicaid Services Hierarchical Condition Category (CMS-HCC) risk score [9], age distribution [<18, 18 to 44, 45 to 64, 65 to 74, and 75 or older]), admission type [elective, emergency, or other], percentage of routine discharge hospitalizations, health insurance type [Medicare, Medicaid, private insurance, or others], and race [white, black, Hispanic, or others]). CMS-HCC risk adjustment was developed by CMS to produce a health-based measure of future medical need which has shown to be a significant predictor of medical costs and has a better predictive accuracy on mortality than the Charlson and Elixhauser methods [10]. A Herfindahl-Hirschman Index (HHI), with the market definition based on area patient flows,[4] was used to adjust for area hospital market concentration. County-level variables potentially affecting access or cost also were included (i.e. total number of residents in the county, percentage of the population in poverty, percentage of the population who are Medicare beneficiaries, percentage of people between age 16 and 64, the unemployment rate, per capita income, and the number of anesthesiologists [MD/DO] per 10,000 residents).[5] The remaining variables are dummy variables for time (T). Ui is facility-level time-invariant unmeasured variable. The error term is indicated as ε_{it}.

Many of the variables available in the NIS included in the inpatient models were not available in the SASD. In the multiple regression models focusing on outpatient surgery, we used all model covariates available in the SASD. The data do not allow identification of the county location of freestanding outpatient facilities. Thus, the outpatient models focusing on the sample of all outpatient facilities account for lagged (year t-1) factors (patient flow, risk score, disposition status, and payment source variables), and a dummy variable for freestanding outpatient facilities (vs. hospital outpatient surgery departments). We addressed the differences (and changes) in access in rural versus urban areas by including an interaction terms of urban/rural indicator and opt-out indicator in the multiple regression models. Alternative models examine dependent variables measured in natural units and log transformations.

We conducted extensive sensitivity analysis to check the robustness of our findings. First, for the NIS, we examined using alternative definitions of access: 1) Removing cases age less than 18 out of total surgical discharges; 2) Removing all transplant Diagnosis-Related Groups (DRGs) and any craniotomy DRGs; and 3) limiting discharges to only hip and knee surgery procedures (DRG 209, 471, 503, 544, 471, or 545) and mean cost per discharge based on the definition. Because many pediatric procedures are performed in children's hospitals where anesthesiologists provide solo care or are part of care team, and given that children are a unique population (with parents making health care decisions), the impact opt-out may be different from the impact on the adult population. Likewise, transplants and craniotomy represent very complex cases where, given current practice patterns, a low percentage of nurse anesthetists would be able to practice without physician supervision for those procedures. Hips and knees were examined separately because they represent a group of very common and fast growing procedures which are often performed in community hospitals.

Second, we examined robustness of our finding by varying covariates included in the models. In the SASD, we estimate separate models by freestanding status, a model focusing on the volume of specific outpatient procedures likely to require general anesthesia, and a model excluding the lagged patient flow variables. To examine whether early opt out have a different impact on outcomes compared to late opt out states, we conducted a set of sensitivity analyses in NIS sample. We repeated the analysis among early opt out states [states with opt out between 2001 and 2005 (i.e., IA, MN, NE, NH, NM, AK, KS, ND, OR, WA, MT, SD, WI) compared with non-opt out states during the period, and late opt out states (states with opt out between 2009 and 2011 (i.e., CA and CO) compared with non-opt out states during the period; in the whole NIS sample, we also ran another model by including opt-out variable (equal 1 after the opt out states opt out) and late opt-out indicator (equal to 1 for CA and CO during the whole study period, 1998 to 2011; equal to zero for other states)]. The coefficients of interaction terms show the differentiated impact of opt-out for late opt-out states comparing to early opt-out states.

Results

The final analytic files included 13,573 facility-year observations in the NIS sample and 9,994 facility-year observations in the SASD sample. Descriptive data for the main outcomes associated with the inpatient file (NIS) and outpatient file(SASD) are shown in Appendix Tables 7 and 8. The results for the inpatient cost models are shown in Table 1. When cost per discharge was the dependent variable, the estimated coefficient of the opt-out variable was positive and statistically significant ($p < 0.01$). The point estimate indicates that the cost per discharge was $1,815 higher in opt-out states relative to non-opt-out states. Similarly, in the log cost models, the estimated coefficient of the opt-out variable was positive and statistically significant. The point estimate indicates that the cost per discharge was about 8.7% higher in opt-out states relative to non-opt-out states.[6]

For the inpatient access models (Table 2), the opt-out variable coefficient was positive but not statistically significant in the model with the number of hospital

discharges as the dependent variable. The magnitude of the point estimate implies an increase in surgical discharges that is small in magnitude – about 40 annually, or about 1.8% (based on the sample mean). Similarly, in the model that used the log of discharges as the dependent variable, the estimated coefficient of the opt-out variable is positive but not statistically significant.

The results for the outpatient access models are shown in Table 3. In the model where the number of surgical procedures is the dependent variable, the estimated coefficient of the opt-out variable was positive but not statistically significant. When the dependent variable is defined as the log of procedures, the estimated coefficient of the opt-out was also positive but not statistically significant.

To assess the robustness of our inpatient model findings, we estimated a number of models with different definitions of "surgical" discharges or different sets of covariates included in the model, as reported in Table 4. Neither early nor late opt-out states had a statistically significant impact on volumes. However, hospitals in late opt-out states (i.e. CA and CO) had a higher cost increase after state opt-out compared to hospitals in early opt-out states. When pediatric surgical discharges were removed from the facility-level total number of annual surgical discharges, the estimates of the opt-out variable coefficient remained positive but not statistically significant, in both the linear and log models. Similarly, when discharges for transplants and any craniotomy DRGs were removed from the total, or when only hip and knee procedure discharges were included, the estimates of the opt-out variable coefficient remained positive but not statistically significant in all models. In addition, dropping groups of covariates from the model specification did not materially alter the results, with one exception. In models that excluded all hospital characteristics, lagged patient flow variables, and county level variables, the estimated opt-out coefficients were negative, and statistically significant ($p < 0.05$) when the dependent variable was the number of surgical discharges.

In the alternative cost models, when all pediatric surgical discharges were removed, or all discharges for transplants and any craniotomy DRGs were removed, the coefficient of the opt-out variable was consistently positive and statistically significant. When only hip and knee procedure discharges were included, the estimated opt-out coefficient was positive but not statistically significant. Similarly, when groups of covariates were dropped from the model specification, the coefficient of the opt-out variable remained consistently positive and statistically significant. Point estimates suggest costs per discharge were about

Table 1 Inpatient Cost Models, Linear and Log Linear

	Mean costs per surgical case		Log Mean costs per surgical case	
	b	t	b	t
Opt out	1815.33***	3.76	0.08*	2.43
Rural hospital	−584.32	−0.51	0.01	0.19
Hospital bed size				
Small (reference)				
Medium	85.99	0.13	−0.03	−0.68
Large	−1037.20	−1.45	−0.10	−1.83
Control/ownership of hospital				
Government or private, collapsed category (reference)				
Government, nonfederal, public,	1403.23	0.99	−0.04	−0.93
Private, non-profit, voluntary	1448.21	0.99	−0.15**	−2.85
Private, invest-own	1770.03	1.11	−0.01	−0.19
Private, collapsed category	3400.20	1.96	0.01	0.17
Teaching hospital	1648.59	1.22	−0.04	−1.30
Hospital HHI based on patient flow	11802.96	1.73	−0.26	−0.56
Lagged (year t-1) facility-level patient summary measures				
Total number of hospitalizations	−0.05	−0.54	−0.00	−0.44
Percentage of cases were female	−2308.72	−0.24	−0.71	−0.93
Mean length of stay	426.60	1.21	0.03	1.11
Percentage of surgical cases	14348.88	1.75	0.54	1.33
Mean (CMS-HCC) risk score	−438.02	−0.16	−0.27	−1.16
Age distribution (%)				
<18	7003.33	0.63	0.96	0.86
18_44 (reference)				
45_64	11426.77	0.91	0.18	0.20
65_74	9031.06	0.47	1.42	1.13
75 or older	8585.06	0.56	0.91	0.86
Admission type (%)				
Elective (reference)				
Emergency	−993.71	−0.50	−0.08	−0.52
Other	1733.18	0.84	0.20	1.85
Percentage of routine discharge hospitalizations	−4511.40	−0.85	−0.47	−1.35
Health insurance type (%)				
Private insurance (reference)				
Medicare	−2590.06	−0.56	−0.15	−0.42
Medicaid	−289.20	−0.06	−0.02	−0.09
Others	559.90	0.21	0.07	0.35
Race (%)				
White (reference)				
Black	5323.13	0.76	−0.11	−0.24
Hispanic	−7994.42	−1.27	−0.38	−1.04
Other	−2340.99	−1.35	−0.19	−1.63

Table 1 Inpatient Cost Models, Linear and Log Linear *(Continued)*

County-level variable				
Total number of residents in the county	0.00	0.77	0.00	0.68
Percentage of people in poverty	42.77	0.38	0.01	0.75
Percentage of people are Medicare beneficiaries	−12526.56	−0.50	−2.32	−1.27
Percentage of people between age 16 to 64	−7064.95	−0.77	−0.31	−0.65
Unemployment rate	1553.06	0.12	−0.73	−0.93
Per capita income	0.10	1.06	0.00	1.63
Number of anesthesiologists [MD/DO] per 10,000 residents	−784.20	−1.39	−0.06	−1.41
Year dummy variables				
2001.year (reference)				
2002.year	466.64	1.66	0.14***	6.16
2003.year	1176.08**	3.62	0.26***	9.19
2004.year	1993.96***	4.18	0.36***	11.54
2005.year	2942.80***	5.06	0.48***	9.88
2006.year	4007.31***	5.60	0.57***	9.93
2007.year	5322.09***	5.76	0.69***	9.80
2008.year	6344.88***	5.84	0.79***	10.12
2009.year	7524.34***	6.37	0.92***	10.61
2010.year	9554.10***	6.17	1.06***	9.39
2011.year	10332.97***	5.79	1.13***	9.21
Constant	−2772.51	−0.16	9.06***	6.87
N	1,339		1,339	
R-squared (within)	0.7226		0.7946	

Notes: [1] t-statistics in parentheses; *p < 0.05; **p < 0.01; ***p < 0.001; [2] Some hospital-year do not have cost-to-charge ratios; therefore, cost measure was not available; [3] interaction term between opt-out and rural hospital status was not statistically significant; therefore, main models do not include interaction terms; [4] Costs were in 2011 dollar adjusted by hospital and related services CPI

$1,760 to $1,980 higher (in the linear models), or about 6.6 to 8.8% higher (in log models), for facilities in opt-out states compared to non-opt-out states.

Several alternative specifications of the outpatient access model were estimated, as summarized in Table 5. In model specifications focusing on freestanding facilities, the estimated coefficient of the opt-out variable is negative and statistically significant, in both the linear and log models. This implies that the opt-out policy reduced the volume of procedures at freestanding outpatient facilities by about 310 procedures, or by about 23%. In the model limited to non-freestanding facilities, the estimated coefficient of the opt-out variable was positive but not statistically significant. When the analysis focused on selected procedures likely to require general anesthesia, the estimated coefficient of the opt-out variable was negative but not statistically significant. Finally, in model specifications dropping groups of covariates, the opt-out coefficient estimates remain positive but not statistically significant.

Discussion

The primary intent of the opt-out laws was to increase access to anesthesia services by increasing the scope of practice of NAs and reducing the barriers to use of NAs. In turn, the hypothesis is that the reduction in barriers will increase access to surgical care. In our study, we do not find evidence to support this belief. In addition to the regression results presented in Tables 1, 2 and 3, we estimated a large number of variations of these base models (Tables 4 and 5).

Overall, the results consistently show no improvement in access to inpatient surgical care associated with the opt-out indicator. In other words, opt out was not associated with increase (or decrease) in access; the opt-out rules had no measurable effect on access. Interestingly, states choosing to opt out were associated with subsequent higher costs per inpatient —about $1,800 higher per surgery, or about 8.7%.

On the surface, the inpatient cost result seems counterintuitive, as opt-out provisions in theory allow lower-priced nurse anesthetists to perform the same services

Table 2 Inpatient Access Models, Linear and Log Linear

	Total number of surgical discharges		Log Total number of surgical discharges	
	b	t	b	t
Opt out	39.78	0.62	0.05	1.08
Rural hospital	−78.00	−0.87	0.05	0.35
Hospital bed size				
Small (reference)				
Medium	20.62	0.77	−0.01	−0.49
Large	226.72	1.39	0.06	1.24
Control/ownership of hospital				
Government or private, collapsed category (reference)				
Government, nonfederal, public,	−151.78	−0.86	0.20	0.53
Private, non-profit, voluntary	112.93	0.69	−0.03	−0.09
Private, invest-own	104.25	1.05	0.27	0.87
Private, collapsed category	15.87	0.10	0.01	0.05
Teaching hospital	75.87	1.12	0.05	0.39
Hospital HHI based on patient flow	254.90	0.61	0.85*	2.15
Lagged (year t-1) facility-level patient summary measures				
Total number of hospitalizations	0.16***	12.43	0.00***	9.02
Percentage of cases were female	−409.79	−0.69	−0.23	−0.21
Mean length of stay	3.98	0.37	0.00	0.01
Percentage of surgical cases	2580.39***	5.43	3.99***	4.46
Mean (CMS-HCC) risk score	−51.14	−0.34	−0.55	−1.55
Age distribution (%)				
<18	293.78	0.49	2.70	1.83
18_44 (reference)				
45_64	−185.31	−0.24	2.07	1.49
65_74	597.26	1.22	2.28	1.81
75 or older	483.46	0.92	0.34	0.31
Admission type (%)				
Elective (reference)				
Emergency	−46.15	−0.40	0.21	1.04
Other	124.02	1.27	0.08	0.49
Percentage of routine discharge hospitalizations	−330.91	−1.27	−0.23	−0.58
Health insurance type (%)				
Private insurance (reference)				
Medicare	−106.02	−0.28	0.23	0.54
Medicaid	163.72	0.61	0.50	1.23
Others	−29.26	−0.14	0.15	0.57
Race (%)				
White (reference)				
Black	−2054.46*	−2.62	−0.21	−0.32
Hispanic	154.64	0.42	0.23	0.40
Other	−168.06*	−2.14	−0.07	−0.79

Table 2 Inpatient Access Models, Linear and Log Linear *(Continued)*

County-level variable				
Total number of residents in the county	−0.00	−0.17	−0.00	−1.24
Percentage of people in poverty	−2.75	−0.31	0.00	0.23
Percentage of people are Medicare beneficiaries	−258.94	−0.24	−1.00	−0.87
Percentage of people between age 16 to 64	−285.91	−0.70	−1.23	−2.03
Unemployment rate	−81.65	−0.07	−4.55*	−2.79
Per capita income	0.01	1.14	0.00	2.03
Number of anesthesiologists [MD/DO] per 10,000 residents	231.51	2.04	−0.02	−0.29
Year dummy variables				
1999.year (reference)	0.00	.	0.00	.
2000.year	78.70*	2.58	−0.01	−0.45
2001.year	90.38*	2.27	0.01	0.22
2002.year	70.76	1.02	0.07	1.33
2003.year	81.98	1.21	0.07	0.85
2004.year	141.51	1.88	−0.01	−0.12
2005.year	122.69	1.53	−0.08	−0.75
2006.year	−2.13	−0.03	−0.15	−1.38
2007.year	44.26	0.49	−0.19	−1.84
2008.year	59.28	0.45	−0.15	−1.14
2009.year	−4.30	−0.03	0.02	0.10
2010.year	−55.14	−0.29	0.01	0.07
2011.year	−183.95	−0.97	−0.06	−0.29
Constant	295.62	0.55	4.94**	3.37
N	2063		2063	
R-squared (within)	0.4010		0.2019	

Notes: [1] t-statistics in parentheses; *p < 0.05; **p < 0.01; ***p < 0.001; [2] Some hospital-year do not have cost-to-charge ratios; therefore, cost measure was not available; [3] interaction term between opt-out and rural hospital status was not statistically significant; therefore, main models do not include interaction terms

as physician anesthesiologists. However, as some recent research has shown, nurse anesthetists take longer to perform the same services. [11] As a result, despite the lower payment per unit for nurse anesthetists, the greater number of units provided may translate into higher anesthesia costs overall. Moreover, recent research suggests that surgery procedures with nurse anesthesia providers working without physician supervision have worse surgery outcomes in terms of complications requiring additional treatment. [6–8] Clearly, surgical procedures with these complications are likely to entail higher overall costs than procedures without complications. [9] Thus, the observed higher costs in opt-out states could be a result of the combined effects of these two issues.

The results for the outpatient access models are less consistent, with some model specifications indicating a reduction in access associated with opt-out status, while other model specifications suggesting no discernable change in access. It is possible that the limited number

of states included in the analysis contributed to this inconsistency. Given the sensitivity of model findings to changes in model specification, the results do not provide support for the belief that opt-out policy improves access to outpatient surgical care, and may even reduce access to outpatient surgical care (among freestanding facilities).

There are some important limitations to this study. First, this is an observational study where states chose to opt out; opt-out was nota random event. There are potential unmeasured confounders associated with opt-out and outcomes. The analytic approach we used eliminates the impact of any unobservables across states that are time-invariant, but does not account for the potential impact of time-varying unobservables. It is possible that the association between opt-out status and higher surgical costs results from differences between opt-out and non-out-out states not accounted for in our analysis. Second, some opt-out states declared opt-out status toward the end of

Table 3 Outpatient Access Linear and Log Models

	Total number of surgical procedures (w/o county variables)		Log of total number of surgical procedures (w/o county variables)	
	b	t	b	t
Opt out	1149.18	1.06	0.06	0.71
Lagged (year t-1) facility-level patient summary measures				
Percentage of female	10380.26	1.28	0.11	0.69
Mean (CMS-HCC) risk score	9003.39	2.17	0.24	1.45
Age distribution (%)				
<18	5126.30	0.48	0.04	0.06
18_44 (reference)				
45_64	8195.99	0.84	0.52	1.18
65_74	−29766.70	−0.86	−0.46	−1.31
75 or older	−13872.42	−1.10	0.76	1.26
Percentage of routine discharge hospitalizations	2073.23	0.52	−0.08	−0.67
Health insurance type (%)				
Private insurance				
Medicare	−1380.08	−0.68	−0.25	−1.79
Medicaid	−10119.71	−0.93	−0.27	−1.04
Others	−10856.39	−1.07	−0.46**	−5.48
Freestanding	−1043.54	−1.04	−0.08	−1.56
Year dummy variables				
1999.year (reference)				
2000.year	−16.36	−0.05	0.05***	11.74
2001.year	−923.90	−1.34	0.02*	3.63
2002.year	−876.51	−1.00	0.09***	9.77
2003.year	7386.10**	4.19	0.61***	21.00
2004.year	9061.60***	16.62	0.76***	36.50
2005.year	10213.33***	20.49	0.79***	41.31
2006.year	11373.59***	22.15	0.84***	43.80
2007.year	32466.04***	59.07	1.58***	78.96
2008.year	63228.57***	202.11	2.26***	73.62
2009.year	62817.03***	271.86	2.18***	207.52
2010.year	62829.63***	143.72	2.15***	162.03
2011.year	62947.40***	89.87	2.12***	91.22
2012.year	63165.88***	57.08	2.14***	74.13
2013.year	64712.58***	27.96	2.21***	17.61
Constant	−57093.83***	−15.05	5.98***	18.56
N	7856		7856	
Squared (within)	0.3581		0.4638	

Note: *$p < 0.05$; **$p < 0.01$; ***$p < 0.001$

the timeline of available data, thereby providing a small number of years post opt-out years for the facility fixed-effects panel models. However, accounting for early vs. late opt-out status indicated later opt-out status was associated with greater increase in cost that the cost increase in early opt-out states, relative to non-opt-out states, but did not alter the finding of no significant improvement in access associated with opt-out. In addition, NIS randomly selected a 20% random sample of national hospitals during out study period. Some hospitals were not included in our sample or contribute fewer years of observation times

Table 4 Sensitivity analyses on NIS sample (Coefficients of opt-out variable)

	Total number of surgical discharges	Log Total number of surgical discharges	Mean costs per surgical case	Log Mean costs per surgical case
Main model	39.78	0.0529	1815.3***	0.0840*
	(0.62)	(1.08)	(3.76)	(2.43)
Subgroup analysis				
Early opt-out[a] vs control	103.9	0.0741	644.5	0.0183
	(1.50)	(1.50)	(1.42)	(0.50)
Late opt-out[b] vs control	−185.4	0.0234	2461.0***	0.120*
	(−1.14)	(0.29)	(4.42)	(2.38)
opt-out variable * late opt-out[c]	−279.9	−0.0687	2202.9**	0.130*
	(−1.87)	(−1.16)	(3.09)	(2.38)
Alternative definitions of surgical case				
Removing cases age <18 out of total surgical discharges	39.91	0.0410	1833.5**	0.0784*
	(0.61)	(0.98)	(3.41)	(2.28)
Removing all transplant DRGs and any craniotomy DRGs	38.84	0.0535	1757.2***	0.0831*
	(0.61)	(1.09)	(3.75)	(2.39)
Include only hip and knee surgery procedures	24.12	0.00109	494.1	0.0292
	(1.55)	(0.03)	(0.63)	(1.27)
Using partial covariates				
Exclude hospital characteristics	33.71	0.0477	1839.3***	0.0762*
	(0.56)	(1.08)	(4.08)	(2.72)
Exclude hospital characteristics and county variables	6.887	0.0364	1903.8**	0.0637*
	(0.12)	(0.70)	(3.06)	(2.10)
Exclude hospital variables, county variables and t-1 year variables	−110.4*	−0.0561	1977.9**	0.0709***
	(−2.03)	(−1.18)	(2.91)	(4.71)

Notes: Costs were in 2011 dollar adjusted by hospital and related services CPI; *$p < 0.05$; **$p < 0.01$; ***$p < 0.001$
[a]Early opt out =1 for those hospitals in states opt out between 2001 and 2005 (i.e. IA, MN, NE, NH, NM, AK, KS, ND, OR, WA, MT, SD, WI)
[b]Late opt out =1 for those hospitals in states opt out between 2009 and 2010 (i.e. CA, CO)
[c]This is the coefficient for the interaction term between opt-out variable and late opt out variable. The model was conducted on whole sample to test whether state opt out in recent year had different impact on outcomes comparing those opt out in early year

Table 5 Sensitivity and subgroup analyses on SASD sample (Coefficients of opt-out variable)

	Total number of surgical procedures	Log of total number of surgical procedures
Main model (sample includes freestanding facilities)	1149.2	0.0601
	(1.06)	(0.71)
Subgroups		
Non-freestanding	1333.9	0.129
	(1.08)	(1.93)
Freestanding	−310.2***	−0.257***
	(−15.71)	(−23.06)
Alternative definition of surgical cases		
Subset of selected procedures per facility usually requiring general anesthesia[2]	−22.84	−0.0916
	(−0.66)	(−0.76)
Using partial covariates		
Exclude t-1 year case mix variables	537.3	0.0496
	(0.34)	(0.48)

Notes: [1] Hospital characteristics and county variables were not available for freestanding facilities; [2] procedures with CPT code of 19301, 19302, 23410, 23412, 23420, 23430, 23470, 23472, 23473, 23474, 23700, 24300, 24341, 24342, 24363, 24370, 24371, 29827, 29882, 29883, 42821, 42826, 47562, 47563, 47600, 47605, 49505, 49507, 49520, 49521, 49525, 49587, 49650, 49651, 58541, 58542, 58543, 58544, 58545, 58546, 58550, 58552, 58553, 58554, 58570, 58571, 58572, 58573, 58670, 58671; *$p < 0.05$; **$p < 0.01$; ***$p < 0.001$

which might reduce to power for the facility-level fixed-effects model. However, given the large sample, it is unlikely to be threat to our main conclusion. Finally, the opt-out status variable is a "black box" in our analysis – it does not measure to what extent either the number of nurse anesthetists or physician anesthesiologists, or their typical workloads, actually changed as a result of the implementation of the opt-out policy. However, our results suggest that, whatever the impact of opt-out on the actual supply of anesthesia services, the net impact of opt-out policy implementation was little or no impact on access to inpatient or outpatient surgical care, and an increase in the cost of inpatient surgical care.

Conclusions

Our results do not support the hypothesis that opt-out laws improve access to inpatient surgical care or reduce its costs. Across a number of specifications for our inpatient discharges models, we find a consistent pattern of point estimates of increased costs with no discernable impact on access. Findings for our outpatient access models are less consistent, but overall, our results suggest opt-out policies were not associated with improvement in access to outpatient surgery.

Endnotes

[1]In NIS, the total number of all surgeries was the sum of all hospitalizations with surgical DRG in a facility (excluding records with patients age younger than 1); In SASD, it was the total number of visits in the facility.

[2]We used the size classification defined by HCUP, for which specific bed-size thresholds for size categories vary across Census regions, and by urban/rural and teaching status (https://www.hcup-us.ahrq.gov/db/vars/hosp_bedsize/nisnote.jsp).

[3]These facility level variables were almost fixed over the sample time period. Dropping the facility variables from the facility fixed-effects model does not change model results.

[4]The market area definition recommended by HCUP was used (see *HCUP Hospital Market Structure File: 2009 Central Distributor SID, NIS, and KID User Guide* [https://www.hcup-us.ahrq.gov/toolssoftware/hms/HMSUserGuide2009.pdf].) Years with missing HHI values were imputed using a time trend.

[5]The source for these data is county-level data from the Area Resource File (ARF).

[6]Estimated as $\beta^* = \left[\exp\left[\hat{\beta} - \frac{1}{2}\,\mathrm{var}\left(\hat{\beta}\right)\right] - 1 \right]$. See Kennedy [12].

Appendix

Table 6 Opt out year-month for states included in our NIS and SASD sample

State	Opt-out date	Included in our sample	
		NIS	SASD
Alaska	Oct. 2003	Yes	No
Arizona	NA	Yes	No
Arkansas	NA	Yes	No
California	Jun. 2009	Yes	Yes
Colorado	Sept. 2010	Yes	Yes
Connecticut	NA	Yes	No
Florida	NA	Yes	Yes
Georgia	NA	Yes	No
Hawaii	NA	Yes	No
Illinois	NA	Yes	No
Indiana	NA	Yes	No
Iowa	Dec. 2001	Yes	No
Kansas	Apr. 2003	Yes	No
Kentucky	Apr. 2012	Yes	yes
Louisiana	NA	Yes	No
Maine	NA	Yes	No
Maryland	NA	Yes	Yes
Massachusetts	NA	Yes	No
Michigan	NA	Yes	No
Minnesota	Apr. 2002	Yes	No
Mississippi	NA	Yes	No
Missouri	NA	Yes	No
Montana	Jan. 2004	Yes	No
Nebraska	Feb. 2002	Yes	No
Nevada	NA	Yes	No
New Hampshire	Jun. 2002	Yes	No
New Jersey	NA	Yes	Yes
New Mexico	Nov. 2002	Yes	No
New York	NA	Yes	No
North Carolina	NA	Yes	No
North Dakota	Oct. 2003	Yes	No
Ohio	NA	Yes	No
Oklahoma	NA	Yes	No
Oregon	Dec. 2003	Yes	No
Pennsylvania	NA	Yes	No
Rhode Island	NA	Yes	No
South Carolina	NA	Yes	No
South Dakota	Mar. 2005	Yes	No
Tennessee	NA	Yes	No
Texas	NA	Yes	No
Utah	NA	Yes	No
Vermont	NA	Yes	No
Virginia	NA	Yes	No
Washington	Oct. 2003	Yes	No
West Virginia	NA	Yes	No
Wisconsin	Jun. 2005	Yes	No
Wyoming	NA	Yes	No

Table 7 Descriptive for the main outcomes in inpatient file (NIS)

Hospital state	Calendar year	Total number of surgical procedures			Log of total number of surgical procedures			Mean costs per surgical case			Log Mean costs per surgical case		
		Mean	Std	N	Mean	Std	N	Mean	Std	N	Mean	Std	N
AK	2010	352.50	318.91	2	5.60	1.07	2	24009.66	1392.48	2	10.09	0.06	2
	2011	389.00	405.88	2	5.57	1.34	2	28491.65	3365.32	2	10.25	0.12	2
AR	2004	1303.41	2157.82	29	5.36	2.50	29	5750.00	2145.57	22	8.59	0.36	22
	2005	1266.71	1802.66	24	5.86	2.01	24	6588.21	2567.39	20	8.71	0.44	20
	2006	1095.63	1635.97	24	5.41	2.20	24	8517.11	9471.11	15	8.80	0.60	15
	2007	609.68	1196.46	22	4.80	2.27	22	8088.49	6913.90	17	8.80	0.61	17
	2008	1643.27	2325.74	22	5.42	2.76	22	8132.00	3451.52	19	8.90	0.50	19
	2009	1400.42	2006.85	19	5.45	2.63	19	9725.37	3875.93	16	9.11	0.39	16
	2010	989.94	1946.63	16	5.03	2.21	16	12334.08	5633.30	15	9.34	0.41	15
	2011	1383.13	2230.16	16	5.94	1.71	16	11072.76	7855.47	12	9.17	0.50	12
AZ	1998	2099.46	2273.16	13	6.36	2.43	13	.	.	0	.	.	0
	1999	2491.25	2883.66	12	6.53	2.41	12	.	.	0	.	.	0
	2000	3115.64	3147.09	14	7.22	1.86	14	.	.	0	.	.	0
	2001	2817.27	2671.47	11	7.33	1.34	11	3893.65	1037.64	10	8.22	0.35	10
	2003	1829.69	2648.37	13	5.96	2.37	13	5872.07	2489.39	12	8.59	0.46	12
	2004	3077.92	4407.92	13	6.09	2.79	13	10111.39	11406.00	12	8.96	0.63	12
	2005	3351.11	4311.27	18	6.52	2.88	18	8077.58	2029.58	11	8.97	0.25	11
	2006	4043.00	4349.95	15	7.05	2.46	15	11028.56	2180.83	12	9.29	0.22	12
	2007	3421.53	4125.20	15	7.15	1.71	15	10193.32	2876.50	13	9.20	0.27	13
	2008	3892.56	4886.74	16	6.31	3.04	16	14195.29	11241.22	16	9.40	0.52	16
	2009	2790.31	2664.93	16	6.98	2.02	16	18316.77	14801.73	15	9.66	0.50	15
	2010	2791.87	2514.98	15	6.96	2.33	15	13640.12	4886.16	15	9.46	0.37	15
	2011	2929.69	3247.85	16	6.88	2.30	16	15769.02	4543.36	15	9.63	0.27	15
CA	1998	2121.70	2167.99	94	6.96	1.54	94	.	.	0	.	.	0
	1999	2330.86	2503.90	95	7.06	1.57	95	.	.	0	.	.	0
	2000	2218.62	2375.59	91	7.02	1.50	91	.	.	0	.	.	0
	2001	2470.48	2350.32	93	6.98	1.93	93	5827.07	2725.23	76	8.59	0.41	76
	2002	2777.43	2780.51	92	7.22	1.68	92	7099.43	2607.84	59	8.81	0.35	59
	2003	2636.85	2417.21	85	7.27	1.42	85	7754.73	3393.70	65	8.88	0.39	65
	2004	2548.71	2434.74	82	7.26	1.31	82	9071.56	4796.00	64	9.03	0.37	64
	2005	2988.06	3147.14	84	7.28	1.53	84	11114.95	5520.25	66	9.24	0.37	66
	2006	2668.75	2479.17	81	7.25	1.50	81	11296.21	5763.61	63	9.25	0.39	63
	2007	3016.74	2996.67	84	7.27	1.63	84	13775.26	7546.54	69	9.43	0.42	69
	2008	2852.38	2782.56	82	7.24	1.62	82	15579.79	8167.87	73	9.56	0.42	73
	2009	3008.26	2974.03	81	7.28	1.54	81	18361.10	11086.31	74	9.69	0.49	74
	2010	2749.08	2502.10	76	7.15	1.74	76	23461.53	17798.25	68	9.89	0.53	68
	2011	2917.49	2701.21	77	7.24	1.77	77	21961.51	8726.40	62	9.92	0.39	62
CO	1998	2118.22	2572.49	18	6.04	2.64	18	.	.	0	.	.	0
	1999	2000.06	2618.33	17	5.89	2.74	17	.	.	0	.	.	0
	2000	1793.05	2551.32	21	5.54	2.72	21	.	.	0	.	.	0
	2001	1959.31	2362.98	16	6.19	2.47	16	5497.33	1593.74	11	8.57	0.31	11
	2002	2199.06	3192.30	18	5.45	3.06	18	6031.03	973.12	11	8.69	0.15	11

Table 7 Descriptive for the main outcomes in inpatient file (NIS) *(Continued)*

	Year												
	2003	1775.06	2425.82	18	5.80	2.57	18	6982.06	1906.24	15	8.82	0.27	15
	2004	2233.00	2843.94	18	6.11	2.73	18	7802.34	1956.12	15	8.93	0.26	15
	2005	2131.39	2924.85	18	5.55	3.19	18	8516.21	3115.39	16	8.96	0.47	16
	2006	1793.11	2699.90	18	5.41	3.01	18	10108.59	4811.35	16	9.06	0.71	16
	2007	2440.00	3039.16	18	6.19	2.65	18	12647.78	5101.15	17	9.38	0.35	17
	2008	2688.25	3054.51	16	6.38	2.66	16	17127.62	11548.88	15	9.60	0.53	15
	2009	2947.40	2995.45	15	7.03	1.78	15	17669.03	5501.60	15	9.74	0.30	15
	2010	2369.47	2769.70	15	6.05	2.82	15	18367.56	6221.43	15	9.74	0.45	15
	2011	2088.00	2184.81	18	6.52	2.17	18	19800.23	5267.59	17	9.86	0.26	17
CT	1998	1629.14	1010.77	7	7.25	0.57	7	.	.	0	.	.	0
	1999	3696.33	4394.93	6	7.74	1.03	6	.	.	0	.	.	0
	2000	3374.83	3147.44	6	7.73	1.00	6	.	.	0	.	.	0
	2001	4053.43	4358.35	7	7.81	1.11	7	5865.99	994.65	7	8.66	0.17	7
	2002	4643.25	4299.35	8	8.09	0.90	8	6811.11	1064.44	8	8.81	0.17	8
	2003	3546.83	3122.36	6	7.77	1.08	6	7541.01	415.77	5	8.93	0.06	5
	2004	3368.30	2431.76	10	7.91	0.68	10	7924.88	1407.79	10	8.96	0.19	10
	2005	3519.13	4567.21	8	7.57	1.15	8	9390.75	1255.57	7	9.14	0.13	7
	2006	4116.50	4043.90	10	7.95	0.92	10	10223.72	1779.58	10	9.22	0.18	10
	2007	3505.22	2348.92	9	7.96	0.69	9	11712.55	2130.87	9	9.35	0.19	9
	2008	5080.00	5647.94	6	7.96	1.21	6	14300.30	2949.97	6	9.55	0.22	6
	2009	4138.86	3933.42	7	7.92	1.01	7	14035.06	3406.36	7	9.53	0.21	7
	2010	4098.14	3510.21	7	8.01	0.88	7	15497.02	3034.58	7	9.63	0.21	7
	2011	3284.75	3282.91	8	7.72	0.95	8	15951.15	2377.51	7	9.67	0.16	7
FL	1998	2554.55	2636.13	106	7.08	1.79	106	.	.	0	.	.	0
	1999	2614.08	3237.07	97	6.95	1.91	97	.	.	0	.	.	0
	2000	2775.69	3191.06	55	6.99	2.01	55	.	.	0	.	.	0
	2001	3008.64	3417.63	55	7.13	1.88	55	5252.91	1226.49	42	8.54	0.23	42
	2002	4004.06	3855.04	51	7.54	1.79	51	6029.14	1587.95	44	8.67	0.28	44
	2003	3290.84	3462.90	58	7.11	2.10	58	7150.79	2201.82	48	8.83	0.31	48
	2004	3335.84	4102.03	55	7.29	1.79	55	8097.76	2484.26	48	8.96	0.30	48
	2005	3245.45	4702.04	51	7.38	1.49	51	9212.34	4003.89	43	9.07	0.31	43
	2006	3552.69	5111.64	51	7.09	1.99	51	10266.39	5588.96	40	9.13	0.44	40
	2007	4014.08	4663.80	50	7.49	1.79	50	10307.93	3107.63	45	9.19	0.38	45
	2008	4171.35	5590.79	49	7.37	1.85	49	11937.08	4949.32	45	9.33	0.32	45
	2009	3520.84	5131.49	50	6.99	2.19	50	12483.18	3539.47	44	9.39	0.29	44
	2010	3629.66	4004.72	44	7.45	1.62	44	16103.68	6455.51	41	9.63	0.33	41
	2011	3433.17	4102.18	46	7.36	1.67	46	16100.65	8814.13	41	9.62	0.32	41
GA	1998	1105.33	1664.79	111	5.61	2.07	111	.	.	0	.	.	0
	1999	1212.11	2133.15	97	5.50	2.09	97	.	.	0	.	.	0
	2000	1449.82	2784.19	57	5.37	2.36	57	.	.	0	.	.	0
	2001	1428.32	2214.31	56	5.67	2.28	56	4565.10	1239.12	34	8.39	0.26	34
	2002	1709.04	3150.41	56	5.41	2.50	56	5581.48	1793.79	33	8.48	0.86	33
	2003	1674.18	3428.28	50	5.55	2.27	50	5784.26	1921.51	24	8.60	0.38	24
	2004	1540.32	2951.55	50	5.50	2.35	50	7671.76	4026.51	30	8.75	0.92	30
	2005	1675.70	2470.76	46	5.86	2.40	46	8251.12	2680.96	34	8.97	0.30	34

Table 7 Descriptive for the main outcomes in inpatient file (NIS) *(Continued)*

	Year												
	2006	1899.24	3001.79	42	5.96	2.29	42	8825.86	2360.98	34	9.05	0.29	34
	2007	2263.03	3518.61	38	6.04	2.43	38	9529.58	3019.18	27	9.12	0.31	27
	2008	1787.58	2382.77	33	5.78	2.48	33	11587.75	4943.59	24	9.28	0.41	24
	2009	1902.58	3117.79	38	5.61	2.51	38	13192.84	7595.41	32	9.39	0.42	32
	2010	1555.05	2097.80	39	5.82	2.29	39	15261.72	11840.58	36	9.48	0.54	36
	2011	1531.57	2266.45	35	5.60	2.50	35	14821.94	5090.16	33	9.55	0.33	33
HI	1998	1140.75	1091.51	4	6.30	1.77	4	.	.	0	.	.	0
	1999	1589.67	1095.95	3	7.12	0.96	3	.	.	0	.	.	0
	2000	1775.67	1192.74	3	7.21	1.04	3	.	.	0	.	.	0
	2001	2012.00	1189.55	3	7.42	0.83	3	.	.	0	.	.	0
	2002	1580.80	1081.55	5	6.03	3.39	5	.	.	0	.	.	0
	2003	915.40	553.97	5	6.64	0.69	5	8995.32	3738.26	4	9.04	0.43	4
	2004	1206.40	1135.34	5	6.63	1.19	5	8027.69	3433.08	5	8.92	0.41	5
	2005	1307.75	1067.76	4	6.91	0.86	4	7571.95	1720.19	3	8.91	0.25	3
	2006	1101.75	779.11	4	6.74	0.90	4	10315.77	2827.16	4	9.21	0.27	4
	2007	1771.25	1367.42	4	7.15	1.08	4	10007.89	658.75	3	9.21	0.07	3
	2008	1147.33	442.97	3	6.99	0.44	3	17131.34	9267.88	3	9.66	0.50	3
	2009	2796.00	.	1	7.94	.	1	19871.55	.	1	9.90	.	1
	2010	1926.75	1060.69	4	7.39	0.75	4	15053.38	7084.85	4	9.55	0.42	4
	2011	.	.	0	.	.	0	.	.	0	.	.	0
IA	1998	849.11	1794.65	53	5.25	1.68	53	.	.	0	.	.	0
	1999	1059.67	2052.33	54	5.30	2.01	54	.	.	0	.	.	0
	2000	1163.16	2206.46	51	5.42	1.92	51	.	.	0	.	.	0
	2001	927.62	1832.94	37	5.32	1.76	37	4748.16	1232.84	25	8.44	0.22	25
	2002	1080.00	2054.53	28	5.36	1.99	28	5224.04	1593.30	16	8.53	0.25	16
	2003	1079.26	2278.38	27	5.20	2.03	27	5596.97	1007.46	17	8.61	0.18	17
	2004	984.92	2188.72	26	4.85	2.24	26	6665.14	2304.46	14	8.76	0.32	14
	2005	912.25	2196.46	28	4.92	2.21	28	7447.16	2289.44	19	8.88	0.28	19
	2006	933.48	1982.12	29	5.04	2.16	29	7978.59	1480.96	21	8.97	0.19	21
	2007	1014.59	2045.78	27	5.04	2.24	27	8824.55	1496.89	19	9.07	0.19	19
	2008	572.59	1409.53	27	4.46	2.11	27	11368.58	3182.80	24	9.30	0.27	24
	2009	634.40	1439.88	25	4.54	2.10	25	16469.25	11479.62	24	9.56	0.50	24
	2010	784.69	1891.69	26	4.50	2.26	26	16279.03	7491.64	25	9.63	0.36	25
	2011	622.75	1059.96	24	4.63	2.15	24	17281.74	5435.92	24	9.71	0.29	24
IL	1998	1915.22	2039.10	74	6.80	1.50	74	.	.	0	.	.	0
	1999	2039.42	2380.00	69	6.72	1.67	69	.	.	0	.	.	0
	2000	2164.01	2692.61	68	6.70	1.68	68	.	.	0	.	.	0
	2001	1943.46	2069.21	65	6.85	1.48	65	5717.47	2415.54	57	8.60	0.31	57
	2002	1987.61	2023.36	46	6.67	1.83	46	6270.24	2823.11	40	8.67	0.37	40
	2003	2138.19	2206.29	42	6.60	2.07	42	6931.04	1482.53	36	8.82	0.23	36
	2004	2040.20	2539.70	40	6.44	2.20	40	8211.13	2369.53	33	8.98	0.26	33
	2005	1917.23	2353.27	43	6.46	1.79	43	8605.82	2595.79	39	9.02	0.28	39
	2006	1980.63	2282.61	40	6.51	1.90	40	10421.62	4419.12	38	9.18	0.36	38
	2007	2510.68	3465.31	41	6.69	1.91	41	12169.86	3928.83	39	9.36	0.29	39
	2008	2012.68	3045.48	44	6.18	2.23	44	15546.74	14632.14	40	9.51	0.43	40

Table 7 Descriptive for the main outcomes in inpatient file (NIS) *(Continued)*

	Year												
	2009	2156.28	3176.05	40	6.23	2.45	40	14185.09	5070.47	38	9.51	0.30	38
	2010	1666.00	2066.70	44	6.21	2.04	44	19032.69	14877.23	44	9.73	0.42	44
	2011	2171.50	2927.36	40	6.22	2.42	40	18344.68	5021.59	40	9.78	0.27	40
IN	2003	1649.25	2370.52	24	6.24	1.65	24	6884.33	2170.24	19	8.79	0.31	19
	2004	1591.21	2183.46	24	6.45	1.43	24	7734.78	1865.94	19	8.92	0.25	19
	2005	1972.68	3039.02	25	6.62	1.45	25	9288.90	5964.20	22	9.02	0.44	22
	2006	1737.81	2383.75	26	6.46	1.55	26	10825.71	8876.06	25	9.15	0.46	25
	2007	1691.65	1601.06	26	6.68	1.50	26	11002.11	3678.46	23	9.24	0.41	23
	2008	2315.56	3771.24	27	6.66	1.62	27	11053.83	4715.52	24	9.19	0.57	24
	2009	1859.04	2602.55	27	6.54	1.58	27	13065.81	5177.26	25	9.36	0.57	25
	2010	2363.33	3663.95	27	6.75	1.71	27	16362.84	8542.15	27	9.58	0.56	27
	2011	1926.80	3586.77	30	6.30	1.80	30	15668.48	5960.95	30	9.57	0.47	30
KS	1998	812.74	2029.40	50	4.62	2.42	50	.	.	0	.	.	0
	1999	761.69	1638.91	51	4.86	2.16	51	.	.	0	.	.	0
	2000	1055.36	2132.07	47	5.16	2.18	47	.	.	0	.	.	0
	2001	1018.44	2134.58	32	4.86	2.43	32	4036.40	1532.23	21	8.24	0.35	21
	2002	851.18	2038.20	28	4.83	2.04	28	4618.32	1501.20	17	8.38	0.37	17
	2003	1161.13	2631.74	24	4.64	2.72	24	5552.28	1640.88	18	8.56	0.39	18
	2004	989.04	2316.78	23	4.40	2.70	23	6669.50	1367.83	11	8.79	0.20	11
	2005	592.18	991.01	17	4.52	2.53	17	6394.52	1722.91	9	8.73	0.26	9
	2006	633.87	1421.98	23	3.95	2.68	23	7227.04	1887.91	15	8.85	0.27	15
	2007	724.00	1212.85	21	4.63	2.56	21	7258.34	2144.50	15	8.84	0.32	15
	2008	617.63	1486.77	24	4.08	2.31	24	10000.85	2734.45	21	9.17	0.29	21
	2009	761.48	1994.03	23	4.12	2.41	23	12874.11	4391.28	22	9.41	0.32	22
	2010	757.86	1782.16	22	4.65	2.26	22	11578.77	3946.00	22	9.30	0.35	22
	2011	674.60	1820.44	25	4.20	2.51	25	14580.75	6887.72	23	9.48	0.49	23
KY	2000	1372.93	2559.16	30	5.44	2.45	30	.	.	0	.	.	0
	2001	1297.93	1838.57	28	5.42	2.62	28	4036.06	1608.75	24	8.23	0.38	24
	2002	1518.56	2360.15	32	5.81	2.20	32	4568.06	1353.64	26	8.39	0.28	26
	2003	1365.83	2290.43	29	5.61	2.29	29	5392.58	1978.43	24	8.52	0.39	24
	2004	1184.62	1804.00	26	5.52	2.20	26	6320.87	2287.17	21	8.70	0.32	21
	2005	1503.11	2660.09	27	5.52	2.30	27	6372.96	2318.52	21	8.70	0.35	21
	2006	1841.32	2983.14	25	5.83	2.31	25	7091.80	3002.84	19	8.74	0.61	19
	2007	1333.26	2458.16	27	5.45	2.41	27	7402.65	2385.76	20	8.70	1.10	20
	2008	1256.75	2090.24	24	5.12	2.78	24	10213.45	3879.04	21	9.16	0.41	21
	2009	1966.50	2974.51	20	5.97	2.47	20	13063.02	10692.82	18	9.33	0.48	18
	2010	1798.45	2655.97	22	5.68	2.66	22	10951.32	5302.18	17	9.14	0.66	17
	2011	1669.30	2789.48	20	5.18	2.85	20	12887.79	3244.17	19	9.43	0.25	19
LA	2008	1181.38	1549.66	26	5.77	2.17	26	9885.81	3275.27	21	9.13	0.43	21
	2009	1156.17	1381.91	24	5.53	2.44	24	11361.36	5101.90	19	9.23	0.50	19
	2010	1306.40	2135.42	25	5.50	2.38	25	12227.67	9150.26	22	9.20	0.66	22
	2011	1416.08	2051.03	25	5.76	2.50	25	13909.64	3844.48	19	9.50	0.28	19
MA	1998	3040.06	3560.46	17	7.45	1.16	17	.	.	0	.	.	0
	1999	2668.40	2537.06	15	7.38	1.20	15	.	.	0	.	.	0
	2000	3492.94	3555.67	16	7.52	1.40	16	.	.	0	.	.	0

Table 7 Descriptive for the main outcomes in inpatient file (NIS) *(Continued)*

	2001	3410.13	3651.13	16	7.42	1.46	16	8413.99	8440.90	12	8.81	0.60	12
	2002	3442.00	3733.66	16	7.58	1.23	16	5895.69	1241.55	9	8.66	0.21	9
	2003	2534.50	2758.85	14	7.08	1.61	14	9383.10	9013.23	11	8.94	0.57	11
	2004	3447.76	4828.80	21	7.28	1.56	21	8081.33	2197.82	18	8.96	0.26	18
	2005	2954.87	3051.40	23	7.25	1.52	23	8492.44	2342.80	21	9.02	0.24	21
	2006	1984.33	2277.51	21	6.67	1.72	21	13118.39	10793.59	18	9.32	0.49	18
	2007	2370.05	3722.28	22	6.76	1.57	22	14091.16	11434.36	19	9.41	0.45	19
	2008	3722.93	5545.08	15	7.41	1.38	15	13294.67	3883.90	15	9.46	0.27	15
	2009	2367.93	2574.38	14	7.19	1.18	14	13486.80	3630.77	13	9.48	0.22	13
	2010	2990.86	3120.01	14	7.20	1.64	14	15322.99	4759.14	13	9.60	0.27	13
	2011	3654.36	5632.16	11	7.50	1.25	11	16360.45	4950.32	11	9.67	0.27	11
MD	1998	2973.22	2512.32	32	7.48	1.26	32	.	.	0	.	.	0
	1999	3517.17	3578.67	23	7.74	0.98	23	.	.	0	.	.	0
	2000	3436.38	2713.03	13	7.82	0.87	13	.	.	0	.	.	0
	2001	4083.83	3087.75	12	7.99	0.90	12	5106.37	949.44	11	8.52	0.20	11
	2002	3958.43	2949.12	14	7.97	0.89	14	5944.15	1251.39	14	8.67	0.21	14
	2003	4126.85	2696.23	13	8.03	0.92	13	6257.75	1462.82	12	8.72	0.23	12
	2004	3628.25	2564.61	12	7.92	0.82	12	7709.09	1974.82	12	8.92	0.26	12
	2005	4483.27	2663.02	11	8.19	0.78	11	6998.57	929.72	9	8.85	0.13	9
	2006	3669.08	3385.82	12	7.83	0.93	12	10206.58	2110.85	12	9.21	0.21	12
	2007	3757.83	2852.34	12	7.71	1.47	12	10210.26	2821.95	11	9.20	0.25	11
	2008	4213.83	3314.87	12	7.72	1.58	12	12733.43	3290.62	11	9.42	0.25	11
	2009	5319.13	3533.63	8	8.25	0.99	8	11155.02	2571.94	7	9.30	0.23	7
	2010	3738.00	3071.34	9	7.83	1.02	9	13287.21	3706.27	9	9.47	0.25	9
	2011	5494.45	5052.51	11	8.11	1.18	11	15155.95	6048.65	11	9.57	0.34	11
ME	1999	1784.18	3545.32	11	6.29	1.69	11	.	.	0	.	.	0
	2000	798.90	762.74	10	6.37	0.80	10	.	.	0	.	.	0
	2001	866.22	841.53	9	6.27	1.15	9	5899.08	784.50	7	8.67	0.14	7
	2002	672.43	981.72	7	5.90	1.09	7	5421.55	1387.84	5	8.57	0.26	5
	2007	455.22	486.18	9	5.54	1.38	9	.	.	0	.	.	0
	2008	577.86	579.34	7	5.60	1.66	7	.	.	0	.	.	0
	2009	390.33	415.61	6	5.30	1.50	6	.	.	0	.	.	0
	2010	315.29	222.46	7	5.55	0.70	7	.	.	0	.	.	0
	2011	357.14	324.29	7	5.53	0.93	7	.	.	0	.	.	0
MI	2001	2437.66	2918.32	29	6.76	1.93	29	4394.89	1119.15	25	8.36	0.26	25
	2002	2678.46	4960.38	28	6.60	1.81	28	5052.02	930.37	23	8.51	0.19	23
	2003	2652.76	5418.02	21	6.49	1.98	21	5558.11	1567.72	19	8.58	0.34	19
	2004	1868.60	2617.99	20	6.67	1.49	20	6615.06	1467.27	14	8.77	0.22	14
	2005	2054.60	3654.68	25	6.32	1.88	25	7694.10	2427.38	18	8.91	0.25	18
	2006	1846.32	2825.92	22	6.31	1.76	22	8437.68	1965.92	16	9.01	0.24	16
	2007	1972.32	3272.58	25	6.07	2.19	25	14935.53	21699.29	18	9.29	0.62	18
	2008	2012.11	2955.49	27	6.06	2.15	27	12527.02	3229.72	22	9.40	0.26	22
	2009	1877.15	2753.51	27	6.14	2.01	27	13048.33	4404.20	23	9.43	0.32	23
	2010	1791.81	2966.56	26	6.00	2.00	26	15506.22	6379.94	21	9.58	0.37	21
	2011	2327.68	4861.48	25	6.03	2.04	25	18401.67	7173.68	21	9.75	0.37	21

Table 7 Descriptive for the main outcomes in inpatient file (NIS) *(Continued)*

MN	2001	1593.49	2871.27	37	5.55	2.41	37	4813.53	1573.53	32	8.44	0.29	32
	2002	1396.35	2597.47	31	5.69	2.13	31	5584.56	2184.26	24	8.56	0.35	24
	2003	1732.46	3046.11	26	5.47	2.43	26	5958.37	2351.46	21	8.60	0.52	21
	2004	1423.04	2633.96	27	5.41	2.27	27	7116.96	1616.54	16	8.85	0.23	16
	2005	1724.23	4070.53	26	5.26	2.47	26	8187.22	3287.80	13	8.96	0.31	13
	2006	1765.89	3706.60	27	5.71	2.20	27	9131.42	2342.33	14	9.09	0.24	14
	2007	1449.47	2417.68	30	5.76	2.12	30	10200.21	2776.88	21	9.20	0.27	21
	2008	1577.71	2661.17	28	5.76	2.30	28	13660.25	6083.18	27	9.45	0.38	27
	2009	1291.23	3283.06	30	5.10	2.33	30	13710.38	4154.01	29	9.49	0.27	29
	2010	1625.16	3344.31	25	5.64	2.31	25	15024.33	4565.17	25	9.58	0.27	25
	2011	1541.65	2585.63	26	5.52	2.46	26	19900.57	8287.35	26	9.83	0.37	26
MO	1998	1384.87	1789.82	38	6.36	1.44	38	.	.	0	.	.	0
	1999	2346.20	3602.97	35	6.36	2.20	35	.	.	0	.	.	0
	2000	2107.66	2901.98	38	6.15	2.43	38	.	.	0	.	.	0
	2001	1291.10	1666.76	21	6.05	1.78	21	4983.54	1252.15	17	8.48	0.27	17
	2002	2832.67	4342.81	18	6.73	1.95	18	6225.39	1784.52	15	8.70	0.29	15
	2003	2191.96	4034.85	25	5.93	2.52	25	7080.02	2561.44	17	8.80	0.36	17
	2004	2332.17	4237.76	24	6.06	2.40	24	7334.60	2871.31	18	8.78	0.64	18
	2005	2535.93	3440.55	29	6.22	2.53	29	9209.76	3689.95	23	9.06	0.37	23
	2006	2255.48	2573.19	27	6.63	1.98	27	10243.57	3248.81	23	9.19	0.31	23
	2007	1200.50	1719.23	28	5.43	2.50	28	9125.08	2427.47	22	9.09	0.25	22
	2008	1814.26	2165.41	27	6.08	2.39	27	11214.30	3697.32	26	9.27	0.35	26
	2009	1825.19	2926.66	27	5.98	2.48	27	11866.57	4808.88	27	9.31	0.38	27
	2010	2080.37	2909.41	27	5.99	2.55	27	15732.51	5576.50	25	9.60	0.35	25
	2011	2894.96	4411.42	24	6.59	2.16	24	14798.95	3745.77	24	9.57	0.25	24
MS	2010	1298.35	2104.14	17	5.23	2.66	17	10981.42	4400.66	14	9.19	0.58	14
	2011	1380.00	2200.31	19	4.68	3.22	19	14807.05	15310.98	15	9.32	0.72	15
MT	2009	996.00	1867.11	7	4.84	2.81	7	13118.94	3808.17	7	9.44	0.30	7
	2010	910.38	1783.19	8	5.23	2.17	8	16332.89	4141.19	8	9.68	0.23	8
	2011	452.80	821.81	5	4.29	2.75	5	14200.83	3843.96	5	9.53	0.27	5
NC	2000	2442.09	3148.80	35	6.90	1.56	35	.	.	0	.	.	0
	2001	2527.59	3508.26	34	6.61	2.03	34	4601.95	1324.24	29	8.40	0.26	29
	2002	1780.33	2997.44	33	6.26	2.05	33	5084.64	1048.73	21	8.52	0.19	21
	2003	2282.53	3427.70	38	6.56	2.05	38	6019.75	2049.56	29	8.66	0.29	29
	2004	2433.35	3271.46	34	6.69	1.94	34	6036.25	1159.98	23	8.69	0.21	23
	2005	2701.42	3844.66	31	6.61	2.23	31	8377.00	4083.28	26	8.96	0.34	26
	2006	2969.15	4299.20	27	6.45	2.56	27	8933.45	2630.25	22	9.06	0.26	22
	2007	2806.31	4039.36	29	6.49	2.44	29	11426.09	5569.56	24	9.27	0.36	24
	2008	2356.43	3188.32	28	6.72	1.86	28	11853.39	4375.17	25	9.33	0.30	25
	2009	2685.00	4077.54	29	6.47	2.18	29	13271.58	6430.74	27	9.42	0.34	27
	2010	2947.85	4413.61	26	6.71	2.10	26	14580.08	7988.63	25	9.49	0.44	25
	2011	2290.96	4080.40	27	5.98	2.43	27	14709.72	3748.94	23	9.57	0.24	23
ND	2011	766.00	1381.47	4	5.01	2.15	4	12425.76	5162.41	4	9.36	0.44	4
NE	2001	562.05	1222.06	20	3.93	2.37	20	.	.	0	.	.	0
	2002	533.53	1360.54	19	4.23	2.06	19	.	.	0	.	.	0

Table 7 Descriptive for the main outcomes in inpatient file (NIS) *(Continued)*

	Year												
	2003	570.63	1396.58	16	4.25	2.12	16	.	.	0	.	.	0
	2004	713.53	1827.72	19	3.51	2.64	19	.	.	0	.	.	0
	2005	510.33	1040.81	15	4.45	2.08	15	.	.	0	.	.	0
	2006	801.33	1110.69	15	4.72	2.56	15	9960.69	3433.49	9	9.15	0.35	9
	2007	639.33	1698.76	15	3.78	2.36	15	9642.63	2243.55	7	9.15	0.26	7
	2008	813.94	1701.11	18	4.48	2.21	18	10768.75	3504.14	15	9.24	0.28	15
	2009	911.50	1960.16	16	5.03	2.01	16	12443.33	2605.78	16	9.41	0.22	16
	2010	719.79	1024.04	14	5.11	2.07	14	15368.49	4066.29	12	9.61	0.26	12
	2011	440.38	700.19	13	4.26	2.29	13	17086.93	6536.34	12	9.67	0.41	12
NH	2003	789.67	954.14	6	6.01	1.25	6	8073.64	1506.33	3	8.98	0.19	3
	2004	1587.75	2546.31	8	6.59	1.24	8	9241.90	1720.66	8	9.11	0.20	8
	2005	1873.50	2401.78	10	6.83	1.29	10	11076.00	1891.01	9	9.30	0.17	9
	2006	1634.78	2675.53	9	6.48	1.39	9	13310.25	1558.80	6	9.49	0.12	6
	2007	2340.38	2876.16	8	6.99	1.45	8	13343.93	2310.80	6	9.49	0.18	6
	2008	1736.75	1766.40	4	6.90	1.32	4	18555.85	2540.10	4	9.82	0.13	4
	2009	2649.80	3523.12	5	7.14	1.43	5	18094.97	4044.47	4	9.78	0.26	4
NJ	1998	4104.00	3571.86	17	7.94	0.93	17	.	.	0	.	.	0
	1999	2952.24	2252.43	17	7.72	0.76	17	.	.	0	.	.	0
	2000	3773.38	3415.28	16	7.94	0.78	16	.	.	0	.	.	0
	2001	3084.86	2365.69	14	7.80	0.70	14	5106.36	1349.19	7	8.51	0.26	7
	2002	4277.36	4395.13	14	7.95	0.92	14	5692.50	1737.38	10	8.61	0.27	10
	2003	3127.31	1839.55	16	7.86	0.68	16	6580.77	3003.24	8	8.73	0.34	8
	2004	4299.23	3217.16	22	8.11	0.76	22	8103.54	4357.98	14	8.91	0.41	14
	2005	3516.14	3766.92	22	7.66	1.26	22	7529.17	1095.34	13	8.92	0.14	13
	2006	3169.64	2372.15	22	7.55	1.53	22	14652.67	12027.58	10	9.40	0.60	10
	2007	3520.62	3285.25	21	7.43	1.78	21	12707.51	8816.48	17	9.33	0.43	17
	2008	3853.06	3194.61	16	7.26	2.26	16	15692.37	12536.29	14	9.48	0.55	14
	2009	3955.79	3702.55	14	7.80	1.26	14	15506.79	9760.97	14	9.54	0.45	14
	2010	4224.00	2393.15	14	8.19	0.59	14	17528.16	12964.92	14	9.63	0.49	14
	2011	3132.64	2052.52	14	7.58	1.44	14	22222.96	18062.96	13	9.81	0.58	13
NM	2009	655.71	527.19	7	5.84	1.68	7	10775.84	4235.77	7	9.24	0.31	7
	2010	696.56	905.38	9	5.05	2.62	9	10790.77	3921.69	7	9.23	0.35	7
	2011	1492.38	2788.29	8	6.12	1.75	8	14892.99	7600.51	6	9.48	0.58	6
NV	2002	2201.25	3100.49	8	6.09	2.68	8	6966.88	1059.68	5	8.84	0.17	5
	2003	2253.29	2768.57	7	5.18	3.54	7	6787.26	2361.39	5	8.76	0.41	5
	2004	4368.00	3669.72	5	7.89	1.26	5	8673.05	2100.31	5	9.05	0.23	5
	2005	1277.33	2140.73	6	5.72	2.14	6	8660.39	3033.09	4	9.03	0.32	4
	2006	2686.33	3136.24	9	6.35	2.91	9	8005.18	3232.06	6	8.89	0.54	6
	2007	2927.75	3811.88	8	6.41	2.97	8	12916.99	3347.11	8	9.44	0.26	8
	2008	1591.73	2078.72	11	5.77	2.85	11	11950.01	3285.93	9	9.36	0.27	9
	2009	2274.13	3016.42	8	6.82	1.60	8	13108.50	2823.15	8	9.45	0.27	8
	2010	2738.36	3289.76	11	6.60	2.20	11	15425.89	4224.43	10	9.61	0.25	10
	2011	2290.71	2654.78	7	6.59	2.05	7	24908.23	20308.00	7	9.94	0.58	7
NY	1998	2132.19	2436.21	52	6.66	2.18	52	.	.	0	.	.	0
	1999	2416.58	2747.45	45	7.07	1.61	45	.	.	0	.	.	0

Table 7 Descriptive for the main outcomes in inpatient file (NIS) *(Continued)*

	Year												
	2000	2853.49	3129.06	45	7.42	1.11	45	.	.	0	.	.	0
	2001	3242.28	4043.79	43	7.33	1.44	43	5590.42	2621.72	37	8.54	0.42	37
	2002	2766.66	3293.78	44	7.18	1.48	44	6597.20	3619.77	36	8.68	0.47	36
	2003	3427.55	3942.44	42	7.16	2.07	42	6155.87	2491.87	37	8.65	0.38	37
	2004	2883.38	3912.49	63	7.06	1.84	63	7947.98	4762.75	52	8.86	0.46	52
	2005	3028.80	3697.53	64	7.10	1.94	64	7771.71	3128.96	53	8.88	0.42	53
	2006	3020.45	4156.70	62	7.14	1.69	62	9034.17	3718.11	55	9.02	0.44	55
	2007	3196.18	3713.86	55	7.25	1.76	55	10117.92	4292.29	49	9.15	0.39	49
	2008	3437.11	4719.26	38	6.87	2.47	38	15607.42	20432.51	37	9.37	0.68	37
	2009	3323.08	4009.90	38	7.52	1.11	38	13472.88	4279.28	32	9.46	0.32	32
	2010	3114.32	3725.60	38	7.22	1.79	38	13776.02	6008.00	33	9.46	0.35	33
	2011	3588.00	6240.09	40	7.04	2.02	40	15140.17	5564.67	36	9.56	0.36	36
OH	2002	2527.00	3307.23	37	7.06	1.32	37	5908.96	1303.04	28	8.66	0.22	28
	2003	2587.85	2724.95	33	7.00	1.95	33	7036.82	1924.44	29	8.81	0.35	29
	2004	2527.94	2588.13	34	7.28	1.19	34	7707.24	1442.44	32	8.93	0.18	32
	2005	2737.21	3092.45	34	7.17	1.42	34	8634.29	1551.10	26	9.05	0.19	26
	2006	2699.14	3322.00	35	6.95	1.62	35	10032.29	4909.26	31	9.16	0.30	31
	2007	2786.47	2714.96	36	7.32	1.30	36	10916.53	2376.28	30	9.28	0.21	30
	2008	2935.29	3930.51	34	7.02	1.65	34	11690.49	2291.54	31	9.35	0.20	31
	2009	2953.63	4831.75	40	7.01	1.57	40	13534.72	4883.91	40	9.46	0.33	40
	2010	2437.24	2835.55	38	6.80	1.79	38	16032.38	8480.62	38	9.61	0.36	38
	2011	2176.49	2657.24	35	6.85	1.48	35	16131.09	4427.39	35	9.65	0.26	35
OK	2005	973.03	2084.27	38	4.45	2.69	38	8844.59	9644.56	29	8.83	0.61	29
	2006	1382.65	2751.57	37	5.02	2.57	37	7603.12	6893.63	28	8.73	0.58	28
	2007	1165.94	2019.20	33	4.99	2.68	33	9764.43	8765.00	27	9.03	0.47	27
	2008	907.56	2022.08	34	4.79	2.56	34	9381.34	5931.77	29	8.99	0.56	29
	2009	1104.82	2458.02	33	5.00	2.39	33	12639.34	11496.96	24	9.24	0.58	24
	2010	1314.17	2576.75	29	5.30	2.37	29	14013.95	13477.54	27	9.30	0.65	27
	2011	823.24	1745.55	29	4.93	2.36	29	14412.94	9515.59	25	9.40	0.59	25
OR	1998	1143.94	1866.50	18	5.91	1.85	18	.	.	0	.	.	0
	1999	1732.29	2261.67	17	6.24	2.11	17	.	.	0	.	.	0
	2000	1630.78	2488.82	18	6.20	2.00	18	.	.	0	.	.	0
	2001	1424.00	2134.01	19	6.03	1.91	19	.	.	0	.	.	0
	2002	2397.56	4019.29	16	6.43	1.77	16	.	.	0	.	.	0
	2003	1203.31	1619.97	16	5.98	1.88	16	7091.79	2519.14	12	8.82	0.32	12
	2004	2312.77	3800.60	13	6.80	1.39	13	.	.	0	.	.	0
	2005	1246.38	2012.70	16	6.18	1.52	16	.	.	0	.	.	0
	2006	2257.20	3245.54	15	6.41	1.89	15	11521.55	2797.04	13	9.32	0.24	13
	2007	1826.40	2653.57	15	6.58	1.46	15	11130.62	2044.44	14	9.30	0.19	14
	2008	1935.00	3184.08	17	6.25	1.83	17	14682.31	3517.72	16	9.57	0.23	16
	2009	2430.36	3640.99	14	6.61	1.81	14	15175.93	3525.53	14	9.60	0.23	14
	2010	1850.64	3201.19	14	6.08	2.35	14	17091.32	4036.51	13	9.72	0.23	13
	2011	1630.07	2867.50	15	5.78	2.36	15	19629.93	8637.12	14	9.80	0.43	14
PA	1998	2004.91	1946.07	47	6.96	1.39	47	.	.	0	.	.	0
	1999	2282.86	2820.36	42	7.14	1.15	42	.	.	0	.	.	0

Table 7 Descriptive for the main outcomes in inpatient file (NIS) *(Continued)*

	Year													
	2000	2262.83	2459.99	42	7.12	1.22	42	.	.	0	.	.	0
	2001	2591.44	3177.39	41	7.15	1.38	41	.	.	0	.	.	0
	2002	2357.03	2555.95	40	7.21	1.16	40	.	.	0	.	.	0
	2003	2845.40	4667.72	40	7.13	1.49	40	.	.	0	.	.	0
	2008	2856.68	4943.77	38	6.67	2.04	38	.	.	0	.	.	0
	2009	2776.63	3268.88	35	6.71	2.06	35	.	.	0	.	.	0
	2010	2782.76	3753.00	41	6.98	1.61	41	.	.	0	.	.	0
	2011	2701.51	4629.25	41	6.84	1.67	41	.	.	0	.	.	0
RI	2001	1331.00	.	1	7.19	.	1	4444.86	.	1	8.40	.	1
	2002	1815.00	.	1	7.50	.	1	7208.26	.	1	8.88	.	1
	2003	4083.75	4135.39	4	7.97	0.91	4	10011.33	.	1	9.21	.	1
	2004	3034.67	1967.73	3	7.88	0.64	3	5181.99	777.22	3	8.55	0.15	3
	2005	2790.67	2302.59	3	7.72	0.77	3	6608.93	2198.37	2	8.77	0.34	2
	2006	1776.33	484.87	3	7.45	0.30	3	8928.95	1255.04	3	9.09	0.15	3
	2007	3505.00	3163.60	2	7.90	1.07	2	8270.36	3117.66	2	8.98	0.39	2
	2008	2340.67	1678.75	3	7.57	0.76	3	9839.77	2289.03	3	9.17	0.25	3
	2009	1961.67	908.60	3	7.51	0.45	3	14115.02	3803.33	3	9.53	0.26	3
	2010	1166.00	147.96	3	7.06	0.13	3	15595.23	1616.71	3	9.65	0.11	3
	2011	2020.50	672.84	4	7.57	0.33	4	15003.24	1753.48	4	9.61	0.12	4
SC	1998	1646.15	2382.98	33	6.17	1.91	33	.	.	0	.	.	0
	1999	1501.39	1956.31	33	6.21	1.85	33	.	.	0	.	.	0
	2000	1490.95	1961.48	19	6.27	1.75	19	.	.	0	.	.	0
	2001	1779.83	2216.75	18	6.59	1.69	18	4621.59	1062.77	16	8.41	0.27	16
	2002	2222.11	2600.56	18	6.55	2.19	18	5644.29	1634.80	17	8.61	0.25	17
	2003	2272.63	2844.52	16	6.54	2.06	16	7215.46	3583.34	16	8.82	0.33	16
	2004	1848.47	2666.79	15	6.22	2.07	15	10264.26	11306.69	12	9.00	0.57	12
	2005	2651.17	2905.95	12	6.91	1.86	12	7889.53	1919.36	9	8.95	0.26	9
	2006	2962.29	3299.72	14	7.04	1.71	14	9703.19	2700.44	12	9.15	0.27	12
	2007	2180.50	2545.26	14	6.80	2.15	14	9584.62	1983.42	13	9.15	0.21	13
	2008	2039.07	2559.10	15	6.73	1.78	15	12803.75	2583.14	14	9.44	0.21	14
	2009	1793.46	2073.91	13	6.53	1.84	13	14592.41	2403.82	11	9.58	0.16	11
	2010	2555.44	3614.53	9	6.70	2.10	9	15033.54	5085.04	9	9.57	0.31	9
	2011	2539.77	2831.04	13	6.61	2.49	13	13914.04	2890.61	13	9.52	0.24	13
SD	2002	831.13	1923.49	8	4.24	2.44	8	4442.12	1683.55	5	8.34	0.36	5
	2003	232.00	432.07	4	3.68	2.13	4	4868.34	1044.80	3	8.48	0.21	3
	2004	2099.40	3852.53	5	5.10	3.54	5	5432.60	1785.25	5	8.54	0.41	5
	2005	119.86	191.03	7	3.73	1.64	7	6187.08	1201.84	4	8.72	0.19	4
	2006	226.89	403.08	9	3.27	2.59	9	7275.17	3033.44	6	8.83	0.38	6
	2007	145.75	243.34	8	3.06	2.38	8	8160.88	2781.22	6	8.95	0.37	6
	2008	179.00	290.30	4	4.20	1.53	4	10415.01	4387.50	3	9.20	0.39	3
	2009	374.40	738.66	5	4.35	1.86	5	9488.79	4516.64	4	9.07	0.50	4
	2010	281.40	498.81	5	4.15	2.16	5	14013.05	3901.63	5	9.52	0.29	5
	2011	1116.33	2205.73	6	3.82	3.53	6	15859.38	3851.55	5	9.65	0.25	5
TN	1998	1833.24	3104.65	72	6.17	1.93	72	.	.	0	.	.	0
	1999	1727.65	3144.11	68	5.91	2.02	68	.	.	0	.	.	0

Table 7 Descriptive for the main outcomes in inpatient file (NIS) *(Continued)*

	Year												
	2000	1470.77	2468.48	31	6.01	1.78	31	.	.	0	.	.	0
	2001	1438.00	2464.06	35	5.64	2.17	35	4562.21	1795.46	29	8.36	0.37	29
	2002	1845.00	3862.56	34	5.15	2.67	34	4310.55	1858.99	22	8.29	0.40	22
	2003	2207.50	4185.64	36	5.89	2.40	36	5381.90	1763.20	30	8.53	0.35	30
	2004	2265.75	4246.16	36	5.93	2.26	36	7562.90	6767.82	32	8.73	0.57	32
	2005	1990.11	3053.85	36	6.01	2.28	36	6936.59	2475.87	28	8.78	0.38	28
	2006	2795.21	3671.37	29	6.41	2.36	29	8230.80	3046.92	25	8.95	0.36	25
	2007	1455.17	2652.67	29	5.32	2.58	29	5339.41	2889.22	26	8.44	0.57	26
	2008	2638.70	4431.94	27	6.03	2.44	27	9429.04	2560.64	22	9.12	0.26	22
	2009	1651.36	2714.76	25	5.78	2.22	25	9848.75	3194.17	24	9.13	0.39	24
	2010	1537.18	2614.39	22	5.38	2.71	22	10252.25	3812.88	20	9.14	0.49	20
	2011	2447.79	4205.03	24	6.43	1.90	24	13518.88	5054.30	20	9.46	0.32	20
TX	2000	2280.67	3318.77	86	6.63	1.83	86	.	.	0	.	.	0
	2001	2366.51	2957.74	88	6.67	1.93	88	.	.	0	.	.	0
	2002	2147.48	2706.98	91	6.41	2.21	91	.	.	0	.	.	0
	2003	2335.74	3213.95	95	6.39	2.19	95	.	.	0	.	.	0
	2004	2265.84	3261.44	93	6.46	1.98	93	.	.	0	.	.	0
	2005	1772.31	2742.68	106	6.04	2.09	106	.	.	0	.	.	0
	2006	1778.82	2528.57	97	6.04	2.23	97	11686.68	10867.66	70	9.10	0.67	70
	2007	1753.61	2467.78	101	5.97	2.27	101	12129.51	11358.05	68	9.21	0.53	68
	2008	1813.89	2547.18	93	6.13	2.19	93	13974.49	12296.02	77	9.34	0.58	77
	2009	1787.28	2829.91	90	6.11	2.10	90	16376.05	13945.55	72	9.50	0.57	72
	2010	1653.68	2405.36	94	6.13	2.05	94	20025.22	16300.70	77	9.67	0.64	77
	2011	2068.35	3832.54	86	6.08	2.10	86	22936.73	17392.40	65	9.83	0.62	65
UT	1998	951.13	1272.27	16	5.66	1.82	16	.	.	0	.	.	0
	1999	1043.24	1710.57	17	5.59	1.93	17	.	.	0	.	.	0
	2000	303.07	341.56	14	5.03	1.27	14	.	.	0	.	.	0
	2001	1192.63	2499.33	16	5.49	1.91	16	3912.22	1205.23	14	8.23	0.31	14
	2002	1711.67	3005.40	15	5.70	2.27	15	4483.40	1303.96	13	8.37	0.27	13
	2003	2156.69	3032.01	13	6.24	2.06	13	5476.93	2136.16	13	8.55	0.35	13
	2004	1291.25	2351.85	12	5.45	2.13	12	5652.46	998.71	12	8.63	0.18	12
	2005	1149.21	1475.50	14	5.87	2.02	14	6114.30	1903.72	12	8.68	0.29	12
	2006	2051.31	3181.74	13	6.12	2.03	13	8116.45	2674.15	11	8.96	0.28	11
	2007	951.67	1642.12	12	5.76	1.68	12	8199.12	2194.26	11	8.98	0.29	11
	2008	1880.54	3130.25	13	6.00	2.09	13	12319.15	10752.92	12	9.24	0.53	12
	2009	1146.50	2418.00	8	5.08	2.18	8	19066.46	24818.49	8	9.47	0.79	8
	2010	2356.40	2982.92	10	6.76	1.83	10	12233.34	4199.51	10	9.36	0.34	10
	2011	2072.78	2315.16	9	6.69	1.83	9	11939.88	2741.62	9	9.36	0.23	9
VA	1999	2163.83	3145.65	47	6.86	1.51	47	.	.	0	.	.	0
	2000	2957.81	4416.64	21	6.99	1.51	21	.	.	0	.	.	0
	2001	2650.17	4247.87	24	6.65	2.07	24	5364.76	1758.76	21	8.55	0.28	21
	2002	2027.21	2361.63	19	7.01	1.15	19	5466.07	1717.03	18	8.57	0.27	18
	2003	3626.33	5260.93	18	7.37	1.31	18	6327.16	1961.95	17	8.71	0.28	17
	2004	3353.11	5117.73	18	7.08	1.69	18	7853.96	3415.77	16	8.90	0.36	16
	2006	3331.60	5168.00	20	6.70	2.24	20	9050.88	2449.50	19	9.08	0.26	19

Table 7 Descriptive for the main outcomes in inpatient file (NIS) *(Continued)*

	2007	3551.24	5334.38	17	6.82	2.07	17	10806.18	4125.97	15	9.22	0.37	15
	2008	2944.38	3510.67	16	6.77	2.06	16	11820.56	3187.60	16	9.35	0.26	16
	2009	3149.15	4461.06	20	6.88	2.18	20	15278.79	12479.85	20	9.50	0.44	20
	2010	3420.63	4320.27	19	6.91	2.25	19	14843.37	8297.78	19	9.52	0.39	19
	2011	2619.26	2948.99	23	6.98	1.61	23	15971.69	5915.47	22	9.62	0.33	22
VT	2001	821.25	680.87	4	6.38	0.99	4	5666.61	615.50	3	8.64	0.11	3
	2002	628.20	570.37	5	6.16	0.81	5	6101.65	1089.40	2	8.71	0.18	2
	2003	775.25	603.56	4	6.46	0.68	4	7457.04	904.78	4	8.91	0.12	4
	2004	1633.14	3181.02	7	6.43	1.24	7	8481.75	1315.27	5	9.04	0.16	5
	2005	1836.50	3429.40	6	6.45	1.42	6	10568.57	2445.73	5	9.25	0.22	5
	2006	1607.57	3159.69	7	6.33	1.37	7	13503.54	4372.78	7	9.47	0.30	7
	2007	2427.50	3864.77	4	6.88	1.46	4	12292.48	2834.93	4	9.40	0.23	4
	2008	686.00	432.75	2	6.42	0.68	2	16488.16	3945.03	2	9.70	0.24	2
	2009	360.50	236.88	2	5.77	0.71	2	16712.07	3012.68	2	9.72	0.18	2
	2010	2827.67	4280.13	3	6.89	1.81	3	19730.94	2612.98	3	9.88	0.13	3
	2011	2011.25	3598.76	4	5.98	2.17	4	25073.62	1485.64	4	10.13	0.06	4
WA	1998	1678.91	2740.89	22	6.05	2.01	22	.	.	0	.	.	0
	1999	1636.73	1930.03	22	6.37	1.84	22	.	.	0	.	.	0
	2000	2030.09	2969.30	23	6.60	1.63	23	.	.	0	.	.	0
	2001	1888.52	2971.38	23	6.57	1.57	23	4905.84	1289.30	18	8.46	0.27	18
	2002	1850.46	2308.31	24	6.20	2.23	24	6189.36	1986.10	16	8.69	0.26	16
	2003	2079.50	2411.59	20	6.39	2.09	20	7138.43	1931.02	16	8.84	0.26	16
	2004	1931.00	2234.20	22	6.55	1.77	22	8257.66	3086.56	17	8.97	0.30	17
	2005	1561.41	1940.25	22	6.49	1.54	22	13840.24	20265.70	17	9.18	0.68	17
	2006	1887.29	3003.83	24	6.38	1.90	24	9767.47	3330.06	19	9.14	0.28	19
	2007	2212.80	3195.13	20	6.37	2.15	20	13778.54	13718.12	18	9.33	0.53	18
	2008	1838.39	2499.92	18	6.25	2.26	18	12219.06	3747.48	18	9.37	0.29	18
	2009	1748.53	2023.22	17	6.37	1.89	17	15604.95	6515.85	17	9.58	0.38	17
	2010	1930.28	2773.72	18	6.43	1.67	18	19868.53	8770.69	17	9.82	0.40	17
	2011	1671.89	2321.80	19	6.29	1.71	19	18375.82	8458.34	17	9.74	0.39	17
WI	1998	1625.94	2337.00	66	6.45	1.51	66	.	.	0	.	.	0
	1999	1492.06	2452.53	65	6.13	1.80	65	.	.	0	.	.	0
	2000	1558.05	2495.54	66	6.23	1.66	66	.	.	0	.	.	0
	2001	1477.54	2870.39	35	6.04	1.77	35	4836.80	1495.99	24	8.44	0.28	24
	2002	1438.72	1895.53	29	6.35	1.57	29	6162.16	1674.11	23	8.70	0.25	23
	2003	1226.64	1772.33	28	5.92	1.73	28	6551.88	1445.91	18	8.76	0.23	18
	2004	1504.37	2333.54	27	6.22	1.58	27	7589.25	1888.95	21	8.90	0.27	21
	2005	1478.83	2072.28	30	6.24	1.63	30	8909.31	2088.56	26	9.07	0.23	26
	2006	1660.79	3368.63	29	5.83	2.07	29	10397.91	1885.77	24	9.23	0.17	24
	2007	1297.37	2005.02	27	5.99	1.80	27	12846.44	9489.97	25	9.35	0.39	25
	2008	1593.83	2328.41	30	6.07	2.07	30	12701.90	2608.61	28	9.43	0.22	28
	2009	1259.47	2216.66	30	5.74	2.12	30	18466.41	15143.07	29	9.67	0.48	29
	2010	1736.61	2211.16	28	6.11	2.21	28	17365.88	10329.55	27	9.69	0.33	27
	2011	1432.87	2180.68	30	5.91	2.19	30	17795.42	5877.10	27	9.73	0.38	27

Table 7 Descriptive for the main outcomes in inpatient file (NIS) *(Continued)*

WV	2000	472.63	557.48	19	4.94	2.21	19	.	.	0	.	.	0
	2001	248.80	278.53	15	4.51	1.88	15	3888.09	534.79	5	8.26	0.13	5
	2002	1351.47	3077.94	19	5.29	2.30	19	4409.61	2031.18	8	8.27	0.57	8
	2003	1049.50	1569.87	18	5.31	2.37	18	5942.96	2070.32	16	8.63	0.36	16
	2004	814.67	1118.55	15	5.64	1.77	15	5359.41	1357.20	6	8.56	0.25	6
	2005	2531.00	3497.98	14	6.77	2.06	14	7780.89	2124.96	9	8.92	0.29	9
	2006	823.38	1262.49	13	5.26	2.11	13	7300.30	1453.31	6	8.88	0.20	6
	2007	1574.67	2429.76	15	5.42	2.68	15	9333.81	3269.12	8	9.09	0.32	8
	2008	1678.00	2495.48	13	5.05	3.14	13	10792.28	5094.92	11	9.17	0.52	11
	2009	919.25	1309.24	12	5.92	1.59	12	10234.95	1996.01	11	9.22	0.19	11
	2010	1210.15	1406.11	13	6.14	1.83	13	14794.36	10101.22	11	9.48	0.45	11
	2011	2780.43	4238.53	7	6.30	2.34	7	19117.61	11847.47	7	9.74	0.48	7
WY	2007	430.00	270.70	4	5.90	0.67	4	12490.09	4404.88	4	9.39	0.35	4
	2008	257.00	318.24	6	4.54	1.86	6	13683.53	3694.38	4	9.50	0.25	4
	2009	414.00	355.24	7	5.56	1.16	7	14386.57	4346.47	7	9.54	0.29	7
	2010	319.14	300.32	7	5.17	1.38	7	13824.34	1395.73	7	9.53	0.11	7
	2011	405.00	254.13	6	5.58	1.35	6	17362.34	5164.73	6	9.72	0.33	6

Table 8 Descriptive for the main outcomes in outpatient file (SASD)

Hospital state	Calendar year	Total number of surgical procedures			Log of total number of surgical procedures		
		Mean	Std	N	Mean	Std	N
CA	2007	3515.62	3625.26	853	7.57	1.32	852
	2008	3432.36	3886.85	831	7.48	1.38	831
	2009	4068.27	4485.46	584	7.73	1.24	584
	2010	4377.43	4874.96	497	7.78	1.27	497
	2011	4527.95	5071.43	458	7.77	1.37	458
CO	2008	4870.29	5532.98	78	7.42	2.09	78
	2009	5103.38	5509.80	74	7.67	1.74	74
	2010	5498.03	5641.74	73	7.80	1.62	73
	2011	5576.49	5952.14	78	7.77	1.66	78
	2012	5473.14	5843.59	78	7.65	1.89	78
FL	2007	5410.50	5283.45	572	8.19	1.03	572
	2008	5337.35	5276.53	587	8.17	1.05	587
	2009	5223.05	4927.84	588	8.17	1.01	588
	2010	5109.85	4912.04	590	8.13	1.04	590
	2011	4832.48	4472.26	605	8.08	1.06	605
	2012	4834.20	4207.72	599	8.13	0.95	599
	2013	4792.27	4237.82	605	8.09	1.05	605
KY	2007	7385.13	8979.66	104	8.13	1.42	104
	2008	13539.70	16737.80	105	8.86	1.21	105
	2009	13416.91	17141.52	131	8.83	1.22	131
	2010	11449.95	14604.36	150	8.67	1.24	150
	2011	10718.50	14358.56	164	8.53	1.39	164
	2012	10301.86	14306.77	177	8.38	1.52	177
	2013	14892.33	20248.58	206	8.69	1.58	206
MD	1998	6807.10	5681.28	52	8.49	0.90	52
	1999	6884.13	5819.98	52	8.47	0.96	52
	2000	7560.06	6166.07	49	8.64	0.82	49
	2001	8000.85	6432.89	48	8.66	0.93	48
	2002	8250.75	6402.70	48	8.74	0.80	48
	2003	17713.54	22895.29	48	9.29	0.96	48
	2004	18459.33	23312.07	48	9.39	0.85	48
	2005	19235.23	23951.71	48	9.43	0.88	48
	2006	20425.46	26811.17	48	9.48	0.86	48
	2007	38515.06	44829.21	52	9.93	1.45	52
	2008	64059.83	71433.03	52	10.52	1.35	52
	2009	65421.62	84632.03	52	10.51	1.35	52
	2010	65719.71	86014.19	51	10.51	1.34	51
	2011	64722.55	89320.17	53	10.26	1.83	53
	2012	64992.65	93877.46	54	10.13	2.11	54
NJ	2008	5504.35	4211.93	79	8.13	1.33	79
	2009	6039.51	4190.19	75	8.28	1.32	75
	2010	6359.12	4434.84	74	8.40	1.12	74
	2011	6489.85	4579.18	74	8.39	1.23	74
	2012	6287.65	4574.22	75	8.26	1.53	75
	2013	6199.96	4668.46	75	8.22	1.48	75

Authors' contribution

For this manuscript, JES led the study and had primary responsibility of the manuscript. RO provided scientific input and writing. PL led the statistical analysis, and TM provided input and editing. CS provided research support and editing. All authors read and approved the final manuscript.

Competing interests

The study was completed by Avalon Health Economics, funded by the American Society of Anesthesiologists (ASA). Thomas Miller is the representative of ASA who supervised the project. Schneider and Scheibling are employees of Avalon Health Economics. Ohsfeldt and Li are contractors to Avalon Health Economics.

Author details

[1]Avalon Health Economics, LLC, 26 Washington Street, 3rd Fl, 07960 Morristown, NJ, USA. [2]Health Policy & Management, Texas A&M University, 212 Adriance Lab Rd, 1266 TAMU, 77843-1266 College Station, TX, USA. [3]Division of General Internal Medicine, University of Pennsylvania, 423 Guardian Dr, Philadelphia, PA 19104, USA. [4]American Society of Anesthesiologists, 1061 American Lane, 60173-4973 Schaumburg, IL, USA. [5]Avalon Health Economics, 26 Washington Street, 3rd Fl., 07960 Morristown, NJ, USA.

References

1. CMS. Medicare Medicaid programs; hospital Conditions of Participation: anesthesia services. Final rule. Fed Regist. 2001;66(219):56762–9.
2. Sun E, Dexter F, Miller TR. The Effect of "Opt-Out" Regulation on Access to Surgical Care for Urgent Cases in the United States: Evidence from the National Inpatient Sample. Anesth Analg. 2016;122(6):1983–91.
3. Census Bureau US. Estimates of the total resident population and resident population age 18 years and older for the United States, States, and Puerto Rico: July 1, 2015 (SCPRC-EST2015-18 + POP-RES). 2015.
4. Dulisse B, Cromwell J. No harm found when nurse anesthetists work without supervision by physicians. Health Aff. 2010;29(8):1469–75.
5. Lewis SR, Nicholson A, Smith AF, Alderson P. Physician anaesthetists versus non-physician providers of anaesthesia for surgical patients. Cochrane Database Syst Rev. 2014; Issue 7. Art. No.: CD010357:1–78.
6. Manchikanti L, Caraway DL, Falco FJ, Benyamin RM, Hansen H, Hirsch JA. CMS proposal for interventional pain management by nurse anesthetists: evidence by proclamation with poor prognosis. Pain Physician. 2012;15(5):E641–64.
7. Daugherty L, Fonseca R, Kumar K, Michaud P. An Analysis of the Labor Markets for Anesthesiology. Santa Monica, CA: RAND Corporation; 2010. http://www.rand.org/pubs/technical_reports/TR688.html.
8. Sun E, Dexter F, Miller TR. The effect of "opt-out" regulation on access to surgical care for urgent cases in the United States: Evidence from the National Inpatient Sample. Anesth Analg. 2016;122(6):1983–91.
9. Sun E, Miller TR, Halzack N. In the United States, "opt-out" States Show no increase in access to anesthesia services for Medicare beneficiaries compared with non–"opt-out" States. Anesth Analg Case Rep. 2016;6(9):283–5.
10. Cullen KA, Hall MJ, Golosinskiy A. Ambulatory Surgery in the United States, 2006. National Health Statistics Reports; no 11. Revised. U.S. Centers for Disease Control and Prevention: Hyattsville, MD; 2009.
11. Pope G, Kautter J, Ellis R, Ash AS, Ayanian JZ, Iezzoni LI, Ingber MJ, Levy JM, Robst J. Risk adjustment of Medicare capitation payments using the CMS-HCC Model. Health Care Financ Rev. 2004;25(4):119–41.
12. Kennedy P. Estimation with correctly interpreted dummy variables in semilogarithmic equations. Am Econ Rev. 1981;71(4):801.

17

Distinct impacts of high intensity caregiving on caregivers' mental health and continuation of caregiving

Narimasa Kumagai

Abstract

Although high-intensity caregiving has been found to be associated with a greater prevalence of mental health problems, little is known about the specifics of this relationship. This study clarified the burden of informal caregivers quantitatively and provided policy implications for long-term care policies in countries with aging populations. Using data collected from a nationwide five-wave panel survey in Japan, I examined two causal relationships: (1) high-intensity caregiving and mental health of informal caregivers, and (2) high-intensity caregiving and continuation of caregiving. Considering the heterogeneity in high-intensity caregiving among informal caregivers, control function model which allows for heterogeneous treatment effects was used.

This study uncovered three major findings. First, hours of caregiving was found to influence the continuation of high-intensity caregiving among non-working informal caregivers and irregular employees. Specifically, caregivers who experienced high-intensity caregiving (20–40 h) tended to continue with it to a greater degree than did caregivers who experienced ultra-high-intensity caregiving (40 h or more). Second, high-intensity caregiving was associated with worse mental health among non-working caregivers, but did not have any effect on the mental health of irregular employees. The control function model revealed that caregivers engaging in high-intensity caregiving who were moderately mentally healthy in the past tended to have serious mental illness currently. Third, non-working caregivers did not tend to continue high-intensity caregiving for more than three years, regardless of co-residential caregiving. This is because current high-intensity caregiving was not associated with the continuation of caregiving when I included high-intensity caregiving provided during the previous period in the regression. Overall, I noted distinct impacts of high-intensity caregiving on the mental health of informal caregivers and that such caregiving is persistent among non-working caregivers who experienced it for at least a year. Supporting non-working intensive caregivers as a public health issue should be considered a priority.

Keywords: Control function approach, High-intensity caregiving, Informal caregiver, Japan, Mental health, State dependence

Background

Co-residential informal caregiving leads to increased stress and lowered psychological health. The intensity of caregiving in co-residential situations appears to be much greater than in extra-residential ones, and this high-intensity caregiving (i.e., 20 or more h per week) leads to especially poor health among family caregivers. "Intensive carers," defined as those who provide more than 20 h of care per week, are more likely to stop working and to have worse mental health outcomes as a result of their caregiving responsibilities [1]. Drawing on British Household Panel Survey data (1991–2000), Hirst showed that individuals who provided high-intensity caregiving had double the risk of psychological distress as did non-caregivers [2].[1] Notably, this effect was greater in women. Colombo et al. argued that high-intensity caregiving is associated with a higher risk of poverty [1].[2] Despite these findings, relatively little is known about the precise impact of high-intensity caregiving on mental health. To address this, I focused on two causal relationships among informal caregivers: between high-intensity caregiving and mental health, and between high-intensity caregiving and continuation of caregiving. The latter relationship was

Correspondence: narimasa@kindai.ac.jp

Faculty of Economics, Kindai University, 3-4-1 Kowakae, Higashiosaka, Osaka 577-8502, Japan examined because a longer duration of high-intensity care appears to exhaust caregivers to a greater degree than does a shorter duration. As such, I wanted to clarify how caregivers' informal caregiving changes with psychological distress during care provision.

In 2006, Japan revised its social long-term care insurance (LTCI) entitlement for mildly disabled older people into a "prevention system," which aims to help those eligible for support to better maintain their independence.[3] Such approaches can be combined with more adequate support strategies for family caregivers [3]. Colombo et al. suggested that supporting family caregivers is effectively a win-win solution, because it involves far less public expenditure for a given amount of care [1]. Indeed, the support of family caregivers is an important public health issue, both in Japan and worldwide.[4] Thus, I aimed to determine whether respite care is useful for supporting the mental health of informal caregivers engaged in high-intensity caregiving. Some previous studies have demonstrated that respite care has a positive effect on caregivers.[5] It is possible that the influence may be greater for caregivers engaged in high-intensity care, while day care appears to be more effective for carers in paid employment (i.e., who are engaged in less intensive care) [4]. Furthermore, the use of a short-term stay service funded by the LTCI has demonstrated positive effects on the well-being of family caregivers. This service is perhaps the most efficient, followed by home-helper services [5]. Greater use of day-care and respite short-stay services have indicated that such services might provide traditional female caregivers with temporary relief from their care burden [6].[6]

As stated before, I investigated the longitudinal associations between high-intensity caregiving and caregivers' mental health, and between high-intensity caregiving and continuation of caregiving in an older adult population. A random-effects probit estimation was employed to reveal the determinants of both caregivers' mental health and continuation of caregiving. However, it must be noted that caregivers often make adjustments in employment status to facilitate caregiving, such as reducing work hours or quitting work altogether [7]. Therefore, it seemed necessary to classify informal caregivers by their employment status (regular employees, irregular employees, and non-working caregivers). In dividing participants by their employment status, I was aware that I would also be dividing participants by their intensity of informal caregiving. This was supported by the fact that a preliminary analysis indicated a difference in hours of caregiving between various employment status groups, even after controlling for other socioeconomic and demographic characteristics. Considering this heterogeneity in high-intensity caregiving among informal caregivers by employment status, I estimated mental health

functions using the control function approach. This approach allows for assessment of heterogeneous treatment effects combined with self-selection of treatment.

This paper is organized as follows. Section 2 provides a literature review of the effects of high-intensity caregiving on caregivers' health and formal care use. Section 3 outlines the characteristics of the nationally representative sample used in this study and the variables of interest, such as caregivers' mental health. In Section 4, I describe the empirical methods and report the estimation results. Section 5 contains conclusions.

Effects of high-intensity caregiving on caregivers' health and formal care use

Caregivers are at risk of becoming patients themselves. Furthermore, most studies have found that caregiver burden is higher for women than for men. This discrepancy may be partially explained by how traditional gender roles place greater pressure on women to commit to the caregiver role [8].[7] Additionally, Brouwer et al. reported that disrupted life schedules and caregivers' health problems were the strongest predictors of subjective burden scores [9].

Objective burden must be considered independently of subjective burden, since caregivers' mental state can alter their perception of their personal burden, regardless of their actual burden [10]. The objective burden of informal caregiving is typically defined as the amount of time spent on this activity. Brouwer et al. found that a greater time spent on caregiving is related to reduced quality of life and probability of having paid employment in the labor force [9].[8] Using a population-based sample, Beach et al. found that an increasing intensity of care was associated with increasingly poor (mental) health for caregivers [11]. Houser and Gibson similarly found that the greater the intensity of caregiving, the greater the magnitude of the health effects due to chronic stress [12]. Additionally, caregiving, particularly intensive caregiving, reduced female labor force participation and hours worked [13–15].

In Japan, informal caregivers can purchase formal care services from LTCI, depending on the eligibility levels of care recipients (i.e., their care needs or support level). Individuals who engage in less intensive caregiving might prefer formal care to informal care—for example, workers with caregiving responsibilities, as it may ease the intensity of informal caregiving and allow them to continue their work. Sugawara and Nakamura found that regular workers are more likely to utilize formal care, whereas non-regular workers tend to provide informal care by themselves [16].[9] Informal care can serve as a substitute for formal long-term care in the sense that elderly parents can receive needed assistance (e.g., in eating or taking a bath) from their children [17].[10] Indeed, Kikuchi confirmed that informal care by a co-residential caregiver had a negative effect on the use of institutional care services [18].

In the present study, changes in work status during care provision were assumed to occur for exogenous reasons, despite the fact that many informal caregivers make simultaneous decisions about formal care use, informal caregiving, labor participation, and living arrangements. Furthermore, due to the limited data on formal care services, the availability of such services was not taken into account in the present study. Instead, I created a proxy variable of formal care use as a dummy variable of respite care, which took on the value of 1 if hours spent on caregiving exceeded work hours in the past year and work hours exceeded hours spent on caregiving this year. Using this dummy variable, I examined whether respite care was useful for informal caregivers in reducing the negative effects of high-intensity caregiving.

Methods
Data
The data used in this study were drawn from five waves of the Longitudinal Survey of Middle-aged and Elderly Persons (LSMEP; 2005–2009) conducted by the Japanese Ministry of Health, Labor and Welfare (MHLW). The LSMEP is a nationally representative sample of the near elderly in Japan (individuals aged 50–59 entered the sample initially). The LSMEP collects information about family situation, health status, and employment status on an annual basis using self-report questionnaires. Samples in the first wave were collected nationwide in November 2005 through a two-stage random sampling procedure.[11]

Samples
I examined regular employees, irregular employees, and non-working caregivers separately, given their different propensities for providing informal care. I further delineated non-working caregivers by social status.[12] Individuals who were not working were categorized as workers during a period of family care leave or unemployment, or as otherwise inactive persons (including homemakers and retirees). I defined informal caregivers who were seeking employment as unemployed. Informal caregivers who did not respond to the questions about labor participation and earned income were defined as "non-working caregivers." Most Japanese companies have a mandatory retirement system—at the time of the 2005 survey, employees were allowed to work until age 60; however, the official employable age was raised from 60 to 65 in 2013.

To explore the effects of high-intensity caregiving on the mental health of informal caregivers, I utilized only those LSMEP respondents who were reported caregivers. To isolate these individuals, I created a respondent-level dataset, and then limited the sample to individuals who had responded to the question on hours of informal caregiving.

The subjects who had not filled out this information were excluded. In total, this sample comprised 15,273 subjects, including 3,445 inactive persons (e.g., homemakers, retirees), 784 workers during a period of family care leave, 486 unemployed individuals, 6,978 irregular employees, and 3,580 regular employees. Because poor mental health status might occur due to unemployment, I excluded unemployed caregivers in the regression analysis.

Main measures
Dependent variables
As a measure of objective mental health measures, the Kessler 6 non-specific distress scale (K6) developed by Kessler et al. [19] was used. The K6 is a six-item psychological screening instrument that was included in the LSMEP. The K6 scale asked respondents how frequently they experienced the following six symptoms: "During the past 30 days, about how often did you feel a) nervous, b) hopeless, c) restless or fidgety, d) so depressed that nothing could cheer you up, e) that everything was an effort, and f) worthless?" For each question, participants answered on a 5-point scale where responses of "none of the time," "a little of the time," "some of the time," "most of the time," or "all of the time" were assigned values of zero, one, two, three, and four, respectively. The responses to the six items were summed to yield a K6 score between 0 and 24, with higher scores indicating a greater tendency towards mental illness. A K6 cut-off point of 13 was established to operationalize the definition of "serious mental distress." Moderate mental distress was defined as $5 \leq K6 < 13$.[13] However, as Oshio [20] argued, because the results were not free from potential biases due to their self-reported nature, I created a dichotomous variable of serious mental illness as well as an ordinal variable (serious = 2, moderate = 1, otherwise = 0).

Primary explanatory variables
A preliminary analysis revealed that non-working caregivers spent more hours on caregiving per week on average than did working caregivers. Specifically, the proportions of individuals who engaged in high-intensity caregiving (20 or more hours per week) were as follows: regular employees, 14.4%; irregular employees, 20.8%; inactive persons, 27.2%; unemployed, 26.5%; and care leave, 50.3%.[14]

It is important to be aware of the non-proportional relationship between hours of caregiving and caregivers' perceived burden. Assessing caregivers' burden with the Zarit Burden Interview, Arai and Ueda confirmed that these two variables are not directly connected [21]. Thus, because longer duration of caregiving does not directly mean that caregivers will have greater burden, simply measuring the presence or absence of high-intensity caregiving might not be an adequate explanatory variable of continuation of caregiving. Therefore, I used three dichotomous variables to measure intensity of caregiving, as follows: (I) 20 or more hours per week = 1, otherwise = 0; (II) more than 20 h and less than 40 h per week = 1, otherwise = 0; and (III) 40 or more hours per week = 1, otherwise = 0. Note that (I) includes (II) and (III).

The LSMEP included items relating to the family member(s) for whom respondents provided care (i.e., father, mother, father-in-law, mother-in-law, and others) at the time of the study. I constructed four binary variables indicating informal care provision for the four family member types (i.e., father, mother, father-in-law, mother-in-law). These dummy variables are the main explanatory variables of interest because a preliminary analysis revealed that the proportion of co-residential caregivers engaged in high-intensity caregiving was relatively higher for care recipient who was a mother or mother-in-law.[15] Furthermore, because co-residential caregivers might commit to more hours of informal care than extra-residential caregivers, and co-residence may reflect having care recipients with higher care needs, co-residential care is often used as a proxy for more intensive care [22, 23].[16] Co-residential adult children have traditionally been the main caregivers in Japan; for example, in 2010, 64% of caregivers for care recipients in the home were co-residential family members.[17] Caregiving for a resident parent is associated with depressive symptoms and sleeping problems; indeed, even just having a parent in need of care increases the likelihood of depression [24].

The effect of respite care was measured by using a time-averaged proxy variable of formal care use. I created this proxy variable to use as a dummy variable of respite care, which took on the value of 1 if hours spent on caregiving exceeded work hours in the previous year and work hours exceeded hours spent on caregiving this year; otherwise it took on the value of 0. [18]

Empirical analysis
Dynamic random-effects probit model and control function (CF) approach
The specifications of the high-intensity caregiving function dictate that the response probability of a positive outcome depends on unobserved effects and past experience. It is important to consider unobserved heterogeneity because ignoring it can lead to overestimation of the degree of state dependence. The random-effects probit model specification allows for unobserved heterogeneity but it treats the initial conditions as exogenous. Estimating a standard uncorrelated random-effects probit model implicitly assumes zero correlation between the unobserved effect and set of explanatory variables.[19] Treatment of the initial conditions in a dynamic random-effects probit (DREP) model is crucial, since misspecification will result in an inflated parameter of the lagged dependent variable term. Additionally, ignoring the initial conditions problem

yields inconsistent estimates [25, 26]. Kumagai and Ogura is a study which overcomes the initial conditions problem [27]. Using the procedure described in [26], they estimated DREP models and revealed that the degree of dependence between previous health stock and current health stock exhibited moderate persistence.[20]

I estimate the DREP models of high-intensity caregiving function in this study. The core econometric specification of this function is as follows:

$$HI_t = f(\beta_C C_t + \beta_{HI} HI_{t-1} + HC'_t\beta_{HC} + D'_t\beta_D + \beta_S S_t + \beta_W W_t + X'_t\beta_X)$$
(1)

where HI is a measure of high-intensity caregiving, C a measure of co-residential caregiving, HC' a vector of the health status of caregivers, D' a vector of demographic variables, S the presence of social relationships (having friends/acquaintances), W the wage rate of caregivers or the relative resources of non-working caregivers, and X' a vector of other socioeconomic variables. β_C, β_{HI}, β_{HC}, β_D, β_S, β_W, and β_X are the coefficients to be estimated. The subscript t indexes time periods. In this analysis, the function f is the probit function when HI is dichotomous. All models included the following covariates: co-residential caregiving; informal care provision for each of the four types of family members; age; marital status (married, divorced, or widowed, with never married as the comparison group); current employment; educational attainment (junior-high education, some post-secondary education, university degree, and graduate degree, with high school completion as the comparison group).

As mentioned above, the subsamples by employment status had differing intensities of informal caregiving. Thus, I am treating the heterogeneity as individual-specific in estimating the effect of explanatory variables on the outcomes of interest.[21] I examined two causal relationships: (1) high-intensity caregiving and mental health of informal caregivers, and (2) high-intensity caregiving and continuation of caregiving. Considering the heterogeneity in high-intensity caregiving among informal caregivers, a method that allows for heterogeneous treatment effects combined with self-selection into treatment is necessary for appropriate analysis of these relationships. Thus, I estimated the following control function model.

When unobservables, $u_{i,t}$ and $\varepsilon_{i,t}$, are assumed to be linearly related to $v_{i,t}$[22] and all unobservables are assumed to be independent of $z_{i,t}$ (i.e., covariates used for modeling the outcome), then $v_{i,t}$ will have a zero mean. Equation (2) can be used to estimate the average treatment effect of high-intensity caregiving. Specifically, the outcome variable of the estimating equation is $MH_{i,t}$ (i.e., the mental health of informal caregivers) and a treatment $HI_{i,t}$ (i.e., a measure of high-intensity caregiving). A dummy variable indicating the treatment condition $HI_{i,t}$ (i.e., $HI_{i,t} = 1$ if informal caregiver i engages in high-intensity caregiving at time t, and 0 otherwise) is directly entered into the regression equation and the outcome variable $MH_{i,t}$ is observed for both $HI_{i,t} = 1$ and $HI_{i,t} = 0$.

$$MH_{i,t} = \eta HI_{i,t} + z_{i,t}{}'\omega + \varepsilon_{i,t},$$

$$HI_{i,t}^* = k_{i,t}{}'\alpha + u_{i,t}, HI_{i,t} = 1 \text{ if } HI_{i,t}^* > 0, \text{ and } HI_{i,t} = 0 \text{ otherwise}$$
(2)

$$E\left(\varepsilon_{i,t} | v_{i,t}\right) = \psi_1 v_{i,t}, \; E\left(u_{i,t} | v_{i,t}\right) = \psi_2 v_{i,t}$$

where $k_{i,t}$ are the covariates used to model treatment assignment. The covariates $z_{i,t}$ and $k_{i,t}$ are unrelated to the error terms.

According to Wooldridge's procedure [28], the control function approach can be used to estimate the following model for a binary treatment variable. After obtaining the generalized residuals ($grHI_{i,t}$) of $HI_{i,t}$ in the regression equation, the control function regression is as follows:

$$MH_{i,t} = \theta_0 + \theta_1 MH_{i,t-1} + \theta_2 HI_{i,t} + z_{i,t}{}'\theta_3 \\ + \theta_4 grHI_{i,t} + \theta_5 (HI_{i,t} \times grHI_{i,t}) + \varepsilon_{i,t} \quad (3)$$

This second-stage regression equation (3) including the generalized residual is without exclusion restrictions due to the residuals' nonlinearity [29].[23] Estimating Eq. (3) allows researcher to analyze whether high-intensity caregiving is associated with worse mental health among informal caregivers. Note that because the effect of moderate or serious mental health was considered persistent for informal caregivers, the lagged mental health variable was used.

Although there are no required exclusion restrictions for endogenous selection models [29, 30], such restrictions are useful for ensuring appropriate identification of the parameters. To control for any factors that might influence the probability of high-intensity caregiving, the initial value of caregiving was included as an exclusion restriction. Notably, there were positive correlations between the initial value of caregiving and high-intensity caregiving among non-working caregivers (0.163, $p < .01$). In contrast, there were no correlations between the initial value of caregiving and serious mental distress among this same employment group. In the preliminary analysis, I observed that the initial value of caregiving had significant ($p < .01$) positive effects on the high-intensity caregiving of both non-working caregivers and irregular employees.

Results and Discussion
Descriptive statistics

Table 1 presents the descriptive statistics of the employment status groups. The proportion of inactive persons who engaged in high-intensity caregiving (20–40 h or 40 h or more) was 27.2% (15.4%, 11.8%), which was higher than the 20.8% (12.8%, 8%) among informal caregivers with part-time work. Of all workers, the proportion of workers taking family care leave who engaged in high-intensity caregiving was the highest among the employment status groups, at 50.3% (22.8%, 27.4%). Regarding the outcomes of interest, the rate of moderate mental distress among inactive persons was 31.6%, which was slightly higher than the 31.1% for informal caregivers with part-time work. In contrast, workers who were taking family care leave had a higher prevalence of severe mental distress (14.3%) than did inactive persons (11.1%).

Most workers taking family care leave were female, and the proportion of these workers who had a drinking habit was the largest among all informal caregivers studied. If there were a simultaneity issue for non-working female caregivers, the relationship between serious mental distress and risky health behavior such as a drinking habit or a smoking habit would likely be positive even after controlling for the other covariates. Considering this possible simultaneity, I did not use lifestyle variables as covariates of the high-intensity caregiving function in further analyses.

As noted above, I constructed a binary variable of co-residential caregiving for each family member type other than spouse. A change from 1 to 0 in this variable indicated a shift from co-residential caregiving to non-residential caregiving.[24] The rate of co-residential caregiving was lowest (0.721) among inactive caregivers, while that of regular employees was 0.825.

Around 7% of inactive persons did not answer the question about their hours of caregiving per week. As such, they were excluded from the remainder of the analyses.

Determinants of high-intensity caregiving

To estimate the determinants of high-intensity caregiving, I estimated random-effects probit models for regular employees, irregular employees, and non-working caregivers. The estimation results for both non-working caregivers and irregular employees showed that co-residential caregiving was significantly positively related to high-intensity caregiving. In contrast, co-residential caregiving had no significant effect on high-intensity caregiving among regular employees. Thus, I focused only on the determinants of high-intensity caregiving among the non-working informal caregivers and irregular employees.[25]

Because there are no available means of dealing with caregiving histories with the initial year missing, left-censored spells are typically omitted from this analysis. To

Table 1 Descriptive statistics of four samples by employment status

Variables	Non-working									Irregular employees			Regular employees		
	Total			Inactive persons			Care leave								
	N	Mean	S.D.	N	Mean	S.D.	N	Mean	S.D.	N	Mean	S.D.	N	Mean	S.D.
Dependent variables															
High-intensity caregiving	4715	0.309	0.46	3445	0.272	0.44	784	0.503	0.50	6978	0.208	0.41	3580	0.144	0.35
High-intensity caregiving (initial)	3957	0.144	0.35	2943	0.131	0.34	618	0.244	0.43	5804	0.085	0.28	2852	0.059	0.24
High-intensity caregiving (20–40 h)	4715	0.165	0.37	3445	0.154	0.36	784	0.228	0.42	6978	0.128	0.33	3580	0.090	0.29
Ultra-high-intensity caregiving (40 h or more)	4715	0.145	0.35	3445	0.118	0.32	784	0.274	0.45	6978	0.080	0.27	3580	0.054	0.23
Sum of K6	4483	4.834	4.71	3277	4.493	4.57	750	5.991	4.97	6540	4.272	4.47	3440	3.903	4.29
Serious mental health ($13 \leq K6$)	4715	0.119	0.32	3445	0.111	0.31	784	0.143	0.35	6978	0.115	0.32	3580	0.082	0.27
Moderate mental health ($5 \leq K6 < 13$)	4715	0.344	0.47	3445	0.316	0.47	784	0.430	0.50	6978	0.311	0.46	3580	0.297	0.46
Explanatory variables															
Co-residential caregiving	4715	0.743	0.44	3445	0.721	0.45	784	0.809	0.39	6978	0.791	0.41	3580	0.825	0.38
Sex (male = 1)	4715	0.145	0.35	3445	0.121	0.33	784	0.121	0.33	6978	0.353	0.48	3580	0.638	0.48
Age	4715	57.56	2.97	3445	57.87	2.91	784	56.72	2.93	6978	57.11	2.99	3580	56.07	2.71
Married	4715	0.737	0.44	3445	0.732	0.44	784	0.754	0.43	6978	0.765	0.42	3580	0.792	0.41
Divorced or widowed	4715	0.010	0.10	3445	0.008	0.09	784	0.010	0.10	6978	0.013	0.11	3580	0.016	0.13
Care recipient															
Father	4715	0.144	0.35	3445	0.139	0.35	784	0.163	0.37	6978	0.173	0.38	3580	0.221	0.41
Mother	4715	0.478	0.50	3445	0.472	0.50	784	0.469	0.50	6978	0.472	0.50	3580	0.532	0.50
Father-in-law	4715	0.083	0.28	3445	0.077	0.27	784	0.106	0.31	6978	0.094	0.29	3580	0.077	0.27
Mother-in-law	4715	0.287	0.45	3445	0.298	0.46	784	0.283	0.45	6978	0.279	0.45	3580	0.211	0.41
Caregiver's income source, health status															
Relative resources or logged wage rate	4715	1.627	2.09	3445	1.712	2.10	784	1.638	2.05	5356	0.818	0.28	2985	0.927	0.15
Dummy for difficulty in daily life activities	4557	0.175	0.38	3339	0.181	0.39	752	0.156	0.36	6690	0.116	0.32	3477	0.078	0.27
Dummy for medication or doctor's consultation	4715	0.297	0.46	3445	0.317	0.47	784	0.224	0.42	6978	0.289	0.45	3580	0.304	0.46
Dummy for hospitalization during the past year	4715	0.024	0.15	3445	0.027	0.16	784	0.011	0.11	6978	0.016	0.13	3580	0.018	0.13
Diabetes	4024	0.093	0.29	2970	0.095	0.29	659	0.064	0.24	5831	0.091	0.29	3183	0.094	0.29
Heart disease (angina, myocardial infarction)	4018	0.041	0.20	2962	0.044	0.20	661	0.024	0.15	5825	0.042	0.20	3183	0.038	0.19
Cerebral stroke	4017	0.022	0.15	2961	0.024	0.15	660	0.006	0.08	5822	0.015	0.12	3180	0.013	0.11
Hypertension	4034	0.234	0.42	2972	0.248	0.43	665	0.203	0.40	5855	0.263	0.44	3195	0.250	0.43
Hyperlipidemia	4026	0.166	0.37	2968	0.175	0.38	661	0.127	0.33	5837	0.163	0.37	3192	0.196	0.40
Cancer	4012	0.032	0.18	2958	0.038	0.19	659	0.009	0.10	5808	0.021	0.14	3173	0.020	0.14
Caregiver's lifestyle															
Having friends/acquaintances	4642	0.829	0.38	3390	0.833	0.37	776	0.825	0.38	6789	0.867	0.34	3527	0.841	0.37
Dummy for current smoker	4715	0.136	0.34	3445	0.118	0.32	784	0.125	0.33	6978	0.226	0.42	3580	0.295	0.46
Dummy for almost every day or every day drinker	4715	0.303	0.46	3445	0.299	0.46	784	0.328	0.47	6978	0.289	0.45	3580	0.258	0.44
Dummy for regular physical activity	4715	0.542	0.50	3445	0.552	0.50	784	0.503	0.50	6978	0.420	0.49	3580	0.426	0.49

High-intensity caregiving (initial) refers to high-intensity caregiving in 2005, when the LSMEP launched
Sources: Longitudinal Survey of Middle-aged and Elderly Persons 2005, 2006, 2007, 2008 and 2009

manage the left-censoring problem in this study, I took into account the initial period choice, because state dependence implies that initial period choices depend endogenously on earlier choices causing left censoring. Thus, I included the initial value of high-intensity caregiving as an explanatory variable in the regression models.

Table 2 shows the estimated determinants of high-intensity caregiving among non-working informal caregivers

Table 2 High-intensity caregiving functions

Independent variables	Non-working	Irregular employees	Regular employees
High-intensity caregiving (−1)			
20–40 h (−1)	0.919***	1.031***	1.013***
	(0.116)	(0.136)	(0.199)
40 h or more (−1)	0.744***	0.538***	0.374*
	(0.104)	(0.116)	(0.194)
High-intensity caregiving (initial)	0.573***	0.550***	0.579***
	(0.115)	(0.134)	(0.189)
m (non-attendance of health checkup)	8.613***	2.081	0.259
	(2.795)	(2.727)	(3.661)
Care leave	0.521***		
	(0.0835)		
Relative resources squared	0.0131**		
	(0.00606)		
Relative resources/wage rate	−0.0538**	−0.134	0.517*
	(0.0222)	(0.126)	(0.275)
Co-residential caregiving	0.285***	0.0753	0.0641
	(0.0753)	(0.0802)	(0.108)
Sex (male = 1)	−0.199*	−0.135*	−0.401***
	(0.106)	(0.0796)	(0.100)
Care recipients			
Father	−0.0517	−0.0366	0.129
	(0.0954)	(0.0935)	(0.107)
Mother	0.137*	0.0564	−0.0185
	(0.0770)	(0.0789)	(0.0988)
Father-in-law	0.274**	−0.0701	0.287*
	(0.121)	(0.116)	(0.151)
Mother-in-law	0.0332	0.0776	−0.162
	(0.0838)	(0.0874)	(0.119)
Health status and Medical care use			
Medication or doctor's consultation	0.243**	0.0613	0.0386
	(0.107)	(0.105)	(0.127)
Hospitalization during the past year	−0.577**	0.263	−0.649*
	(0.233)	(0.247)	(0.390)
Difficulty in daily life activities	−0.00896	0.0340	−0.289*
	(0.0863)	(0.103)	(0.171)
Hypertension	−0.201*	−0.0996	0.00882
	(0.104)	(0.100)	(0.122)
Hyperlipidemia	−0.182**	−0.118	0.00838
	(0.0906)	(0.0903)	(0.104)
Constant	−4.304***	−3.358***	−1.365
	(1.160)	(1.133)	(1.502)
$\ln\sigma_u^2$	−1.266***	−0.716***	−1.815**
	(0.384)	(0.274)	(0.913)

Table 2 High-intensity caregiving functions *(Continued)*

σ_u	0.531***	0.699***	0.403**
	(0.101)	(0.095)	(0.184)
Intra-class correlation $(\sigma_u^2/(1 + \sigma_u^2))$	0.220	0.328	0.140
Likelihood-ratio test of $\rho = 0$ [chi^2(1)]	11.32	28.96	1.62
Prob $\geq$ chi^2	0.00	0.00	0.10
Log likelihood	−1501.54	−1610.13	−733.07
N	2879	3580	2063

High-intensity caregiving (initial) refers to high-intensity caregiving in 2005.
m(X) means time-average of time-variant explanatory variable (X)
Age, educational attainment, marital status, residence, having cancer, cerebral stroke, diabetes, heart disease, and friends were included as covariates
Standard errors in parentheses. *** $p < 0.01$, ** $p < 0.05$, * $p < 0.1$

and irregular employees. Among both groups, past high-intensity caregiving (20–40 h and 40 h or more) and the initial value of high-intensity caregiving had significant ($p < .01$) positive effects on current high-intensity caregiving. Notably, the coefficients for high-intensity caregiving of 20–40 h were larger than were those of ultra-high-intensity caregiving (i.e., 40 h or more); this indicated that caregivers who experienced high-intensity caregiving 20–40 h more likely to continue that high-intensity caregiving than were caregivers who had experienced ultra-high-intensity caregiving. Considering the non-proportional relationship between hours of caregiving and caregivers' burden found by Arai and Ueda (2003), the perceived burden of caregivers who experienced high-intensity caregiving (20–40 h) might be the heaviest among all informal caregivers. This finding was considered in the specification of the continuation of caregiving function described below. It should be noted that being male had a marginally significant negative effect on the likelihood of high-intensity caregiving at the 10% significance level.

Among non-working informal caregivers, taking care leave, co-residential caregiving, medication or doctor's consultation, and caregiving for a father-in-law had positive effects on high-intensity caregiving. Furthermore, both relative resources and the squared term of relative resources were significantly related to high-intensity caregiving ($p < .05$). Relative resources—namely, the difference between logged spouse's income and logged respondent's income—had a value of 0 if the respondent was single. The quadratic function of relative resources had a minimum value of −0.055 at 2.05, which would mean that there is a high likelihood of high-intensity caregiving among non-working caregivers with a large difference between the logged spouse's income and logged respondent's income.

The relative resources squared (*rrs*) is considered a proxy variable of the shadow price of informal care for non-working caregivers (inactive or taking care leave) because individuals with higher income tend to spend less hours in informal caregiving. Therefore, the *rrs* includes the opportunity costs of informal caregivers, which shows the monetary value of the alternative use of hours of caregiving as market work or leisure time. The Pearson correlation between *rrs* and household income ratio (*hir*) is 0.501, and *hir* was not statistically significant at the 10% level when using *rrs* and *hir* as explanatory variables of the high-intensity caregiving function, suggesting that multicollinearity may exist between them. The *hir* is the ratio of household income to the poverty line. The poverty line, for example 1.25 million yen in 2009, was obtained from the Comprehensive Survey of Living Conditions. The *rrs* was associated with both the household income status and socioeconomic status, although the definition of socioeconomic status is an arbitrary one.[26] Non-working caregivers with less education were not likely to be accepted in the labor force, and tended to engage in high-intensity caregiving in their household. The estimation results of random-effects models of *rrs* are shown in the Appendix. The Hausman tests supported the random-effects models.

In contrast, having hyperlipidemia and being hospitalized during the past year had negative effects on high-intensity caregiving ($p < .05$). Being married also had negative effects on high-intensity caregiving (see Appendix), suggesting that the "never married" group (i.e., the comparison group) were more likely to engage in high-intensity caregiving. The proportion of inactive persons who were never married was 0.26.

I determined the intra-class correlation coefficients (ICCs) from an error-components panel data model using the equation $\text{ICC} = \sigma_u^2/(1 + \sigma_u^2)$, where σ_u^2 represents the variance of the unobserved individual effect. ICCs are used to measure the proportion of the total unexplained variation that can be attributed to individual effects. Here, the ICC represents the correlations between high-intensity caregiving across the different periods of observation; an ICC value close to unity indicates a high persistence of high-intensity caregiving.

The estimation results of the DREP model for irregular employees showed that unobserved heterogeneity was a strong source of persistence in high-intensity caregiving; specifically, unobserved heterogeneity accounted for 32.8% of the unexplained variance in high-intensity caregiving. Considering the population distribution of unobserved heterogeneity, I obtained population-averaged parameters as $\beta_a = \beta/\sqrt{(1 + \sigma_u^2)}$. The averaged parameter of lagged high-intensity caregiving (20–40 h) among irregular employees was 0.845 (1.031/1.220), while that among non-working caregivers was 0.812 (0.919/1.132). The averaged parameters of lagged high-intensity caregiving (40 h or more) were relatively smaller, at 0.441 among irregular employees and 0.657 among non-working caregivers. The degree of state dependence between previous and current high-intensity caregiving (20–40 h) exhibited moderate persistence.

The averaged parameter of co-residential caregiving among non-working caregivers was 0.285; in other words, almost 25% of the persistence of high-intensity caregiving was increased by co-residential caregiving overall. Furthermore, almost 71% of the persistence of high-intensity caregiving was increased by co-residential caregiving for a father-in-law and having a doctor's consultation. The time average of non-attendance of health checkup had a positive and significant ($p < .01$) effect on high-intensity caregiving. This suggests that non-working caregivers who had not received health checkups during the current period had a high likelihood of engaging in high-intensity caregiving.[27] These tendencies were not found for irregular employees.

Effects of high-intensity caregiving on caregivers' mental health
The dependent variable of the mental health function was serious mental distress as measured by the K6. The independent variables of the first-stage pooled probit model were age, care leave, co-residential caregiving, caregivers' health status, relation of care recipients, educational attainment, having friends or acquaintances, hospitalization, marital status, medication or doctor's consultation, residence, sex, and relative resources or wage rate. The initial value of caregiving was also included as an exclusion restriction. The estimation results of the DREP models showed that high-intensity caregiving was associated with worse mental health among non-working caregivers. Indeed, there were distinct impacts of high-intensity caregiving on mental health of informal caregivers. However, high-intensity caregiving did not have any effect on serious mental health among irregular employees.

Table 3 shows that both the generalized residual and the interaction (HI × GR) were not significant ($p > .05$), and that high-intensity caregiving was an exogenous variable of caregivers' mental health. The averaged parameter of high-intensity caregiving was 1.086 (1.234/ 1.137) among non-working caregivers. This result indicates that caregivers who had engaged in high-intensity caregiving would have a current mental health status of serious mental distress when their mental health was moderate ($5 \leq \text{K6} < 13$) in the past period.[28]

The averaged parameter of the lagged mental health of non-working caregivers was 0.438. This indicates that the degree of state dependence between previous mental health and current serious mental distress reflected moderate persistence. All the initial values of mental health—which ranged from serious (2) to light (0)—were significantly related with current mental health at the 1% level. Depressive symptoms were considered persistent for non-working caregivers.

Table 3 Caregivers' mental health functions

	Non-working	Irregular employees
Dependent variables	Serious mental distress (13 ≤ K6)	
Independent variables		
Mental health (−1) (1 = moderate, 2 = serious)	0.498***	0.381***
	(0.0697)	(0.0609)
Mental health (initial)	0.478***	0.346***
	(0.0863)	(0.0718)
m(proxy of formal care use)	−115.3***	−49.58*
	(36.30)	(28.14)
High-intensity caregiving (HI)	1.234**	−0.208
	(0.496)	(1.148)
Generalized residual (GR)	−0.684*	0.0828
	(0.372)	(0.922)
HI × GR	0.00418	0.143
	(0.395)	(0.810)
Care leave	−0.181	
	(0.163)	
Health status		
Difficulty in daily life activities	0.487***	0.279**
	(0.108)	(0.111)
Hospitalization during the past year	0.605**	0.188
	(0.252)	(0.274)
Diabetes	0.159	0.223
	(0.156)	(0.139)
Heart disease	0.299	0.487***
	(0.200)	(0.170)
Cerebral stroke	−0.236	−0.0761
	(0.302)	(0.348)
Hypertension	−0.0266	0.160
	(0.144)	(0.118)
Hyperlipidemia	−0.0348	0.0595
	(0.135)	(0.107)
Having friends/acquaintances	−0.184	−0.360***
	(0.114)	(0.116)
Constant	1.466	0.313
	(1.503)	(1.212)
$\ln\sigma_u^2$	−1.231**	−1.438**
	(0.531)	(0.634)
σ_u	0.540***	0.487***
	(0.143)	(0.154)
Intra-class correlation ($\sigma_u^2/(1 + \sigma_u^2)$)	0.226	0.192
Likelihood-ratio test of $\rho = 0$ [chi^2(1)]	6.19	3.88
Prob ≥ chi^2	0.00	0.02

Table 3 Caregivers' mental health functions *(Continued)*

Log-likelihood	−637.77	−830.43
N	2785	3448

Mental health (initial) refers to high-intensity caregiving in 2005. m(X) means the time-average of a time-variant explanatory variable (X)
Age, care recipients, educational attainment, marital status, medication or doctor's consultation, residence, sex, and having cancer were included as covariates
Standard errors in parentheses. *** $p<0.01$, ** $p<0.05$, * $p<0.1$

To investigate the hypothesis that respite care was useful in alleviating mental distress among informal caregivers who were engaged in high-intensity caregiving, a time-averaged proxy variable of formal care use was used. Among non-working caregivers, when this variable was included as a covariate of random-effects, it was significantly negatively related to mental distress ($p < .01$). This suggests that respite care was indeed useful in alleviating mental distress for non-working caregivers.

There was a high likelihood of high-intensity caregiving among non-working caregivers who had not received a health checkup during the current period. Therefore, we might consider that caregivers whose time discount rate is high do not give much thought to their future health status and therefore are more likely to engage in high-intensity caregiving. Unobservables such as higher time discount rates could have increased the rate of high-intensity caregiving, which in turn would correlate to unobservables that worsened the mental health of caregivers.

Effects of high-intensity caregiving on continuation of caregiving

Given the findings of the previous analysis that high-intensity caregiving was associated with worse mental health among non-working caregivers, I focused on the impact of current high-intensity caregiving on continuation of caregiving only in this group. More specifically, since the transition from non-working to part-time work was infrequent among informal caregivers, I extracted those who were not working at time t and did not provide high-intensity care at time $t-1$ before running the regression. During the sample period, about 6% of non-working caregivers in period t transitioned to part-time work in the next period. In contrast, 29% of workers in period t transitioned to non-working caregivers in the next period.

Table 4 shows the estimation results of the continuation of caregiving functions among non-working caregivers. The dependent variable of continuation of caregiving was informal caregiving in the next period, which includes non-residential caregiving. To control for factors influencing the probability of high-intensity caregiving among non-working caregivers when analyzing continuation of caregiving, I

Table 4 Continuation of caregiving of non-working caregivers

Independent variables		HI not provided in previous period
Co-residential caregiving	−0.0101	−0.0417
	(0.122)	(0.129)
Co-residential caregiving (initial)	0.456***	0.573***
	(0.104)	(0.121)
m(proxy of formal care use)	−62.58**	−68.33**
	(26.23)	(29.21)
High-intensity caregiving (HI)	1.047*	1.232**
	(0.537)	(0.570)
Generalized residual (GR)	−0.462	−0.363
	(0.422)	(0.434)
HI × GR	0.0907	−0.281
	(0.485)	(0.520)
Relative resources squared	0.00917	0.00598
	(0.00878)	(0.00931)
Relative resources	0.0229	0.0374
	(0.0327)	(0.0351)
Sex (male = 1)	−0.120	−0.104
	(0.157)	(0.167)
Care recipients		
Father	0.0599	0.0339
	(0.135)	(0.144)
Mother	0.408***	0.469***
	(0.111)	(0.122)
Father-in-law	−0.143	−0.117
	(0.166)	(0.178)
Mother-in-law	0.284**	0.317**
	(0.118)	(0.129)
Health status		
Difficulty in daily life activities	−0.0223	−0.0518
	(0.124)	(0.140)
Diabetes	0.0400	0.0541
	(0.167)	(0.184)
Heart disease	−0.168	−0.0844
	(0.225)	(0.242)
Cerebral stroke	−0.0348	0.0627
	(0.327)	(0.340)
Hypertension	0.216	0.231
	(0.152)	(0.164)
Hyperlipidemia	0.0545	−0.0108
	(0.123)	(0.132)
Having friend	0.206*	0.274**
	(0.124)	(0.134)
Constant	1.492	0.926

Table 4 Continuation of caregiving of non-working caregivers (Continued)

	(1.330)	(1.445)
$\ln\sigma_u^2$	−0.422	−0.376
σ_u	0.809***	0.828***
	(0.141)	(0.157)
Intra-class correlation ($\sigma_u^2/(1 + \sigma_u^2)$)	0.396	0.407
Likelihood-ratio test of $\rho = 0$ [chi^2(1)]	18.10	15.70
Prob ≥ chi^2	0.00	0.00
Log-likelihood	−1005.92	−857.71
N	1743	1454

Co-residential caregiving (initial) refers to high-intensity caregiving in 2005. Age, educational attainment, hospitalization, marital status, medication or doctor's consultation, residence, and having cancer were included as covariates
Standard errors in parentheses. *** $p<0.01$, ** $p<0.05$, * $p<0.1$

included respondents' answer to the question "Do you sometimes try to rest to maintain your health?" as an exclusion restriction.[29] I observed a negative correlation between this exclusion restriction variable and high-intensity caregiving among non-working caregivers (−0.039, $p < .05$). In contrast, there were no correlations between this variable and continuation of caregiving.

The second-stage estimation results of the DREP models showed that current high-intensity caregiving was significantly associated with continuation of caregiving ($p < .05$). Because the averaged parameter of high-intensity caregiving was 0.949 (1.232/1.299) when high-intensity caregiving was not provided during the previous period, caregiving was considered persistent for non-working caregivers. Notably, there was a high likelihood of continuation of caregiving when the care recipient was a mother or mother-in-law, regardless of the provision of high-intensity caregiving during the previous period. However, non-working caregivers did not tend to continue high-intensity caregiving for more than three years because current high-intensity caregiving was not associated with the continuation of caregiving when high-intensity caregiving provided during the previous period was included in the regression. The time-averaged proxy variable of formal care use was significantly and negatively related to continuation of caregiving, indicating that current respite care has a negative effect on continuation of informal caregiving. This suggests that caregivers might elect to use formal care when formal care services are readily available in the next period.

Conclusions

The results of the present study offered robust support for a causal relationship between high-intensity caregiving and mental health problems. This suggests that supporting family caregivers is an important public health issue. While little was known until now about the specifics of the negative relation between high-intensity caregiving and caregivers' mental health in Japan, the present study shed some light on this area.

Three major findings were uncovered: First, hours of caregiving is thought to influence the continuation of high-intensity caregiving among non-working informal caregivers and irregular employees. Specifically, caregivers who experienced high-intensity caregiving (20–40 h) tended to continue with it to a greater degree than did caregivers who experienced ultra-high-intensity caregiving (40 h or more). Second, there were distinct impacts of high-intensity caregiving on the mental health of informal caregivers. High-intensity caregiving was associated with worse mental health among non-working caregivers, but had no effect on the serious mental distress of irregular employees. Caregivers who had engaged in high-intensity caregiving tended to exhibit serious mental distress currently when they exhibited mental health in the previous period. Furthermore, the time-averaged proxy variable of formal care use was significantly negatively related to mental distress; this suggests that respite care was useful for non-working caregivers. Finally, non-working caregivers did not tend to continue high-intensity caregiving for more than three years, regardless of co-residential caregiving. This is because current high-intensity caregiving was not associated with the continuation of caregiving when I included high-intensity caregiving provided during the previous period in the regression. In sum, caregiving tends to persist among non-working caregivers who experienced high-intensity caregiving for a year. Thus, supporting non-working intensive caregivers should be a priority public health issue.

Although a shift from caregiving to employment has been observed when formal care services are readily available, due to the limited data, I did not fully control for simultaneity between informal caregiving, the eligibility levels of care recipients, and formal care use. This simultaneity problem should be examined in further analyses.

Endnotes

[1] Hirst specifically examined changes in experienced distress levels between caregivers and non-caregivers surrounding transitions into and out of caregiving [2].

[2] Intensive caregivers tend to have lower incomes compared to non-intensive caregivers. Notably, intensive care is predominately provided by the spouse of the care recipient, and most intensive caregivers are 50–64 years old [1].

[3] The Japanese government introduced a community-based, prevention-oriented long-term care (LTC) benefit targeted at low-care-needs seniors in 2006. Since April 2006, there are seven levels of care needs certification under public LTCI: the two lowest levels are "assistance required" (*yo-shien* in Japanese) and the remaining five levels refer to "care required" (*yo-kaigo* in Japanese). Similarly, in 2008, Germany introduced "carrot-and-stick" financial incentives for sickness funds that proved successful at rehabilitating and moving LTC users from institutions to lower-care settings [1].

[4] In Japan, spending on public LTC increased 40% over the six years from 2006 to 2012. A further increase in LTC expenses is expected as the Japanese population continues to age.

[5] In Japan, respite care, or short-stay care (i.e., having the care recipient spend a few nights at a time in a nursing home) is widely used (350,000 stays per month), but the number of institutional beds is inadequate because of high demand [31].

[6] Female caregivers, who were expected to have home-making skills according to family-bound gender roles, were the least likely to use formal visiting homecare services [6].

[7] According to [1], across the Organization for Economic Cooperation and Development (OECD) member countries, more than one in ten adults over 50 years of age provide (usually) unpaid help with personal care to people with functional limitations. Close to two-thirds of such caregivers are women.

[8] As they suggested, the objective burden of informal care does not include how caregivers experience their caregiving tasks.

[9] Because long-term care is time consuming, the flexibility of non-regular work might be preferable for informal caregivers [16].

[10] In contrast, informal care might serve as a complement to formal care that cannot be replaced by family or other informal caregivers, such as outpatient care requiring professional practice.

[11] First, 2,515 districts were randomly selected from the 5,280 districts used in the MHLW's nationwide, population-based "Comprehensive Survey of the Living Conditions of People on Health and Welfare," conducted in 2004. These 5,280 districts had been randomly selected from about 940,000 national census districts. Second, 40,877 residents aged 50–59 years as of October 30, 2005 were randomly selected from each selected district proportionate to its population size. A total of 34,240 individuals responded to the first survey wave (response rate: 83.8%), while 32,285 subjects returned the questionnaires for the second wave (response rate: 92.2%). The third to fifth waves of the survey were conducted in 2007–2009 and consisted of 30,730 (response rate: 95.4%), 29,605 (96.2%), and 28,736 (97.3%)

respondents, respectively. No new respondents were added after the first wave.

[12]Socially disadvantaged families may be more likely to engage in caregiving and have fewer labor market opportunities [1].

[13]Prochaska et al. [32] identified a K6 ≥ 5 as the optimal lower threshold cut-off for moderate mental distress according to a receiver operating characteristic curve. Prochaska et al. also found that mental distress was more prevalent among those with lower education levels, those who were unemployed and looking for work, those who were not married, binge drinkers and current and former smokers, those who were not regularly physically active, and those who were obese.

[14]Regarding the hours of informal caregiving in 2007 (2010), the proportion of main caregivers who provided "2 h or more per day" for care recipients with a care level of 3 was 0.577 (0.663), while the proportion who provided "almost all day" was 0.309 (0.338) [Comprehensive Survey of the Living Conditions of People on Health and Welfare, 2007, 2010].

[15]This tendency was the same for caregivers who were not co-residing with the care recipient.

[16]Co-residential caregiving is also likely to involve considerable transition costs, such that caregivers are more likely to remain caregivers in the future [33].

[17]In 2010, 41% of co-residential females in their 50s or 60s were the primary caregivers according to the Comprehensive Survey of Living Conditions 2010 by the MHLW (Available from http://www.mhlw.go.jp/toukei/saikin/hw/k-tyosa/k-tyosa10/4-3.html) (in Japanese).

[18]Although family caregivers could rely only on home help, day care, and other home and community-based services, this is not enough to relieve their burden so long as caring is regarded as a full-time duty [31]. Furthermore, based on a survey of 2,530 family caregivers, Suzuki et al. found that there is insufficient provision of short-term stays, day services, and home-helper services [5].

[19]Assuming that initial conditions are exogenous, the random effects variance is restricted to zero. This indicates that there is no unobserved heterogeneity in participation probabilities.

[20]Higher income was found to be positively related to latent health stock, while low educational attainment, difficulty in daily life activities, and care for family members were negatively related [27]. They used health stock as a dummy variable, which took on the value of 1 if the latent health stock was good and 0 otherwise.

[21]The discrete-factor random-effects estimator approach provides econometricians with an easy method of jointly estimating two (or more) behaviors of interest [34].

[22]This assumption enables a specific correlation structure between unobservables that affects the treatment and the unobservables that affect potential outcomes.

[23]Vella proposed that a generalized residual has two important characteristics: it has a mean zero over the whole sample, and it is uncorrelated with the explanatory variables in the first-step probit model [29].

[24]For informal caregiving overall, a shift from 1 to 0 indicated a shift from informal caregiving to no longer being an informal caregiver (i.e., beginning use of formal care use or the death of the care recipient).

[25]It should be noted here that 575 of the inactive persons changed from previous non-working status to current working status, while 263 changed from previous working status to current non-working status. However, the dataset is weakly balanced because each panel contains the same number of observations but not the same time points.

[26]Because the rrs is distributed in a biased manner among non-working caregivers, the explanation of the rrs depends on hir, sending living expenses for non-housemates (slc), and high or low socioeconomic status (hses or lses). The coefficient of lses was −0.56, and its magnitude was about 1.43 times that of hir. When censoring the caregivers whose rrs was zero (N = 1460), the coefficient of lses of the random-effects tobit model was −0.99, and its magnitude was about 2.28 times that of hir (not shown in Table 6). About half of the informal caregivers belonged to the lses. The lses includes non-married, non-working caregivers whose educational attainment is low (less than high school). The hses consists of non-working caregivers who are married and whose educational attainment is high (university level or above).

[27]Using a subset of non-working informal caregivers who had received health checkups before a change in medication, I examined whether a change in medication or a doctor's consultation had a negative effect on health checkup attendance. No such effect was found ($p > .05$). I also confirmed that high-intensity caregiving had no negative effect on non-working informal caregivers' health checkup attendance ($p > .05$).

[28]The generalized residual was significant at the 5% level when including "unemployed" in the non-working group; thus, it may be that poor mental health due to unemployment can cause people to choose to stay in home and provide informal care.

[29]The independent variables of the first-stage pooled probit model were age, care leave, co-residential caregiving, caregivers' health status, care recipients, educational attainment, having friends or acquaintances, hospitalization, marital status, medication or doctor's consultation, residence, sex, relative resources or wage rate, and the exclusion restriction.

Appendix

Table 5 High-intensity caregiving functions (continuation of Table 2)

Independent variables	Non-working	Irregular employees	Regular employees
Age and Marital status			
Age	0.0187	0.0269**	−0.006
	(0.0129)	(0.0126)	(0.0169)
Married	−0.349***	0.0361	−0.0957
	(0.101)	(0.104)	(0.148)
Educational attainment			
Junior high school	−0.00893	−0.101	0.0893
	(0.106)	(0.108)	(0.151)
Vocational school	−0.0298	0.190*	−0.0753
	(0.111)	(0.114)	(0.150)
Junior college or technical college	0.121	0.0536	−0.120
	(0.0921)	(0.107)	(0.156)
University	−0.0657	−0.0973	−0.157
	(0.106)	(0.0986)	(0.105)
Graduate school	−0.145	0.000837	0.284
	(0.513)	(0.388)	(0.302)
Residence			
Rental housing	0.0491	0.227*	0.197
	(0.137)	(0.121)	(0.163)
Company residence	−0.371	0.560	0.254
	(0.522)	(0.425)	(0.450)
Other residences	−0.169	0.357	0.510
	(0.263)	(0.225)	(0.335)
Health status and Medical care use			
Diabetes	−0.0372	−0.151	−0.0755
	(0.122)	(0.125)	(0.148)
Heart disease	0.0851	0.0306	0.320*
	(0.166)	(0.167)	(0.187)
Cerebral stroke	0.0890	0.203	−0.681
	(0.222)	(0.259)	(0.545)
Cancer	−0.0948	−0.00433	0.435
	(0.212)	(0.238)	(0.300)
Having friend/acquaintances	−0.0823	0.0586	0.121
	(0.0867)	(0.103)	(0.122)

Divorced or widowed was dropped because of collinearity
Standard errors in parentheses. *** $p < 0.01$, ** $p < 0.05$, * $p < 0.1$

Table 6 Relative resources squared and household income status

	Random-effects model		Fixed-effects model	
Dependent variable	Relative resources squared			
Independent variables	[1]	[2]	[3]	[4]
Low socioeconomic status	−0.561**	−0.447*	−1.855**	−1.855**
	(0.241)	(0.250)	(0.752)	(0.752)
High socioeconomic status		0.744*		0.147
		(0.423)		(0.705)
Household income ratio	0.392***	0.390***	0.311***	0.311***
	(0.0108)	(0.0109)	(0.0125)	(0.0125)
Sending living expenses for non-housemates	0.886***	0.859***	−0.0298	−0.0327
	(0.256)	(0.256)	(0.399)	(0.399)
Constant	6.288***	6.179***	7.560***	7.549***
	(0.188)	(0.198)	(0.405)	(0.409)
R-squared	0.255	0.256	0.243	0.243
Hausman test				
chi^2 (Prob > chi^2)	[1] vs [3] 182.10 (0.00)		[2] vs [4] 179.95 (0.00)	
N	4097	4097	4097	4097

Standard errors in parentheses. *** $p < 0.01$, ** $p < 0.05$, * $p < 0.1$

Abbreviations
DREP model: Dynamic random-effects probit model; K6: Kessler 6 non-specific distress scale; LSMEP: Longitudinal Survey of Middle-aged and Elderly Persons; LTCI: Long-term care insurance; MHLW: Ministry of Health, Labor and Welfare

Acknowledgments
I am grateful for the helpful comments of anonymous reviewers, professors Seiritsu Ogura and Haruko Noguchi. I would also like to express my appreciation for the financial support from Japan's Ministry of Education, Culture, Sports, Science, and Technology (JSPS KAKENHI Grant Number JP15K03528).

Competing interests
The author has no competing interests.

References
1. Colombo F, Llena-Nozal A, Mercier J, Tjadens F. Help wanted? providing and paying for long-term care. Paris: OECD; 2011.
2. Hirst M. Career distress: a prospective, population-based study. Soc Sci Med. 2005;61(3):697–708.
3. Tjadens F, Colombo F. Long-term care: valuing care providers. Eurohealth. 2011;17(2–3):13–7.
4. Davies B, Fernandez J, Nomer B. Equity and efficiency policy in community care: needs, service productivities, efficiencies, and their implications. Farnham: Ashgate Publishing; 2000.
5. Suzuki W, Ogura S, Izumida N. Burden of family care-givers and the rationing in the long-term care insurance benefits of Japan. Singapore Econ Rev. 2008;53:121–44.
6. Tokunaga M, Hashimoto H, Tamiya N. A gap in formal long-term care use related to characteristics of caregivers and households, under the public universal system in Japan: 2001–2010. Health Policy. 2015;119(6):840–9.
7. Guberman N, Maheu P, Maille C. Women as family caregiver: why do they care? The Gerontologist. 1992;32(5):607–17.

8.   Bauer JM, Sousa-Poza A. Impacts of informal caregiving on caregiver employment, health, and family. J Popul Ageing. 2015;8(3):113–45.

9.   Brouwer WBF, van Exel JA, van den Berg B, Dinant HJ, Koopmanschap MA, van den Bos GA. Burden of caregiving: evidence of objective burden, subjective burden, and quality of life impacts on informal caregivers of patients with rheumatoid arthritis. Arthritis Rheumatol. 2004;51(4):570–7.

10. Crocco EA, Eisdorfer C. Research in caregiving. In: Talley RC, Fricchione GL, Druss BG, editors. The challenges of mental health caregiving: research - practice ? policy. New York: Springer; 2014. p. 205–21.

11. Beach SR, Schulz R, Yee JL. Negative and positive health effects of caring for a disabled spouse: longitudinal findings from the caregiver health effects study. Psychol Aging. 2000;15(2):259–71.

12. Houser A, Gibson M. Valuing the unvaluable: The economic value of family caregiving, 2008 Update. AARP Public Policy Institute. 2008. http://assets.aarp.org/rgcenter/il/i13_caregiving.pdf. Accessed 6 Apr 2013.

13. Heitmueller A. The chicken or the egg? Endogeneity in labour market participation of informal carers in England. J Health Econ. 2007;26(3):536–59.

14. Carmichael F, Charles S, Hulme C. Who will care? Employment participation and willingness to supply informal care. J Health Econ. 2010;29:182–90.

15. Lilly MB, Laporte A, Coyte P. Do they care too much to work? The influence of caregiving intensity on the labour force participation of unpaid caregivers in Canada. J Health Econ. 2010;29:895–903.

16. Sugawara S, Nakamura J. Can formal elderly care stimulate female labor supply? The Japanese experience. J Jpn Int Econ. 2014;34:98–115.

17. Hanaoka C, Norton EC. Informal and formal care for elderly persons: How adult children's characteristics affect the use of formal care in Japan. Soc Sci Med. 2008;67:1002–8.

18. Kikuchi J. Does formal care substitute for family care in Japan? (Kaigo Service ha Kazoku niyoru Kaigo wo Daitaisuruka?). In: Ihori T, Kaneko Y, Noguchi H, editors. New risk and social security (Aratana Risk to Syakaihosyo). Tokyo: University of Tokyo Press; 2012. p. 211–30.

19. Kessler RC, Andrews G, Colpe LJ, Hiripi E, Mroczek DK, Normand SL, Walters EE, Zaslavsky AM. Short screening scales to monitor population prevalences and trends in non-specific psychological distress. Psycho Med. 2002;32(6):959–76.

20. Oshio T. How is an informal caregiver's psychological distress associated with prolonged caregiving? Evidence from a six-wave panel survey in Japan. Qual Life Res. 2015;24(12):2907–15.

21. Arai Y, Ueda T. Paradox revisited: still no direct connection between hours of care and caregiver; burden. Int J Geriatr Psych. 2003;18(2):188–9.

22. Ettner SL. The opportunity costs of elder care. J Hum Resour. 1996;31:189–205.

23. Carmichael F, Charles S. The opportunity costs of informal care: does gender matter? J Health Econ. 2003;22:781–803.

24. Amirkhanyan A, Wolf D. Parent care and the stress process: Findings from panel data. J Gerontology Series B: Psycho Sci Soci Sci. 2006;61(5):S248–255.

25. Hsiao C. Analysis of panel data. Cambridge: Cambridge University Press; 1986.

26. Wooldridge JM. Simple solutions to the initial conditions problem in dynamic nonlinear panel data models with unobserved heterogeneity. J Appl Eco. 2005;20:39–54.

27. Kumagai N, Ogura S. Persistence of physical activity in middle age: a nonlinear dynamic panel approach. Eur J Health Econ. 2014;15:717–35.

28. Wooldridge JM. Control function methods in applied econometrics. J Hum Resour. 2015;50(2):420–45.

29. Vella F. Estimating models with sample selection bias: A survey. J Hum Resour. 1998;33(1):127–69.

30. Heckman J, Navarro-Lozano S. Using matching, instrumental variables, and control functions to estimate economic choice models. Rev Econ Stat. 2004;86(1):30–57.

31. Tamiya N, Noguchi H, Nishi A, Reich MR, Ikegami N, Hashimoto H, Shibuya K, Kawachi I, Campbell JC. Population ageing and wellbeing: lessons from Japan's long-term care insurance policy. Lancet. 2011;378:1183–92.

32. Prochaska JJ, Sung H-Y, Max W, Shi Y, Ong M. Validity study of the K6 scale as a measure of moderate mental distress based on mental health treatment need and utilization. Int J Method Psych. 2012;21(2):88–97.

33. Michaud P-C, Heitmueller A, Nazarov Z. A dynamic analysis of informal care and employment in England. Labour Econ. 2010;17:455–65.

34. Gilleskie D. Dynamic models: Econometric considerations of time. In: Culyer A, editor. Encyclopedia of health economics Vol. 1. San Diego: Elsevier; 2014. p. 209–16.

18

Is health care a necessary or luxury product for Asian countries? An answer using panel approach

S. M. Abdullah[1*], Salina Siddiqua[2†] and Rumana Huque[1†]

Abstract

A number of studies have estimated the income elasticity of health care expenditure to identify whether health care is a necessary or luxury product. However, the issue has received less attention in developing countries, especially in Asian economies. The current study for the first time has used the panel data covering 36 Asian countries for the period 1995–2013 for revealing the nature of health care as a product. Along with conventional econometric techniques we have addressed the issue of cross section dependence and used Westerlund (2007) panel cointegration test which is robust against cross section dependence and heterogeneity for detecting the presence of panel cointegration. By applying Fully Modified OLS (FMOLS) and Dynamic OLS (DOLS) it was found that the long run elasticity of Health Care Expenditure (HCE) with Gross Domestic Product (GDP) is less than unit implying that the health care can be regarded as necessary in nature for these countries.

Keywords: Income elasticity, Health care expenditure, Panel cointegration, Panel unit root, Cross section dependence, FMOLS, DOLS

JEL Classification: I10, C51

Background

Macro level health spending has significant beneficial effects on health outcomes [1–3]. Data from 47 African countries [4] and 133 low and middle income countries [1] showed that increased health spending led to reduced infant and under-5 child mortality rates. Hence, the share of health expenditure, the determinants of resources a country devotes to medical care, and the relationship between national income and national health care expenditures have drawn attention of health economists worldwide. A large number of studies have estimated the income elasticity of health care expenditure to identify whether health care is a necessary or luxury product, and found varying results. While income elasticity coefficient of health care expenditure was found unity in 21 Organization of Economic Cooperation and Development (OECD) countries reflecting health care

not a luxury [5], it was found less than unity in 13 MENA (Middle East and North Africa) countries characterizing health care as a necessary product [6]. However, majority of these studies have focused mainly on developed countries, including OECD countries [5, 7–9], United States [10], Middle East and African countries [6, 11], and European Countries [12, 13].[1] The issue has been discussed little in developing countries, especially in Asian economies. In recent years only Hassan et. al [14] analysed this relation using South Asian Association for Regional Cooperation (SAARC) countries' experience. One major limitation of many of the previous studies is that of using a single year of data to obtain cross-country estimates of the natural correlation [11, 15–17], making the regression results spurious. More recently, researchers have used panel data on Health Care Expenditure (HCE) and Gross Domestic Product (GDP) measured across countries and across time [18–23], which offers a number of advantages over cross-sectional study. Using multiple years of data enables researchers to include country-specific fixed effects for each country, thereby controlling for a wide range of

* Correspondence: abdullahsonnet@gmail.com
†Equal contributors
[1]Department of Economics, University of Dhaka, Dhaka 1000, Bangladesh
Full list of author information is available at the end of the article

time-invariant country characteristics, This avoids potential bias for the estimated relationship between HCE and GDP while retaining the cross sectional dependence and panel heterogeneity as important issues. In addition, the stationarity of the concerned variables are of vital importance when dealing with long panel. Considering these drawbacks of earlier studies, this study examined the impact of income on health care expenditure at macro level using a long panel of 36 Asian countries[2] for the period 1995 to 2013 while addressing the issue of heterogeneity and cross sectional dependence.

The paper is organized in the following sections: section 2 describes the source of data and methodological procedures applied in this paper. In Section 3, results of econometric estimations have been discussed and section 4 concludes.

Methods

We aimed to estimate income elasticity of health care expenditure and detect whether health care is a necessary or luxury product in Asian countries. Thus, we estimated the responsiveness of health care expenditure with respect to the change in income while controlling for other variables related to health status improvement. We estimated the following model by using appropriate econometric methods such as Fully Modified OLS (FMOLS) and Dynamic OLS (DOLS):

$$lnHCE_{i,t} = \beta_0 + \beta_1 lnGDP_{i,t} + \beta_2 HSI_{i,t} + \varepsilon_{i,t}$$

where, i = 1, 2, ----- N and t = 1, 2, ----- T indexes cross section and time series units respectively. $lnHCE_{i,t}$ is the natural logarithm of health care expenditure (measured in current US \$) for country i at time t and $lnGDP_{i,t}$ is the natural logarithm of GDP (measured in current US \$) and used as proxy of income. $HSI_{i,t}$ stands for health status improvement of country i at time t which is proxied by using infant mortality and life expectancy for all countries. Finally, $\varepsilon_{i,t}$ is the error term with all unobserved factors.

In the above model, β_1 is the coefficient which measures the impact of income on health care expenditure. As the higher the income the higher is the health care expenditure, this coefficient is expected to carry a positive sign. However, its magnitude determines whether health care is a necessary or luxury product. More specifically, as the standard theory of microeconomics suggests if,

$$0 \leq \frac{\delta lnHCE_{i,t}}{\delta lnGDP_{i,t}} = \beta_1 \leq 1, \text{ then health care would be necessary product}$$

$$\frac{\delta lnHCE_{i,t}}{\delta lnGDP_{i,t}} = \beta_1 > 1, \text{ then health care would be luxury product}$$

Data and statistical software

We have used two secondary data sources to develop the panel data set, namely World Development Indicators (WDI) and Health Nutrition and Population Statistics (HNPS) from World Bank database. A total of 36 Asian countries have been studied for the period of 1995 to 2013. The variables that we have used are, Health Care Expenditure, Gross Domestic Product and Health Status Improvement measured through Infant Mortality (IM) and Life Expectancy (LE). We used EViews 9 and STATA 14 softwares to carry out the econometric analysis.

Cross section dependence test

The existence of common shocks among sample countries could result in creating contemporaneous correlation, popularly known as cross section dependency, among the different countries included in the panel. As the size of the panel unit root test usually becomes distorted because of the presence of cross sectional dependence, it is crucial to diagnose this issue before estimating panel data models. We tested the following null hypothesis: the residuals from the standard panel regression are contemporaneously uncorrelated. Therefore, we diagnosed whether the pair - wise covariance among residuals are zero or not. Symbolically:

$$H_0 : \rho_{ij} = \rho_{ji} = Cov(\varepsilon_{it}, \varepsilon_{jt}) = 0, \text{ for all } t, \ i \neq j$$

$$H_1 : \rho_{ij} = \rho_{ji} = Cov(\varepsilon_{it}, \varepsilon_{jt}) \neq 0, \text{ for all } t, \ i \neq j$$

In order to test the above hypothesis, we applied four different tests namely Breuch – Pagan Lagrange Multiplier (LM) [24], Pesaran Cross Sectional Dependence (CD), Pesaran Scaled LM [25] and Baltagi, Feng and Kao Bias Corrected Sclaed LM [26]. However, Pesaran CD is regarded as the most general one as it is suitable for stationary and as well as non – stationary panels. It also consists of reasonable small sample properties.

Panel unit root test

Panel based unit root test are more preferred to individual time series ones given the better power properties of the former test. Cross – sectional independence is a crucial assumption for all the readily available panel unit root tests. However, Im, Pesaran and Shin (IPS) panel unit root test by Im et al. [27] relaxes the restrictive assumptions of no serial correlation and panel homogeneity. Im et al. [28] proposed demeaning procedure (subtracting group mean from the data) to denounce the contemporaneous correlation of the data. Therefore, we have used IPS panel unit root test along with Levin, Lin and Chu (LLC) panel unit root test by Levin et al. [29], ADF – Fisher and PP – Fisher panel unit root test by Choi [30] to detect the stationarity of the variables. In order to carry out these tests first for each variable, we estimated an auroregressive (AR) process, and then an Augmented Dickey Fuller (ADF) test regression was fitted for each cross-section unit. For detecting the stationarity of the variables, the statistical significance of the autoregressive coefficient attached with lagged level dependent variable in test regression is tested. Therefore, if the ADF test regression takes the following form:

$$\Delta y_{i,t} = \alpha y_{i,t-1} + \sum_{j=1}^{p_i} \beta_{i,j} \Delta y_{i,t-j} + x'_{i,t} \delta + \varepsilon_{i,t}$$

then the appropriate null hypothesis for testing the panel unit root would be $H_0 : \alpha_i = 0$, *for all i*. In the above regression y_{it} denotes the variable of concern for which stationary property would be tested and $x_{i,t}$ stands for other control variables.

Panel cointegration test

Several panel cointegration tests are available, including Pedroni [31, 32], McCoskey and Kao [33], Kao [34] and Westerlund [35]. We employed Pedroni [31, 32] and Westerlund [35] panel cointegration test for detecting the existence of cointegrating relationship among the variables. The reason is that the first one allows for heterogeneity while the second one is robust against heterogeneity and cross correlation in panel.

Pedroni panel coinetgration test

The Pedroni [31, 32] is an Engle – Granger based panel cointegration test. Pedroni's proposed test for panel cointegration considers heterogeneous intercept and trend coefficient across cross country. We estimated the following regression to conduct the test:

$$HCE_{i,t} = \alpha_i + \phi_i t + \gamma_1 GDP_{i,t} + \gamma_2 HSI_{i,t} + e_{i,t}$$

where, i = 1, 2, ----- N and t = 1, 2, ----- T, and HCE, GDP and variables i.e. infant mortality and life expectancy under HSI are assumed to be integrated of order one, I(1). We obtained the residuals from the above regression and performed an ADF test on the residuals to estimate whether they are I(1) using the following test regression for each country:

$$\Delta e_{i,t} = \rho_{it} e_{i,t-1} + \sum_{j=1}^{p_i} \psi_{i,j} \Delta e_{i,t-1} + v_{i,t}$$

Based on various methods, Pedroni provided a total of eleven statistics in two groups; panel statistic (within dimension) and group statistic (between dimension). The following hypothesis is tested against the alternatives:

$H_0 : \rho_i = 0$ (*No Cointegration*)

Homogeneous Alternative, $H_1 : (\rho_i = \rho) < 1 \forall i$
Heterogeneous Alternative, $H_1 : \rho_i < 1 \forall i$

In particular panel statistic is concerned with homogeneous alternative while group statistics is concerned with

the other. However, all these statistics are distributed as asymptotically normal.

Westerlund panel cointegration test

There are cases where theory suggests existence of long run relationship among variables, panel cointegration tests have failed to reject the null hypothesis of *"no cointegration"*. It occurs due to the failure of *"common – factor restriction"* (Banerjee et. al [36]). By depending on structural dynamics (rather than error dynamics) Westrelund [35] have developed a set of panel cointegration test which do not require any common factor restriction. These tests are general enough to be robust against heterogeneity and cross section dependence. The cointegration test assumes the following data generating process:

$$\Delta HCE_{i,t} = \delta'_i d_t + \alpha_i HCE_{i,t-1} + \lambda'_i x_{i,t-1}$$
$$+ \sum_{j=1}^{p_i} \alpha_{ij} \Delta HCE_{i,t-1} + \sum_{j=-q_i}^{p_i} \gamma_{ij} \Delta x_{i,t-1} + e_{i,t}$$

Where, i = 1, 2, ----- N and t = 1, 2, ----- T indexes cross sectional units and time series. In the above process, x is a vector of independent variables that includes GDP and HSI measured in terms of infant mortality and life expectancy and finally d_t contains deterministic components. Here, α_i is referred to as error correction parameter. If $\alpha_i < 0$ then there will be error correction and hence cointegration while if $\alpha_i = 0$, reflects that the error correction is absent and consequently there is no cointegration.

Westerlund [35] proposed four panel statistics, among which two (Panel Statistic) test the alternative hypothesis that panel is cointegrated as a whole while the other two (Group Statistic) test that at least one is cointegrated. Thus, the null and alternative hypothesis tested is formulated in the following way:

Panel Statistic : $H_0 : \alpha_i = 0$ *against* $H_1^P : \alpha_i < 0 \forall i$

Group Statistic : $H_0 : \alpha_i = 0$ *against* $H_1^G : \alpha_i < 0$ *for at least some i*

Estimation of cointegrating relationship

In our data GDP and HSI i.e. infant mortality and life expectancy can become endogenous and also the error terms can be serially correlated which would result in the dependence of OLS estimators on nuisance parameters. In order to solve these problems two estimators namely FMOLS and DOLS can be introduced. Phillips and Hansen [37] proposed a semi parametric correction for the problem of long run correlation among cointegrating equation and stochastic regressors innovations resulting in FMOLS estimators. It is asymptotically unbiased. On the other hand Saikkonen [38] and Stock and Watson [39] advanced an asymptotically efficient estimator which eliminates the feedback in the cointegrating system by augmenting the cointegrating regression with lags and leads of independent variables. The resulting estimator is known as DOLS estimator.

With a view to explain the idea of FMOLS estimator consider the following fixed effect model:

$$HCE_{i,t} = \alpha_i + x_{i,t}'\beta + u_{i,t}$$

Where, i = 1, 2,———, N and t = 1, 2, ———, T indexes cross section and time series units respectively, $HCE_{i,t}$ is the health care expenditure (an I(1) process), β is (2*1) vector of parameters, α_i are intercepts and $u_{i,t}$ are the stationary disturbance terms. Here $x_{i,t}$ are assumed to be (2*1) vector of independent variables (GDP and HSI measured with infant mortality and life expectancy) which are I(1) for all cross section units. It is assumed that it follows an autoregressive process of following form:

$$x_{i,t} = x_{i,t-1} + \varepsilon_{i,t}$$

Innovation Vector, $w_{i,t} = \left(u_{i,t}, \ \varepsilon_{i,t}\right)$

Given that $w_{i,t} = (u_{i,t}, \ \varepsilon_{i,t}) \sim I(0)$ the variables are said to be cointegrated for each members of the panel with cointegrating vector β. The asymptotic distribution of the OLS estimator is condition to the long run covariance matrix of the innovation vector. The FMOLS estimator is derived by making endogeneity correction (by modifying variable $HCE_{i,t}$) and serial correlation correction (by modifying long run covariance of innovation vector, $w_{i,t}$). The resulting final estimator is expressed as follows:

$$\hat{\beta}_{FMOLS} = \left[\sum_{i=1}^{N}\sum_{t=1}^{T}(x_{it}-\overline{x}_i)(x_{it}-\overline{x}_i)' \right]^{-1}$$

$$* \left[\sum_{i=1}^{N}\left(\sum_{t=1}^{T}(x_{it}-\overline{x}_i)\widehat{HCE}_{it} - T\hat{\Delta}_{\varepsilon u} \right) \right]$$

The cointegrating regression is augmented by lead and lagged differences of GDP and other independent variables in DOLS framework for controlling endogeneity (by following Saikkonen, [38]). For controlling serial correlation, lead and lagged difference of the HCE has also been included in the model (by following Stock and Watson, [39]). Thus, the estimated regression equation under DOLS framework was as follows:

$$HCE_{i,t} = \alpha_i + \beta_i x_{i,t} + \sum_{k=-p_1}^{p_2}\delta_k \Delta HCE_{i,t-k}$$

$$+ \sum_{k=-q_1}^{q_2}\lambda_k \Delta x_{i,t-k} + u_{i,t}$$

Results

With a view to determining the appropriate estimation method, we need to check the stationary of the variables and also their order of integration. However, cross sectional dependence or cross sectional correlation of the variables is a fact that should be detected for the variables to decide which panel unit root test would be applied.

Table 1 contains the test results for Cross Sectional Dependence of different variables, and suggests that it is possible to reject the null hypothesis for all the variables at 1% level of significance. Therefore, the residuals from the standard panel regression would be contemporaneously correlated and this should be addressed while panel stationarity would be tested.

Table 1 Test Results for Cross Sectional Dependence of the Variables

Variables and Test Names		Breusch - Pagan LM	Pesaran - Scaled LM	Bias Corrected Scaled LM	Pesarn CD
H_0: No Cross - Section Dependence					
GDP (Current US $)	Statistic	10994.69[a]	291.99[a]	290.99[a]	104.58[a]
	Prob.	0.000	0.000	0.000	0.000
Health Care Expenditure (Current US $)	Statistic	10541.35[a]	279.22[a]	278.22[a]	102.40[a]
	Prob.	0.000	0.000	0.000	0.000
Infant Mortality	Statistic	10563.79[a]	279.85[a]	278.85[a]	100.50[a]
	Prob.	0.000	0.000	0.000	0.000
Life Expectancy	Statistic	11418.19[a]	303.92[a]	302.92[a]	106.79[a]
	Prob.	0.000	0.000	0.000	0.000

Note: [a] Indicates 1% level of significance

Therefore, we have used IPS panel unit root test to detect the stationarity of the variables along with some other tests e.g. Levin, Lin and Chu (LLC) test (Levin et al., [29]), ADF - Fisher Test and PP – Fisher test (Choi, [30]).

Table 2 and Tables 7, 8 and 9 in Appendix contain the panel unit root test results for each of the variables. All the tests are concerned with the null hypothesis of *"Panels Contain Individual Unit Root"* except LLC that tests the null hypothesis of *"Panel Contains Common Unit Root"*. The tests have been carried out with two different test regression specifications; one with constant and the other with constant and trend. It is evident from the test results that GDP and HCE are difference stationary i.e. I(1) variable according to all tests. With regards to infant mortality, it is also found to be difference stationary in intercept and trend specification under IPS, ADF – Fisher and PP – Fisher test. Thus it can be treated as an I(1) variable. Life expectancy was found to be difference stationary in intercept specification under IPS, in intercept and trend specification under LLC and in both specification under ADF - Fisher test. Since all the variables have been found to be integrated of a unique order we have identified the long run relationship among them by establishing the panel cointegration.

In order to check the existence of cointegration among the variables along with Pedroni [31, 32] Engle Granger based panel cointegration test, we applied Westerlund [35] error correction based panel cointegration test. The later one is already established in the literature for its robustness against panel with heterogeneity and cross sectional dependence. Hence, application of this test allowed us to check issue of existence of cointegartion among health care expenditure and income while controlling for health status improvement measured with infant mortality and life expectancy in a more

comprehensive manner. Both the tests have been performed with three different deterministic specifications.

Table 3 and Table 10 in Appendix contain the test results of panel cointegration. For testing the cointegration among health care expenditure, income and infant mortaility when neither constant nor trend was used as deterministic specification, the null hypothesis of *"no cointegration"* was rejected by all 11 statistic under Pedroni [31, 32] test. All the 4 statistic of Westerlund [35] test have also found to be significant. In the same specification when cointegration was checked among health care expenditure, income and life expectancy a total of 7 statistic in Pedroni [31, 32] and 2 among 4 statistic of Westerlund [35] was found to be statistically significant. When the deterministic specification was changed to allow the presence of constant, only 7 and 6 of 11 statistic for infant mortality and life expectancy respectively have found to be able to reject the non existence of cointegration under Pedroni [31, 32] test. By using the similar deterministic specification Westerlund [35] test was able to reject the null for both variables under 2 statistic out of 4. The conclusion of Westerlund [35] test has remained the same when the deterministic specification allows for both the constant and trend. While Pedroni [31, 32] test was carried out by using the later deterministic specification, 4 statistic have found to be significant when panel cointegration was checked with infant mortality while the number was 6 if it was tested with life expectancy. Thus, it can be argued that there might exists a long run cointegrating relationship among health expenditure, income and health status improvement which is substituted by using infant mortality and life expectancy.

With a view to estimate the cointegrating vector we have applied two different methods, FMOLS and DOLS. Each of the methods provides three different estimators namely, pooled, pooled weighted and grouped mean.

Table 2 Panel Unit Root Test Results of the Variables

Variables	Im – Pesaran – Shin (IPS) Test for Panel Unit Root Null: Panels Contain Unit Roots(Individual)			
	Intercept		Intercept and Trend	
	IPS W – Stat	Prob.	IPS W - Stat	Prob.
GDP (Current US $)	20.06	1.000	6.15	1.000
D(GDP)	−4.79[a]	0.000	−12.43[a]	0.000
Health Care Expenditure (Current US $)	21.23	1.000	6.07	1.000
D(Health Care Expenditure)	−3.70[a]	0.000	−12.61[a]	0.000
Infant Mortality	−20.81[a]	0.000	0.36	0.642
D(Infant Mortality)	−2.18	0.014	−5.04[a]	0.000
Life Expectancy	−1.62	0.052	−10.72[a]	0.000
D(Life Expectancy)	−15.08[a]	0.000	−20.25[a]	0.000

Note: [a]Indicates 1% level of significance

Table 3 Westerlund Panel Cointegration Test

Westerlund (2007) ECM Panel Cointegration Test, H_0: No Cointegration

Statistic	HCE, GDP and IM		HCE, GDP and LE	
	Stat.	Prob.	Stat.	Prob.
Deterministic Specification: No Constant & Trend				
Gt	−2.702[a]	0.000	−2.788[a]	0.000
Ga	−7.807[b]	0.015	−6.778	0.148
Pt	−16.120[a]	0.000	−12.352[a]	0.000
Pa	−11.134[a]	0.000	−2.579	0.461
Deterministic Specification: Constant Only				
Gt	−2.912[a]	0.000	−3.074[a]	0.000
Ga	−7.555	0.934	−6.475	0.994
Pt	−18.933[a]	0.000	−18.24[a]	0.000
Pa	−6.287	0.326	−6.512	0.244
Deterministic Specification: Constant & Trend				
Gt	−2.921[a]	0.003	−3.096[a]	0.000
Ga	−5.376	1.000	−4.293	1.000
Pt	−18.059[a]	0.000	−16.477[a]	0.001
Pa	−5.223	1.000	−5.665	1.000

Note: [a] and [b] Indicates 1% and 5% level of significance respectively

The pooled FMOLS estimator is the extension of Phillips and Hansen [37] FMOLS estimator offered by Phillips and Moon [40] which provides the estimators after correcting deterministic components in regressand and regressors. In order to allow different long run variances across the cross section for heterogeneous panels, Pedroni [41] and Kao and Chiang [42] proposed pooled weighted FMOLS. Finally the grouped mean FMOLS estimator developed by Pedroni [41, 43] is derived by averaging the individual cross section FMOLS estimates. In contrast to FMOLS, augmentation of model with lags and leads of differenced regressand and regressors in

DOLS helps it to overcome the problem of asymptotic endogeneity and serial correlation. Kao and Chiang [42], Mark and Sul [44, 45] and Pedroni [43] extended the standard DOLS estimation developed by Saikkonen [38] and Stock and Watson [39]. Kao and Chiang [42] proposed pooled DOLS where the augmented cointegrating regression allows the short run dynamics to be cross section specific. By allowing heterogenous long run variance, Mark and Sul [44, 45] developed pooled weighted DOLS. Finally, Pedroni [43] developed the grouped mean DOLS estimates by averaging the individual cross section DOLS estimates.

Table 4 contains the estimation results of long run relationship between health care expenditure and GDP and infant mortality as a measure of health status improvement. It is evident that the elasticity of health care expenditure with respect to income in Asian countries is less than unit. The elasticity coefficient varies from 0.73 to 0.83 when the model was estimated using FMOLS while the range was found to be 0.67 to 0.80 while estimating using DOLS method. The Wald test was observed to be significant in all cases. Thus, health care in Asian countries can be argued as a necessary and normal product. The elasticity coefficient of infant mortality was found to be negative and significant in almost all cases. Therefore, there is an inverse relationship between health care expenditure and infant mortality in Asian countries. Thus, the higher the health care expenditure, the lower the infant mortality or vice − versa.

Table 5 contains the results of cointegrating relationship between health care expenditure and GDP and another indicator of health status improvement measured by life expectancy. The elasticity coefficient of health care expenditure with respect of income was also found to be less than one. Here the elasticity measure varied in between 0.84 to 0.92 in FMOLS method and 0.77 to 0.91 in DOLS method. The coefficient has been

Table 4 Estimation of Cointegrating Regression with Infant Mortality as proxy for Health Status Improvement

Variables	FMOLS			DOLS		
	Pooled	Weighted	Grouped	Pooled	Weighted	Grouped
Cointegrating Regression						
Log of GDP	0.832[a]	0.730[a]	0.816[a]	0.742[a]	0.807[a]	0.676[a]
	(0.040)	(0.009)	(0.042)	(0.081)	(0.025)	(0.127)
Log of IM	−0.366[a]	−0.431[a]	−0.675[a]	−0.477[a]	−0.389[a]	−0.861
	(0.087)	(0.001)	(0.190)	(0.136)	(0.054)	(0.758)
Wald Test, H_0: Coefficient of Log of GDP equal to One						
t − Stat.	−4.166[a]	−28.637[a]	−4.355[a]	−3.155[a]	−7.666[a]	−2.534[b]
χ^2 Stat.	17.357[a]	820.080[a]	18.973[a]	9.957[a]	58.782[a]	5.719[b]

Note: In DOLS (Pooled) and FMOLS (Pooled) estimation coefficient of covariance was computed using sandwich method and in DOLS (Grouped) estimation individual heteroscedasticity and autocorrelation consistent standard errors and covariances were used. Numbers in the parenthesis indicate standard error.
[a] Indicates 1% and [b] indicates 5% level of significance

Table 5 Estimation of Cointegrating Regression with Life Expectancy as proxy for Health Status Improvement

Variables	FMOLS			DOLS		
	Pooled	Weighted	Grouped	Pooled	Weighted	Grouped
Cointegrating Regression						
Log of GDP	0.924^a	0.841^a	0.924^a	0.774^a	0.917^a	0.831^a
	(0.033)	(0.009)	(0.031)	(0.085)	(0.027)	(0.100)
Log of LE	0.912	1.489^a	5.464^a	3.906^a	1.416^b	10.419^a
	(0.629)	(0.001)	(1.459)	(1.496)	(0.673)	(3.530)
Wald Test, H_0: Coefficient of Log of GDP equal to One						
t – Stat.	-2.20^b	-16.091^a	-2.436^b	-2.632^a	-3.023^a	-1.674^c
χ^2 Stat.	4.883^b	258.944^a	5.938^b	6.930^a	9.140^a	2.805^c

Note: In DOLS (Pooled) and FMOLS (Pooled) estimation coefficient of covariance was computed using sandwich method and in DOLS (Grouped) estimation individual heteroscedasticity and autocorrelation consistent standard errors and covariances were used. Numbers in the parenthesis indicate standard error.
[a] Indicates 1%, [b] indicates 5% and [c] indicates 10% level of significance

observed to remain positive and significant in all cases. Thus, for Asian countries health care expenditure increases less than proportionately with the increase in income. The coefficient of life expectancy was found to be significant in almost all cases. Therefore, with respect to increase in life expectancy, health care expenditure increases in these countries.

Thus, unlike many OECD and developed countries such as USA, Canada, Germany and Italy where health care expenditure has been identified as luxury good, for Asian Countries it is revealed to be a necessary one. The findings contradict Hassan et. al [14] but in line with what have been found in Dreger and Reimers [5], Mehrara et. al [6] and Penas et. al [8].

Discussion and conclusion

By exploiting data for the period of 1995 to 2013, the study finds that long run elasticity of health care expenditure in relation to income is less than unit in 36 Asian countries, ensuring that the health care can be treated as a necessary product as a whole for the sample countries. In general the responsiveness was found to be higher when life expectancy was used instead of infant mortality as proxy of health status improvement. Our finding is different from that of Hassan et. al [14] which suggested health care as luxury products for South Asian Association for Regional Cooperation (SAARC) countries. However, the latter study has ignored the issue of cross correlation which may mislead the findings. Moreover, the way the coefficients had been analyzed made the reasoning and policy implications rather weak.

The contribution of this paper to the literature on the relationship between health care expenditure and income is twofold. First, it has covered almost all the countries in Asia, and analyzed the issue in a more rigorous manner in the sense of addressing cross correlation and heterogeneity problem that potentially exists in the panel and brought the findings in front to realize how health care should be treated in those countries. Second, from methodological point of view, as the study has addressed the issue of cross sectional correlation and panel heterogeneity, the findings are more reliable. The current work has examined the existence of long run relationship between health care expenditure and income using a panel cointegration technique which is robust against cross sectional correlation and panel heterogeneity along with conventional panel cointegration test. The estimation technique- FMOLS and as well as DOLS- has been used which is robust against asymptotic endogeneity and serial correlation.

The study has a number of areas to improve. As cross section dependence was detected it would have been better if second generation panel unit root tests were used when identifying the integration order of the variables. However, demeaning of data has taken care of the severity of problem to some extent. Throughout the analysis the parameters have been assumed to be stable, thus should there be any structural instability the findings may vary. Further research is required addressing the above issues.

Endnotes
[1] A summary of previous studies have presented in Table 6 in Appendix

[2] List of Countries: Bahrain, Bangladesh, Bhutan, Brunei, Cambodia, China, India, Indonesia, Iran, Israel, Japan, Jordan, Kazakhstan, Korea Rep., Kuwait, Kyrgyzstan, Laos, Lebanon, Malaysia, Mongolia, Maldives, Nepal, Oman, Pakistan, Philippines, Qatar, Saudi Arabia, Singapore, Srilanka, Tajikistan, Thailand, Turkmenistan, United Arab Emirates, Uzbekistan, Vietnam and Yemen

Appendix

Table 6 Summary of Existing Studies

Study	Data	Method	Elasticity of Income/Findings
Abel – Smith (1967) [15]	30 Countries from Africa, Europe, America, South East Asia, Eastern Mediterranean, Western Pacific, 1961	Cross – Sectional (Survey)	>1
Kleiman (1974) [51]	16 Countries, 1968		>1
Maxwell (1981) [52]	10 Countries, 1975		>1
Gertler & van der Gaag (1990) [48]	25 Countries, 1975		>1
Getzen (1990) [49]	United States, 1966–1987		>1
Schieber (1990) [53]	Canada, France, The Federal Republic of Germany, Italy, Japan, The United Kingdom, and The United States, 1960–1987	Country Specific Time Series, Compound Annual Rate of Growth	>1
Getzen & Poullier (1992) [50]	19 OECD Countries, 1965–1986	Country Specific Time Series, Forecasting Model and Coparison of Mean Absolute Error (MAE)	>1
Fogel (1999) [47]	United States	Long Term Trend Analysis	>1
Newhouse (1977) [66]	13 OECD Countries, 1968–1972	Cross – Sectional, Regression Model Estimation	>1
Leu (1986) [60]	19 OECD Countries	Cross – Sectional	>1
Parkin et. al (1987) [17]	18 OECD Countries, 1980	Cross – Sectional, Estimation of Linear, Semi – Log, Exponential and Double Log Model	>1
Gbesemete & Gerdtham (1992) [11]	30 African Countries, 1984	Cross – Sectional, WLS, RESET Test	Income elasticity close to unity
Hitiris & Posnett (1992) [21]	20 OECD Countries, 1960–1987	Panel Data, Estimation of Linear and Log Linear Models	Income elasticity close to unity
Gerdtham et. al (1992) [20]	19 OECD Countries, 1987	Cross Section, General to Specific Approach	>1
Hansen & King (1996) [55]	20 OECD Countries, 1960–1987	Time Series, Unit Root and Cointegration	HCE, GDP are Stationary
Blomqvist & Carter (1997) [58]	24 OECD Countries, 1960–1991	Time Series, OLS, Unit Root, Cointegration and Long Run Estimation	Reservation about having an elasticity coefficient as greater than 1
Hitiris (1997) [12]	10 European Community Countries (1960–1991)	Panel Data, GLS, Pooled OLS	>1
McCoskey & Selden (1998) [33]	20 OECD Countries	Panel Data, Panel unit Root	HCE, GDP are Stationary
Roberts (2000) [13]	10 European Community Countries (1960–1993)	Panel Data, GLS, Unit Root and Long Run Relationship	Short Run Income Elasticity is significantly less than Unity
Okunade & Murthy (2002) [56]	USA, 1960–1997	Time Series, Unit Root and Cointegration	>1
Bhat & Jain (2004) [59]	OECD Countries	Panel Data	>1
Clemente et. al (2004) [57]	22 OECD Countries	Country Specific Time Series, Cointegration and Long Run Analysis	>1
Sen (2005) [23]	15 OECD Countries, 1990–1998	Panel Data Fixed Effect Model, GLS, WLS and IV Estimation	Elasticity varied between 0.21 to 0.51
Dreger & Reimers (2005) [5]	21 OECD Countries, 1975–2001	Panel Unit Root and Panel Cointegration	Health Care Expenditures are not Luxury Good. Income elasticity is not different from unity.
Wang & Rettenmaier (2006) [61]	50 States in the United States, 1980–2000	Panel Data, Unit Root with Structural Break, Cointegration	>1
Chakroun (2009) [54]	17 OECD Countries, 1975–2003	Panel Threshold Regression	

Table 6 Summary of Existing Studies *(Continued)*

			Health Care is a Necessity rather than a Luxury
Baltagi & Moscone (2010) [18]	20 OECD Countries 1971–2004	Panel Data, Panel Unit Root, Corss Section Dependence, Common Correlated Effect Pooled Estimator (CCEP), Panel Fixed Effect, Spatial MLE	<1
Mehrara *et. al* (2012) [6]	13 MENA (Middle East & North Africa), 1995–2005	Panel Data, Panel Unit Root and Panel Cointegration	<1
Liu et. al (2011) [22]	22 OECD Countries, 1960–2002	Semiparametric Panel Varying Coefficient Model	Relationship between HCE and Income is subject to Structural Change. Full Sample Income Elasticity was greater than unity.
Hassan *et. al* (2014) [14]	South Asian Association for Regional Cooperation (SAARC), 1995–2010	Panel Data, Panel Unit Root Test, Panel Cointegration, Panel Long Run Estimation	HCE are Luxury Goods in SAARC Countries
Penas *et. al* (2013)	31 OECD Countries, 1970–2009	Panel Data, Panel Unit Root, LSDV and NLLS Estimation	Difference in Short term and Long Term. Elasticities, Long run Elasticity is close to unity
Jewell *et. al* (2003) [7]	20 OECD Countries, 1960–1997	Panel Data, Panel Unit Root Test with Structural Breaks	HCE, GDP are Stationary when allowing for Structural Breaks

Note: Adapted and Extended by using, Getzen [46], Penas *et. al* [8] and Mehrara *et. al* [6]

Table 7 Panel Unit Root Test Results of the Variables

Variables	Levin, Lin & Chu Test for Panel Unit Root *Null: Panels Contain Unit Roots(Common)*			
	Intercept		Intercept and Trend	
	LLC t – Stat	Prob.	LLC t - Stat	Prob.
GDP (Current US $)	17.35	1.000	−1.23	0.1090
D(GDP)	−6.36[a]	0.000	−14.12[a]	0.000
Health Care Expenditure (Current US $)	20.28	1.000	−0.43	0.332
D(Health Care Expenditure)	−4.98[a]	0.000	−10.69[a]	0.000
Infant Mortality	−32.60[a]	0.000	−3.92[a]	0.000
D(Infant Mortality)	−3.49[a]	0.000	−7.52[a]	0.000
Life Expectancy	−4.98[a]	0.000	−1.54	0.060
D(Life Expectancy)	−12.32[a]	0.000	−19.43[a]	0.000

Note: [a]Indicates 1% level of significance

Table 8 Panel Unit Root Test Results of the Variables

Variables	ADF Fisher Test for Panel Unit Root (Choi, 2001) Null: Panels Contain Unit Roots(Individual)			
	Intercept		Intercept and Trend	
	ADF – Chi Z - Stat	Prob.	ADF – Choi Z - Stat	Prob.
GDP (Current US $)	17.79	1.000	6.66	1.000
D(GDP)	−4.45[a]	0.000	−11.03[a]	0.000
Health Care Expenditure (Current US $)	18.40	1.000	7.02	1.000
D(Health Care Expenditure)	−3.15[a]	0.000	−11.13[a]	0.000
Infant Mortality	−14.46[a]	0.000	2.39	0.991
D(Infant Mortality)	−1.46	0.072	−3.78[a]	0.000
Life Expectancy	−2.18	0.014	−1.15	0.123
D(Life Expectancy)	−11.65[a]	0.000	−13.95[a]	0.000

Note: [a]Indicates 1% level of significance

Table 9 Panel Unit Root Test Results of the Variables

Variables	PP- Fisher Test for Panel Unit Root (Choi, 2001) Null: Panels Contain Unit Roots(Individual)			
	Intercept		Intercept and Trend	
	PP – Chi Z - Stat	Prob.	PP – Choi Z - Stat	Prob.
GDP (Current US $)	21.15	1.000	8.75	1.000
D(GDP)	−7.78[a]	0.000	−14.65[a]	0.000
Health Care Expenditure (Current US $)	21.33	1.000	10.34	1.000
D(Health Care Expenditure)	−7.59[a]	0.000	−13.89[a]	0.000
Infant Mortality	−23.52[a]	0.000	3.90	1.000
D(Infant Mortality)	−2.46[a]	0.006	−4.94[a]	0.000
Life Expectancy	−7.97[a]	0.000	4.74	1.000
D(Life Expectancy)	−1.926	0.027	1.84	0.967

Note: [a]Indicates 1% level of significance

Table 10 Pedroni Panel Cointegration Test

Pedroni (1999, 2004) Engle – Granger Based Cointegration Test, H_0: No Cointegration

	Panel Statistic				Group Statistic	
	IM		LE		IM	LE
	Stat.	W-Stat	Stat.	W-Stat	Stat.	Stat.
Deterministic Specification: No Constant & Trend						
V-Stat	3.069[a]	1.629[a]	−2.61	0.407	-	-
	(0.001)	(0.051)	(0.995)	(0.341)	-	-
Rho-Stat	−4.214[a]	−3.116[a]	−0.372	−2.349[a]	−1.659[b]	−1.227
	(0.000)	(0.000)	(0.354)	(0.009)	(0.048)	(0.109)
PP-Stat	−5.164[a]	−5.469[a]	−4.595[a]	−4.942[a]	−7.727[a]	−8.896[a]
	(0.000)	(0.000)	(0.000)	(0.000)	(0.000)	(0.000)
ADF-Stat	−4.58[a]	−6.337[a]	−4.582[a]	−5.999[a]	−8.271[a]	−9.302[a]
	(0.000)	(0.000)	(0.000)	(0.000)	(0.000)	(0.000)
Deterministic Specification: Constant Only						
V-Stat	0.573	−0.024	2.113[b]	−0.061	-	-
	(0.283)	(0.509)	(0.017)	(0.524)	-	-
Rho-Stat	−0.701	−1.813[b]	0.071	−1.57[c]	0.093	0.292
	(0.241)	(0.034)	(0.528)	(0.058)	(0.537)	(0.615)
PP-Stat	−1.826[b]	−6.580[a]	−1.015	−6.389[a]	−7.881[a]	−8.119[a]
	(0.033)	(0.000)	(0.154)	(0.000)	(0.000)	(0.000)
ADF-Stat	−1.328[c]	−9.675[a]	−1.129	−8.969[a]	−11.31[a]	−10.507[a]
	(0.092)	(0.000)	(0.129)	(0.000)	(0.000)	(0.000)
Deterministic Specification: Constant & Trend						
V-Stat	−2.933	−3.527	2.113[b]	−0.061	-	-
	(0.998)	(0.999)	(0.017)	(0.524)	-	-
Rho-Stat	3.022	1.37	0.071	−1.57[b]	3.023	0.292
	(0.998)	(0.914)	(0.528)	(0.058)	(0.998)	(0.615)
PP-Stat	0.316	−5.997[a]	−1.015	−6.389[a]	−8.391[a]	−8.119[a]
	(0.624)	(0.000)	(0.154)	(0.000)	(0.000)	(0.000)
ADF-Stat	0.653	−8.513[a]	−1.129	−8.969[a]	−8.197[a]	−10.507[a]
	(0.743)	(0.000)	(0.124)	(0.000)	(0.000)	(0.000)

Note: [a],[b] and [c] Indicates 1%, 5% and 10% level of significance respectively

Acknowledgement
Authors of the paper are greatly indebted to Professor Joakim Westerlund and Dr. Damiaan Persyn for sharing their codes to perform econometric exercise which made the journey of completion of the work easier.

Authors' contributions
All the authors in the current work have contributed uniformly. SMA developed the research problem formulated the model design and performed the econometric exercise. SS took the responsibility to do the survey of existing literature and finding the research gap and contributed to the result explanations. RH synthesized research gap with the methodology and have given effort to bring the issue into perspective and contributed to prepare the draft. All authors have read and approved the manuscript.

Competing interests
The authors declare that they have no competing interests.

Author details
[1]Department of Economics, University of Dhaka, Dhaka 1000, Bangladesh.
[2]Department of Development Studies, University of Dhaka, Dhaka 1000, Bangladesh.

References
1. Farag M, Nandakumar AK, Wallack S, Hodgkin D, Gaumer G, Erbil C. Health expenditures, health outcomes and the role of good governance. Int J Health Care Finance Econ. 2013;13(1):33–52.
2. Allen S, Badiane O, Sene L, Ulimwengu J. Government expenditures, health outcomes and marginal productivity of agricultural inputs: The case of Tanzania. J Agric Econ. 2014;65(3):637–62.
3. Elola J, Daponte A, Navarro V. Health indicators and the organization of health care systems in western Europe. Am J Public Health. 1995;85(10):1397–401.
4. Anyanwu JC, Erhijakpor AE. Health expenditures and health outcomes in Africa. Afr Dev Rev. 2009;21(2):400–33.
5. Dreger C, Reimers HE. Health care expenditures in OECD countries: a panel unit root and cointegration analysis. 2005.
6. Mehrara M, Fazaeli AA, Fazaeli AA, Fazaeli AR. The Relationship between Health Expenditures and Economic Growth in Middle East & North Africa (MENA) Countries. Int J Buss Mgt Eco Res. 2012;3(1):2012.
7. Jewell T, Lee J, Tieslau M, Strazicich MC. Stationarity of health expenditures and GDP: evidence from panel unit root tests with heterogeneous structural breaks. J Health Econ. 2003;22(2):313–23.
8. Lago-Peñas S, Cantarero-Prieto D, Blázquez-Fernández C. On the relationship between GDP and health care expenditure: a new look. Econ Model. 2013;32:124–9.
9. MacDonald G, Hopkins S. Unit root properties of OECD health care expenditure and GDP data. Health Econ. 2002;11(4):371–6.
10. Wang Z, Rettenmaier AJ. A note on cointegration of health expenditures and income. Health Econ. 2007;16(6):559–78.
11. Gbesemete KP, Gerdtham UG. Determinants of health care expenditure in Africa: a cross-sectional study. World Dev. 1992;20(2):303–8.
12. Hitiris T. Health care expenditure and integration in the countries of the European Union. Appl Econ. 1997;29(1):1–6.
13. Roberts J. Spurious regression problems in the determinants of health care expenditure: a comment on Hitiris (1997). Appl Econ Lett. 2000;7(5):279–83.
14. Hassan SA, Zaman K, Zaman S, Shabir M. Measuring health expenditures and outcomes in saarc region: health is a luxury? Qual Quant. 2014;48(3):1421–37.
15. Abel-Smith B, World Health Organization. An international study of health expenditure and its relevance for health planning. 1967.
16. Newhouse JP. Medical-care expenditure: a cross-national survey. J Hum Resour. 1977;12(1):115–25.
17. Parkin D, McGuire A, Yule B. Aggregate health care expenditures and national income: is health care a luxury good? J Health Econ. 1987;6(2):109–27.
18. Baltagi BH, Moscone F. Health care expenditure and income in the OECD reconsidered: Evidence from panel data. Econ Model. 2010;27(4):804–11.
19. Chakroun M. Health care expenditure and GDP: An international panel smooth transition approach. Int J Econ. 2010;4(1):189–200.
20. Gerdtham UG, Søgaard J, Andersson F, Jönsson B. An econometric analysis of health care expenditure: a cross-section study of the OECD countries. J Health Econ. 1992;11(1):63–84.
21. Hitiris T, Posnett J. The determinants and effects of health expenditure in developed countries. J Health Econ. 1992;11(2):173–81.
22. Liu D, Li R, Wang Z. Testing for structural breaks in panel varying coefficient models: with an application to OECD health expenditure. Empir Econ. 2011;40(1):95–118.
23. Sen A. Is health care a luxury? New evidence from OECD data. Int J Health Care Finance Econ. 2005;5(2):147–64.
24. Breusch TS, Pagan AR. The Lagrange Multiplier Test and Its Applications to Model Specification in Econometrics. Rev Econ Stud. 1980;47(1):239–53.
25. Pesaran MHHM. General diagnostic tests for cross section dependence in panels. CESifo Working Papers. 2004;1233:255–60.
26. Baltagi BH, Feng Q, Kao C. A Lagrange Multiplier test for cross-sectional dependence in a fixed effects panel data model. J Econ. 2012;170(1):164–77.
27. Im KS, Pesaran MH, Shin Y. Testing for unit roots in heterogeneous panels. J Econ. 2003;115(1):53–74.

28. Im KS, Pesaran MH, Shin Y. Testing for unit roots in heterogeneous panels. Mimeo: Department of Applied Economics, University of Cambridge; 1997.

29. Levin A, Lin CF, Chu CSJ. Unit root tests in panel data: asymptotic and finite-sample properties. J Econ. 2002;108(1):1–24.

30. Choi I. Unit root tests for panel data. J Int Money Financ. 2001;20(2):249–72.

31. Pedroni P. Critical values for cointegration tests in heterogeneous panels with multiple regressors. Oxf Bull Econ Stat. 1999;61(s 1):653–70.

32. Pedroni P. Panel cointegration: asymptotic and finite sample properties of pooled time series tests with an application to the PPP hypothesis. Economet Theor. 2004;20(03):597–625.

33. McCoskey S, Kao C. A residual-based test of the null of cointegration in panel data. Econ Rev. 1998;17(1):57–84.

34. Kao C. Spurious regression and residual-based tests for cointegration in panel data. J Econ. 1999;90(1):1–44.

35. Westerlund J, Edgerton DL. A panel bootstrap cointegration test. Econ Lett. 2007;97(3):185–90.

36. Banerjee A, Dolado J, Mestre R. Error-correction mechanism tests for cointegration in a single-equation framework. J Time Ser Anal. 1998;19(3):267–83.

37. Phillips PC, Hansen BE. Statistical inference in instrumental variables regression with I (1) processes. Rev Econ Stud. 1990;57(1):99–125.

38. Saikkonen P. Estimation and testing of cointegrated systems by an autoregressive approximation. Economet Theor. 1992;8(01):1–27.

39. Stock JH, Watson MW. A simple estimator of cointegrating vectors in higher order integrated systems. Econometrica. 1993;61(4):783–820.

40. Phillips PC, Moon HR. Linear regression limit theory for nonstationary panel data. Econometrica. 1999;67(5):1057–111.

41. Pedroni P. Fully Modified OLS for Heterogeneous Cointegrated Panels. 2000.

42. Kao C, Chiang MH. On The Estimation and Inference of A Cointegrated Regression In Panel Data. 2000.

43. Pedroni P. Purchasing power parity tests in cointegrated panels. Rev Econ Stat. 2001;83(4):727–31.

44. Mark N, Sul D. A computationally simple cointegration vector estimator for panel data, Ohio State University manuscript. 1999.

45. Mark NC, Sul D. Cointegration Vector Estimation by Panel DOLS and Long-run Money Demand. Oxf Bull Econ Stat. 2003;65(5):655–80.

46. Getzen TE. Health care is an individual necessity and a national luxury: applying multilevel decision models to the analysis of health care expenditures. J Health Econ. 2000;19(2):259–70.

47. Fogel RW. Catching up with the economy. The American Economic Review. 1999;89(1):1–21.

48. Gertler P, & Van der Gaag J. The willingness to pay for medical care: evidence from two developing countries. Baltimore, Maryland, Johns Hospital University Press. 1990. ix, 139 p.

49. Getzen TE. Macro forecasting of national health expenditures. Advances in health economics and health services research. 1990;11:27–48.

50. Getzen TE, & Poullier JP. International health spending forecasts: concepts and evaluation. Social Science & Medicine. 1992;34(9):1057–1068.

51. Kleiman E. The determinants of national outlay on health. In: Perlman, M. (Ed.), The Economics of Health and Medical Care. Macmillan, London. 1974.

52. Maxwell RJ. Health and wealth: An international study of health-care spending. Lexington Books, MA. 1981.

53. Schieber GJ. Health expenditures in major industrialized countries. Health care financing review. 1990;11(4):159–169.

54. Chakroun M. Health care expenditure and GDP: An international panel smooth transition approach (No. 14322). University Library of Munich, Germany. 2009.

55. Hansen P, & King A. The determinants of health care expenditure: a cointegration approach. Journal of health economics. 1996;15(1):127–137.

56. Okunade AA, & Murthy VN. Technology as a 'major driver'of health care costs: a cointegration analysis of the Newhouse conjecture. Journal of health economics. 2002;21(1):147–159.

57. Clemente J, Marcuello C, Montañés A, & Pueyo F. On the international stability of health care expenditure functions: are government and private functions similar?. Journal of Health Economics. 2004;23(3):589–613.

58. Blomqvist ÅG, & Carter RA. Is health care really a luxury?. Journal of Health Economics. 1997;16(2):207–229.

59. Bhat R, & Jain N. Analysis of public expenditure on health using state level data. Indian Institute of Management: Ahmedabad (India). 2004.

60. Leu RE. The public-private mix and international health care costs. Public and private health services. 1986;(7):41.

61. Wang Z, & Rettenmaier AJ. A note on cointegration of health expenditures and income. Health Economics. 2007;16(6):559–578.

Permissions

The contributors of this book come from diverse backgrounds, making this book a truly international effort. This book will bring forth new frontiers with its revolutionizing research information and detailed analysis of the nascent developments around the world.

We would like to thank all the contributing authors for lending their expertise to make the book truly unique. They have played a crucial role in the development of this book. Without their invaluable contributions this book wouldn't have been possible. They have made vital efforts to compile up to date information on the varied aspects of this subject to make this book a valuable addition to the collection of many professionals and students.

This book was conceptualized with the vision of imparting up-to-date information and advanced data in this field. To ensure the same, a matchless editorial board was set up. Every individual on the board went through rigorous rounds of assessment to prove their worth. After which they invested a large part of their time researching and compiling the most relevant data for our readers.

The editorial board has been involved in producing this book since its inception. They have spent rigorous hours researching and exploring the diverse topics which have resulted in the successful publishing of this book. They have passed on their knowledge of decades through this book. To expedite this challenging task, the publisher supported the team at every step. A small team of assistant editors was also appointed to further simplify the editing procedure and attain best results for the readers.

Apart from the editorial board, the designing team has also invested a significant amount of their time in understanding the subject and creating the most relevant covers. They scrutinized every image to scout for the most suitable representation of the subject and create an appropriate cover for the book.

The publishing team has been an ardent support to the editorial, designing and production team. Their endless efforts to recruit the best for this project, has resulted in the accomplishment of this book. They are a veteran in the field of academics and their pool of knowledge is as vast as their experience in printing. Their expertise and guidance has proved useful at every step. Their uncompromising quality standards have made this book an exceptional effort. Their encouragement from time to time has been an inspiration for everyone.

The publisher and the editorial board hope that this book will prove to be a valuable piece of knowledge for researchers, students, practitioners and scholars across the globe.

List of Contributors

Martin Bierbaum and Oliver Schöffski
Friedrich-Alexander-Universität Erlangen-Nürnberg (FAU), Nuremberg, Germany

Benedikt Schliemann and Clemens Kösters
Department of Trauma, Hand and Reconstructive Surgery, University Hospital Münster, Münster, Germany

Beáta Gavurová
Department of Banking and Investment, Faculty of Economics, Technical University of Košice, Němcovej 32, 04001 Košice, Slovak Republic

Viliam Kováč
Department of Finance, Faculty of Economics, Technical University of Košice, Němcovej 32, 04001 Košice, Slovak Republic

Ján Fedačko
1st Department of Internal Medicine, Louis Pasteur University Hospital in Košice, Trieda Slovenského národného povstania 1, 04011 Košice, Slovak Republic
Centre of Excellence in Atherosclerosis Research, Pavol Jozef Šafárik University in Košice, Trieda Slovenského národného povstania 1, 04011 Košice, Slovak Republic

Javad Javan-Noughabi
Health Management and Economics Research Center, Iran University of Medical Sciences, Tehran, Iran
Department of Health Economics, School of Health Management and Information Sciences, Iran University of Medical Sciences, Tehran, Iran

Zahra Kavosi
Health Human Resources Research Center, Shiraz University of Medical Sciences, Shiraz, Iran

Ahmad Faramarzi
Department of Health Management and Economics, School of Public Health, Tehran University of Medical Sciences, Tehran, Iran

Mohammad Khammarnia
Health Promotion Research Center, Zahedan University of Medical Sciences, Zahedan, Iran

David G. Lugo-Palacios
Centre for Health Economics, University of Manchester, 4.306 Jean McFarlane Building, Oxford Road, M13 9PL, Manchester, UK

Brenda Gannon
Centre for the Business and Economics of Health, The University of Queensland, Faculty of Business, Economics and Law, QLD, St Lucia 4072, Australia

Olaf C. Jensen, Lulu Hjarnoe and Despena Andrioti
Centre of Maritime Health and Society, Institute of Public Health, Faculty of Health Sciences, University of Southern Denmark, Niels Bohrs vej 9, 6700 Esbjerg, Denmark

Mads D. Faurby
Centre of Maritime Health and Society, Institute of Public Health, Faculty of Health Sciences, University of Southern Denmark, Niels Bohrs vej 9, 6700 Esbjerg, Denmark
Faurby Consulting, Aebleparken 190, 3rd floor, 5270 Odense N, Denmark

Derek Asuman and Charles Godfred Ackah
Institute of Statistical, Social and Economic Research, University of Ghana, E.N. Omaboe Building, Legon, Ghana

Ulrika Enemark
Section for Health Promotion and Health Services Research, Department of Public Health, Aarhus University, Bartholins Alle 2, 8000 Aarhus C, Denmark

Beata Gavurova and Tatiana Vagasova
Faculty of Economics, Technical University of Kosice, Nemcovej 32, 040 01 Kosice, Slovakia

Xiaodong Zheng
College of Economics and Management, China Agricultural University, Beijing, China

Xiangming Fang
College of Economics and Management, China Agricultural University, Beijing, China
School of Public Health, Georgia State University, 140 Decatur Street, Atlanta, GA 30303, USA

Deborah A. Fry and Tabitha Casey
Moray House School of Education, University of Edinburgh, Edinburgh, Scotland

Gary Ganz and Catherine L. Ward
Department of Psychology, University of Cape Town, Cape Town, South Africa

Celia Hsiao
Save the Children South Africa, Johannesburg, South Africa

Dosse Mawussi Djahini-Afawoubo and Esso-Hanam Atake
Department of Economic Sciences, University of Lomé (Togo), Lome, West africa, Togo

Beat Hulliger and Martin Sterchi
Institute for Competitiveness and Communication, University of Applied Sciences and Arts Northwestern Switzerland (FHNW), Riggenbachstrasse 16, 4600 Olten, Switzerland

Murad Ali and Megersa Debela
Department of Economics, Haramaya University, College of Business and Economics, Dire Dawa, Ethiopia

Tewfik Bamud
Department of Economics, Hawasa University, College of Business and Economics, Awasa, Ethiopia

Martin Emmert, Nina Meszmer, Lisa Jablonski, Lena Zinth and Oliver Schöffski
School of Business and Economics, Health Services Management, University of Erlangen-Nuremberg, Lange Gasse 20 90403 Nuremberg, Nuremberg, Germany

Fatemeh Taheri-Zadeh
Media, Information and Design Department of Information and Communication, University of Applied Sciences and Arts, Hannover, Germany

I. Mosweu and P. McCrone
King's Health Economics, Institute of Psychiatry, Psychology & Neuroscience, King's College London, The David Goldberg Centre, De Crespigny Park, Denmark Hill, London SE5 8AF, UK

R. Moss-Morris
Department of Psychology,Institute of Psychiatry Psychology & Neuroscience, King's College London, London, UK

L. Dennison
School of Psychology, University of Southampton, Southampton, UK

T. Chalder
Department of Psychological Medicine, King's College London, Cutcombe Road, London SE5 9RJ, UK

W. Kip Viscusi
Vanderbilt University Law School, 131 21st Avenue South, Nashville, TN 37203, USA

Patricia H. Born
Florida State University, College of Business, Tallahassee, FL, USA

J. Bradley Karl
East Carolina University, College of Business, Greenville, NC, USA

Edward Kwabena Ameyaw and Francis Appiah
Department of Population and Health, Faculty of Social Sciences, University of Cape Coast, Cape Coast, Ghana

Raymond Elikplim Kofinti
Department of Economics, Faculty of Social Sciences, University of Cape Coast, Cape Coast, Ghana

John E. Schneider
Avalon Health Economics, LLC, 26 Washington Street, 3rd Fl, 07960 Morristown, NJ, USA

Robert Ohsfeldt
Health Policy & Management, Texas A&M University, 212 Adriance Lab Rd, 1266 TAMU, 77843-1266 College Station, TX, USA

Pengxiang Li
Division of General Internal Medicine, University of Pennsylvania, 423 Guardian Dr, Philadelphia, PA 19104, USA

Thomas R. Miller
American Society of Anesthesiologists, 1061 American Lane, 60173-4973 Schaumburg, IL, USA

Cara Scheibling
Avalon Health Economics, 26 Washington Street, 3rd Fl., 07960 Morristown, NJ, USA

Narimasa Kumagai
Faculty of Economics, Kindai University, 3-4-1 Kowakae, Higashiosaka, Osaka 577-8502, Japan

S. M. Abdullah and Rumana Huque
Department of Economics, University of Dhaka, Dhaka 1000, Bangladesh

Salina Siddiqua
Department of Development Studies, University of Dhaka, Dhaka 1000, Bangladesh

Index

www.ingramcontent.com/pod-product-compliance
Lightning Source LLC
Chambersburg PA
CBHW080406190526
45161CB00003B/152